TSRA Operative Di

David D. Odell, MD MMSc
University of Pittsburgh
Cardiothoracic Surgery Resident
Advanced Thoracic Surgery Fellow
TSRA President 2013-2014

Damien J. LaPar, MD MSc
University of Virginia
Cardiothoracic Surgery Fellow
TSRA President 2014-2015

Section Editors

Shawn S. Groth, MD MS
Brigham and Women's Hospital
Cardiothoracic Surgery Resident
University of Pittsburgh
Advanced Thoracic Surgery Fellow
Thoracic Surgery Section

Michael P. Robich, MD MPH
Cleveland Clinic Foundation
Cardiothoracic Surgery Fellow
Adult Cardiac Surgery Section

Muhammed Aftab, MD
Texas Heart Institute, Baylor University
Cardiothoracic Surgery Resident
Congenital Cardiac Surgery Section

Copy Editor

Ernest G. Chan, BS
Stony Brook School of Medicine
4th Year Medical Student

Thoracic Surgery Residents Association
www.tsranet.org

Copyright

TSRA Review of Cardiothoracic Surgery

Copyright © 2014 by the Thoracic Surgery Residents Association, Damien J. LaPar, David D. Odell.

TSRA / TSDA
633 N. Saint Clair Street
Suite 2320
Chicago, IL 60611
www.tsranet.org

Disclaimer

The material presented herein is to the best of our knowledge, accurate and factual to date. The text is provided as a basic outline of a dictated description of the stated operative procedure. The text is not intended to serve as a guide for the actual performance of the operation and this book should not be construed as a surrogate for formalized operative instruction. Further, the descriptions contained in this book represent one safe approach to an operation. The TSRA and the authors make no claims regarding the superiority of these described approaches relative to other operative strategies as we recognize that alternate strategies may be safely and efficaciously employed by practicing surgeons.

All rights reserved. This book is protected by copyright. No part of this book may be reproduced in any form or by any means, electronic or mechanical, including photocopying or the use of any information storage and retrieval system without written permission from the copyright owners.

Cover artwork by: Carmina Mery, Ramón Mery, and Mari Pili Guzmán (age 3)

"To Kelly and Jacqueline"

- Damien J. LaPar

"To Alessia, Pietra and Wilson for your unwavering support and love."

- David D. Odell

Foreword

With this publication, the TSRA extends its record of outstanding contributions to Thoracic Surgical Education. It provides the reader with a concise and clearly focused overview of the steps of a given operative procedure, and provides excellent advice on potential pitfalls of the procedure. Such pearls are invaluable. By providing templates for the dictation of operative notes, it serves as an excellent resource for the student of Thoracic Surgery as one learns such a large number of procedures.

This volume helps to address an important gap in Thoracic Surgical Education and once again points to the valuable contributions that the TSRA has made to our specialty. It will go a long way in helping with the education Thoracic Surgical Residents at all levels.

David A. Fullerton, MD
President, TSDA

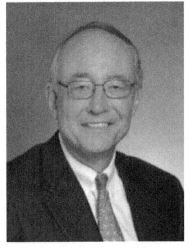

Preface

The Thoracic Surgery Residents Association (TSRA) was established in 1997 under the guidance of the Thoracic Surgery Directors Association (TSDA) to create a unified voice to represent residents during cardiothoracic surgery training. The organization has developed as a core mission a focus on improving the quality, accessibility and utility of resident education. In 2010, we released the *TSRA Review of Cardiothoracic Surgery*. This would be the first of a series of publications, written by residents, which have sought to address areas of perceived need in cardiothoracic education. The *Review* provided a series of short reference chapters introducing key knowledge and concepts in an easily digestible point-of-care format. The book was a phenomenal success and has now been downloaded in pdf format more than 9000 times and been translated into several languages. The TSRA followed this publication with the release in 2013 of the *Primer in Cardiothoracic Surgery* a book focused on basic concepts within the field of CT surgery which form the foundation for further learning. At the other end of the continuum of learning, the *TSRA Clinical Scenarios in Cardiothoracic Surgery* provided a compilation of common, high-yield, and important scenarios which might arise in the course of a surgeon's training or practice.

The current publication seeks to provide a resource which may be used in the surgeon's daily practice as a resource for the review of the major steps of an operation as well as a guide to the appropriate documentation of the conduct of that operation. We hope that the text will be useful for both practicing surgeons and residents in training. While the list of operations included in the text is extensive it is by no means intended to be inclusive of the entire breadth of the field of cardiothoracic surgery. Additionally, the text provides descriptions of one approach to the operations included. We acknowledge that the approach to a given operation may vary among surgeons, and institutions. This text is not intended to establish a uniform 'correct' approach, nor is it intended as a surrogate for formal residency training.

We strove to attain a high level of technical accuracy with the operative descriptions contained in this text with four levels of peer review. Each chapter was carefully reviewed by an established faculty member, a section editor as well as the two main editors. Our main goal was to ensure that the operative dictations contained descriptions of a safe approach to practice. Despite this rigorous review process, the reader will likely notice differences between the described operations and the practice in their institutions. The book is intended to be a dynamic resource and space has been left at the end of each section for the reader to make notes highlighting their individual approach to the operation. We welcome feedback from the reader and encourage the submission of additional operative descriptions beyond what is included in the text to David D. Odell, MD MMSc (daviddodell@gmail.com) and Damien J. LaPar, MD MSc (dlapar@virginia.edu). We hope you enjoy the book and find it a useful resource.

DDO and DJL

Contributors

Contributors

Muhammad Aftab, MD
Baylor College of Medicine/Texas Heart Institute
Aortic Root Replacement With Homograft For Aortic Root Abscess (Native And Or Prior Bentall), Infra-Cardiac Total Anomalous Pulmonary Venous Return (TAPVR), Aortic Coarctation Repair With Extended End-To-End Anastomosis, Modified Blalock-Taussig Shunt (Using Interposition Gore-Tex Tube Graft), Bidirectional Glenn Procedure, Extra-Cardiac (Non-Fenestrated) Completion Fontan Procedure, Arterial Switch Procedure, Tetralogy Of Fallot Repair - Infundibular Sparing (Transatrial Repair), Pulmonary Valve Replacement And Reconstruction Of Right Ventricle Outflow Tract, Pediatric Lung Transplantation: Bilateral Sequential Lung Transplantation

Magdy M. El-Sayed Ahmed, MD
Texas Heart Institute
Pediatric Lung Transplantation: Bilateral Sequential Lung Transplantation

Gorav Ailawadi, MD
University of Virginia
Coronary Artery Bypass Grafting With Cardiopulmonary Bypass

Luis F. Alberton, MD
North Shore Long Island Jewish Health System
Laparoscopic Nissen Fundoplication

Uthman Aluthman, MD
University of Calgary
Coronary Artery Bypass Grafting With Mammary and Vein Grafts - Off Pump

Parth Amin, MD
Loyola University Medical Center
Elephant Trunk Part 1, Elephant Trunk Part 2, Endovascular Management of Acute Type B Dissection

Mara B. Antonoff, MD
Washington University
Lung Procurement, Lung Transplantation

Anelechi Anyanwu, MD, MSc, FRCS
Mount Sinai Medical Center
Repair of Post-Infarction Ventricular Septal Defect, Pulmonary Embolectomy

Nicholas Baker, MD
University of Pittsburgh Medical Center
Mediastinoscopy

Contributors

Jamil Bashir, MD
St. Paul's Hospital
Biatrial Cox-Maze Ablation for Atrial Fibrillation, Permanent Pacemaker Insertion

Kfir Ben-David, MD
University of Florida
Esophageal Stent Placement

Thomas Birdas, MD
Indiana University School of Medicine
Open Thoracostomy (Eloesser Flap and Clagett Window)

Mark Bleiweis MD
University of Florida
Repair of Partial Anomalous Pulmonary Venous Return

Andrew I.M. Campbell
British Columbia's Children's Hospital
Ventricular Septal Defect: Perimembranous, Completion Lateral Tunnel Fontan, Ross Procedure for the Correction of Congenital Aortic Stenosis

Thomas Caranasos MD
University of Florida
Repair of Partial Anomalous Pulmonary Venous Return, Esophageal Stent Placement

Stephen D. Cassivi, MD, MSc
Mayo Clinic
Transcervical Thymectomy

Mohiuddin Cheema, MD
Cedars Sinai Medical Center
Endovascular Repair of Descending Thoracic Aortic Aneurysm (TEVAR)

Frederick Y. Chen, MD, PhD
Brigham and Women's Hospital
Aortic Valve Replacement for Aortic Insufficiency Or Aortic Stenosis

Jordy C. Cox, MD
University of California San Francisco
Open Ivor-Lewis Esophagectomy

Jonathan D'Cunha, MD, PhD
University of Pittsburgh Medical Center
Tracheostomy

Contributors

Joseph A. Dearani, MD
Mayo Clinic
Repair of Obstructive Hypertrophic Cardiomyopathy: (Septal Myomectomy), Cone Repair for Ebstein Malformation

Daniel T. DeArmond, MD
University of Texas Health Science Center
VATS Evacuation of Hemothorax

Walter F. DeNino, MD
Medical University of South Carolina
Valve Sparing Root Replacement, Carinal Pneumonectomy

Chadrick E. Denlinger, MD
Medical University of South Carolina
Carinal Pneumonectomy

Jessica S. Donington, MD
New York University School of Medicine
Chamberlain Procedure, Trans-sternal Thymectomy

Desmond M. D'Souza, MD
Cleveland Clinic
Lung Volume Reduction Surgery

Michelle C. Ellis, MD
University of Michigan
Coronary Artery Bypass Grafting With Aortic Valve Replacement, Transhiatal Esophagectomy

Nicholas Engstrom, MD
Oregon Health and Sciences Center
Diagnositic Thoracoscopy

Lloyd M. Felmly
Medical University of South Carolina
Carinal Pneumonectomy

Joss Fernandez, MD
Missouri Heart Center, Columbia, MO
Endovascular Management of Acute Type B Dissection

Amy Fiedler, M.D
Brigham and Women's Hospital
Aortic Valve Replacement for Aortic Insufficiency or Aortic Stenosis

Contributors

Charles D. Fraser Jr, MD
Texas Children's Hospital/Baylor College of Medicine
Arterial Switch Procedure

James J. Gangemi, MD
University of Virginia
Complete Atrioventricular Canal Repair

Jose P. Garcia, MD
Massachusetts General Hospital
Orthotopic Heart Transplantation

Erin Gillaspie, MD
Mayo Clinic
Open Lobectomies

Leonard N. Girardi, MD
New York Presbyterian –Weill Cornell Medical Center
Thoracoabdominal Aneurysm Repair

David Graham, MD
Children's Medical Center of Dallas
Repair of Supravalvular Aortic Stenosis, Pleural Decortication, Pleural Biopsy (Open/Thoracoscopic) (Open/Thoracoscopic)

Eugene Grossi, MD
New York University Langone Medical Center
Mitral Valve Replacement

Jonathon W. Haft, MD
University of Michigan
Coronary Artery Bypass Grafting With Aortic Valve Replacement

M. Scott Halbreiner, MD
Cleveland Clinic
Minimally Invasive Directed Coronary Artery Bypass

Michael E. Halkos, MD, MSc
Emory University
Aortic Root Replacement (Endocarditis)

Contributors

Jeffrey S. Heinle, MD
Texas Children's Hospital/Baylor College of Medicine
Infra-Cardiac Total Anomalous Pulmonary Venous Return (TAPVR), Extra-Cardiac (Non-Fenestrated) Completion Fontan Procedure, Pulmonary Valve Replacement and Reconstruction of Right Ventricle Outflow Tract, Pediatric Lung Transplantation: Bilateral Sequential Lung Transplantation

Joshua L. Hermsen, MD
Seattle Children's Hospital
Repair of Truncus Arteriousus (TA)

Jonathan C. Hong, MD
St. Paul's Hospital
Permanent Pacemaker Insertion, Completion Lateral Tunnel Fontan

John S. Ikonomidis, MD, PhD
Medical University of South Carolina
Total Arch/Hemiarch Replacement with DHCA – Dissection, Valve Sparing Root Replacement

David M. Jablons, MD
University of California San Francisco
Open Ivor-Lewis Esophagectomy

Mathéau A. Julien, MD, PhD
Tufts Medical Center
DeVega Tricuspid Valve Repair

Narongrit Kantathut, MD
Cleveland Clinic
Aortic Valve Surgery with Upper Hemisternotomy Approach

Sunjay Kaushal, MD, PhD
University of Maryland Medical Center
Pediatric Heart Transplantation

Michael O. Kayatta, MD
Emory University
Aortic Root Replacement (Endocarditis)

Mark J. Kerns, MD
St. Paul's Hospital
Biatrial Cox-Maze Ablation for Atrial Fibrillation

Contributors

Kemp Kernstine, MD, PhD
University of Texas Southwestern
Pleural Decortication (Open/Thoracoscopic), Pleural Biopsy (Open/Thoracoscopic)

Zarrish S. Khan, MD
New York Presbyterian –Weill Cornell Medical Center
Thoracoabdominal Aneurysm Repair, Open Modified McKeown Esophagectomy

Ali Khoynezhad, MD, PhD
Cedars Sinai Medical Center
Endovascular Repair of Descending Thoracic Aortic Aneurysm (TEVAR)

Teresa M. Kieser, MD
University of Calgary
Coronary Artery Bypass Grafting With Mammary and Vein Grafts - Off Pump

Samuel S. Kim, MD
University of Arizona
Segmentectomy

Paul Kirshbom, MD
Yale University
Partial AV Canal Repair

Sean Kwan, MD
North Shore Long Island Jewish Health System
Laparoscopic Nissen Fundoplication

Geoffrey T. Lam, MD
New York University School of Medicine
Chamberlain Procedure, Trans-sternal Thymectomy

Damien J. Lapar, MD, MSc
University of Virginia
Coronary Artery Bypass Grafting With Cardiopulmonary Bypass

Ala Al-Lawati, MD
British Columbia's Children's Hospital
Ross Procedure for the Correction of Congenital Aortic Stenosis

Juan M. Lehoux, MD
Texas Children's Hospital/Baylor College of Medicine

Contributors

Supra-Cardiac Total Anomalous Pulmonary Venous Return (TAPVR), Aortic Coarctation Repair With Extended End-To-End Anastomosis, Tetralogy of Fallot: Transventricular Repair
Ryan M. Levy, MD
University of Pittsburgh Medical Center
VATS Pericardial Window, Open Transthoracic Diaphragm Plication, Mediastinoscopy

Jules Lin, MD
University of Michigan
Transhiatal Esophagectomy

Chaim Leker Locker, MD
Mayo Clinic
Redo Sternotomy and Difficult Sternal Closure
Gabriel Loor, MD
University of Minnesota
Transcatheter Aortic Valve Implantation (TAVI): (Transfemoral-Transapical Approach)

James D. Luketich, MD
University of Pittsburgh Medical Center
Minimally Invasive Ivor-Lewis Esophagectomy, Laparoscopic Paraesophageal Hernia Repair
Robroy MacIver, MD, MPH
University of Minnesota
Patent Ductus Arteriosus Ligation

George Makdisi, MD
Mayo Clinic
Unexpected Intraoperative Complications, Redo Sternotomy and Difficult Sternal Closure, Bronchial and Arterial Sleeve Resection, Chest Wall Tumor Resection and Chest Wall Reconstruction, Extrapleural Pneumonectomy for Mesothelioma
Fahd Makhdom, MD
McGill University
Repair of Atrial Septal Defect- Secundum Atrial Septal Defect

Hari Mallidi, MD, FRCSC
Baylor College of Medicine/ Texas Heart Institute
Donor Heart Procurement

Tomas D. Martin, MD
University of Florida
Hemiarch Replacement with DHCA – Aneurysm

Carlo O. Martinez, MD

University of Texas Health Science Center
VATS Evacuation of Hemothorax

David P. Mason, MD
Cleveland Clinic
Lung Volume Reduction Surgery

Douglas J. Mathisen, MD
Massachusetts General Hospital
Rigid Bronchoscopy, Tracheal Resection and Reconstruction

E. Dean McKenzie
Texas Children's Hospital/Baylor College of Medicine
Tetralogy of Fallot: Transventricular Repair, Tetralogy of Fallot Repair - Infundibular Sparing (Transatrial Repair)

D. Michael McMullan, MD
Seattle Children's Hospital
Repair of Truncus Arteriousus (TA)

Justin R. Van Meeteren, DO
Mayo Clinic
Repair of Obstructive Hypertrophic Cardiomyopathy: (Septal Myomectomy)

Carlos M. Mery, MD, MPH
Texas Children's Hospital/Baylor College of Medicine
Supra-Cardiac Total Anomalous Pulmonary Venous Return (TAPVR), Aortic Coarctation Repair with Extended End-To-End Anastomosis, Modified Blalock-Taussig Shunt (Using Interposition Gore-Tex Tube Graft), Bidirectional Glenn Procedure

Stephanie Mick, MD
Cleveland Clinic
Aortic Valve Surgery with Upper Hemisternotomy Approach

Jacob Moremen, MD
Indiana University School of Medicine
Open Thoracostomy (Eloesser Flap and Clagett Window)

Raghav Murthy, MD
Children's Medical Center of Dallas, Texas
Pulmonary Artery Banding, Repair Of Supravalvular Aortic Stenosis

James H. Neel, MD
University of Louisville
Repair of Post-Infarction Ventricular Aneurysm (Dor Endoventricular Circular Patch Plasty (EVCPP))

Contributors

Andrew B. Nguyen, MD
University of Pittsburgh Medical Center
Laparoscopic Paraesophageal Hernia Repair

Khanh Nguyen, MD
Mount Sinai Medical Center
Total Anomalous Pulmonary Venous Return (TAPVR) - Cardiac Type

Francis C. Nichols III, MD
Mayo Clinic
Extrapleural Pneumonectomy for Mesothelioma

David D. Odell, MD, MMSc
University of Pittsburgh Medical Center
Minimally Invasive Ivor-Lewis Esophagectomy

Bharat Pancholy, MD
Rush University Medical Center
Flexible Bronchoscopy

Michael K. Pasque, MD
Washington University
Lung Procurement

G. Alexander Patterson MD
Washington University
Lung Transplantation

Subroto Paul, MD
New York Presbyterian –Weill Cornell Medical Center
Open Modified McKeown Esophagectomy

Amit Pawale, MD, FRCS
Mount Sinai Medical Center
Repair of Post-Infarction Ventricular Septal Defect, Pulmonary Embolectomy, Total Anomalous Pulmonary Venous Return (TAPVR) - Cardiac Type

Paul A. Perry, MD
University of California Davis
Resection of Atrial Myxoma

Duc Thinh Pham, MD
Tufts Medical Center

DeVega Tricuspid Valve Repair

Allan Pickens, MD
Emory University
VATS Thymectomy

Timothy J Pirolli, MD
Stanford University
Esophagogastroduodonoscopy

Eitan Podgaetz, MD, MPH
University of Minnesota
VATS Wedge Resection, VATS Sympathectomy

Ourania Preventza, MD
Baylor College of Medicine/Texas Heart Institute
Aortic Root Replacement with Homograft for Aortic Root Abscess (Native And Or Prior Bentall)

Wissam Raad, MD, MRCS
Albert Einstein College of Medicine
Division of Vascular Ring
Ramachandra Reddy, MD, MBA
Mount Sinai Medical Center
Pulmonary Embolectomy
J. Matthew Reinersman, MD
Mayo Clinic
Transcervical Thymectomy

Otis Rickman, DO
Vanderbilt University Medical Center
Tunneled Catheter Placement

R. Taylor Ripley, MD
Memorial Sloan-Kettering Cancer Center
Pancoast Tumor

Michael P. Robich, MD
Cleveland Clinic
Septal Myectomy

Valerie W. Rusch, MD
Memorial Sloan-Kettering Cancer Center
Pancoast Tumor

Contributors

Joseph Sabik, MD
Cleveland Clinic
Minimally Invasive Directed Coronary Artery Bypass

Sameh M. Said, MD
Mayo Clinic
Mitral Valve Repair for Bileaflet Prolapse, Cone Repair for Ebstein Malformation

Sandeep Sainathan, MD
Yale University
Aortic Valve Replacement with Aortic Root Enlargement, Partial AV Canal Repair

Ismael Alejandro Salas De Armas, MD
Baylor College of Medicine/Texas Heart Institute
Aortic Coarctation Repair with Extended End-To-End Anastomosis, Modified Blalock-Taussig Shunt (Using Interposition Gore-Tex Tube Graft), Bidirectional Glenn Procedure, Tetralogy of Fallot Repair - Infundibular Sparing (Transatrial Repair)

Manu S. Sancheti, MD
Emory University
VATS Thymectomy

Peter Sassalos, MD
University of Michigan
Norwood Procedure

Hartzell V. Schaff, MD
Mayo Clinic
Mitral Valve Repair for Bileaflet Prolapse

Lara Schaheen, MD
University of Pittsburgh Medical Center
Tracheostomy

Jeffrey Schwartz, MD
Loyola University Medical Center
Elephant Trunk Part 1, Elephant Trunk Part 2

Vinod Sebastian, MD
Children's Medical Center of Dallas, Texas
Pulmonary Artery Banding, Repair of Supravalvular Aortic Stenosis

Fawwaz R. Shaw, MD
University of Washington
Aortic Root Replacement for Ascending Aortic Aneurysm

Contributors

Ahmad Y. Sheikh, MD
Stanford University
Esophagogastroduodonoscopy

Robert Shen, MD
Mayo Clinic
Chest Wall Tumor Resection and Chest Wall Reconstruction, Open Lobectomies

Ming Si, MD
University of Michigan
Norwood Procedure

Mark S. Slaughter, MD
University of Louisville
Repair of Post-Infarction Ventricular Aneurysm (Dor End ventricular Circular Patch Plasty (EVCPP))

Nicholas Smedira, MD
Cleveland Clinic
Septal Myectomy

Brian Solomon, MD
New York University Langone Medical Center
Mitral Valve Replacement

Tae H. Song, MD
Massachusetts General Hospital
Orthotopic Heart Transplantation

John R. Spratt, MA, MD
University of Minnesota
Patent Ductus Arteriosus Ligation, VATS Wedge Resection, VATS Sympathectomy

Cameron T. Stock, MD
Massachusetts General Hospital
Rigid Bronchoscopy, Tracheal Resection and Reconstruction

John M. Stulak, MD
Mayo Clinic
Unexpected Intraoperative Complications

Jennifer L. Sullivan, MD
University of Pittsburgh Medical Center

Contributors

VATS Pericardial Window, Open Transthoracic Diaphragm Plication

Julia C. Swanson, MD
University of Virginia
Complete Atrioventricular Canal Repair

Scott J. Swanson, MD
Brigham and Women's Hospital
Repair of Anterior Restrosternal (Morgagni) and Posterolateral (Bochdalek) Diaphragm Hernias, Pleurectomy and Decortication

Keerit Tauh, MD
British Columbia's Children's Hospital
Ventricular Septal Defect: Perimembranous

Christo I. Tchervenkov, MD
McGill University
Repair of Atrial Septal Defect- Secundum Atrial Septal Defect

Tom P. Theruvath, MD, PhD
Medical University of South Carolina
Total Arch/Hemiarch Replacement with DHCA – Dissection

Brandon Tieu, MD
Oregon Health and Sciences Center
Diagnositic Thoracoscopy

Michael Tong, MD, MBA
Cleveland Clinic
LVAD – Heartware, LVAD – Heart Mate II, Total Artificial Heart

Dimitrios Topalidis, MD
University of Minnesota
Transcatheter Aortic Valve Implantation (TAVI): (Transfemoral-Transapical Approach)

Alexandra Tuluca, MD
Baylor College of Medicine/ Texas Heart Institute
Donor Heart Procurement

Ramanan Umakanthan
Texas Children's Hospital/Baylor College of Medicine
Extra-Cardiac (Non-Fenestrated) Completion Fontan Procedure, Pulmonary Valve Replacement and Reconstruction of Right Ventricle Outflow Tract, Pediatric Lung Transplantation: Bilateral Sequential Lung Transplantation

Contributors

Edward D. Verrier, MD
University of Washington
Aortic Root Replacement for Ascending Aortic Aneurysm

William H Warren, MD
Rush University Medical Center
Flexible Bronchoscopy

Brody Wehman, MD, MSc
University of Maryland Medical Center
Pediatric Heart Transplantation

Samuel Weinstein, MD, MBA
Albert Einstein College of Medicine
Division of Vascular Ring

Abby White, DO
Brigham and Women's Hospital
Repair of Anterior Restrosternal (Morgagni) and Posterolateral (Bochdalek) Diaphragm Hernias, Pleurectomy and Decortication

Dennis Wigle, MD, PhD
Mayo Clinic
Bronchial and Arterial Sleeve Resection

James E. Wiseman, MD
University of Arizona
Segmentectomy

Leora T. Yarboro, MD
University of Virginia
Coronary Artery Bypass Grafting + Mitral Valve Repair vs. Replacement

J. Nilas Young, MD
University of California Davis
Resection of Atrial Myxoma

Kenan W. Yount, MD, MBA
University of Virginia
Coronary Artery Bypass Grafting + Mitral Valve Repair vs. Replacement

David D. Yuh MD
Yale University
Aortic Valve Replacement with Aortic Root Enlargement

Contributors

Sanford Zeigler, MD
Stanford University
Total Arch Replacement with Deep Hypothermic Circulatory Arrest for Aneurysm

Thomas J. Zeyl, MD
University of Florida
Hemiarch Replacement with DHCA – Aneurysm

Elena M. Ziarnik, MD
Vanderbilt University Medical Center
Tunneled Catheter Placement

Table of Contents

I. GENERAL THORACIC SURGERY — 1

1. Flexible Bronchoscopy — 2
- Essential Operative Steps — 2
- Potential Complications and Pitfalls — 2
- Template Dictation — 3

2. Rigid Bronchoscopy — 5
- Essential Operative Steps — 5
- Potential Complications and Pitfalls — 5
- Template Dictation — 5

3. Esophagogastroduodonoscopy — 8
- Essential Operative Steps — 8
- Potential Complications and Pitfalls — 8
- Template Dictation — 8

4. Mediastinoscopy — 10
- Essential Operative Steps: — 10
- Potential Complications and Pitfalls: — 10
- Template Dictation — 11

5. Chamberlain Procedure — 13
- Essential Operative Steps — 13
- Potential Complications and Pitfalls — 13
- Template Dictation — 13

6. Diagnositic Thoracoscopy — 15
- Essential Operative Steps — 15
- Potential Complications and Pitfalls — 15
- Template Dictation — 15

7. Tunneled Catheter Placement — 18
- Essential Operative Steps — 18
- Potential Complications and Pitfalls — 18
- Template Dictation — 19

8. Open Thoracostomy (Eloesser Flap and Clagett Window) — 21
- Essential Operative Steps — 21
- Potential Complications and Pitfalls — 21

I. General Thoracic Surgery

Template Dictation ... 21

9. Pleural Biopsy (Open/Thoracoscopic) ... 24
    Essential Operative Steps ... 24
    Potential Complications and Pitfalls ... 25
    Template Dictation ... 25

10. Pleurectomy and Decortication ... 27
    Essential Operative Steps ... 27
    Potential Complications and Pitfalls ... 28
    Template Dictation ... 28

11. Pleural Decortication (Open/Thoracoscopic) ... 31
    Essential Operative Steps ... 31
    Potential Complications and Pitfalls ... 33
    Template Dictation ... 33

12. Open Transthoracic Diaphragm Plication ... 36
    Essential Operative Steps ... 36
    Potential Complications and Pitfalls ... 36
    Template Dictation ... 36

13. Repair of Anterior Restrosternal (Morgagni) and Posterolateral (Bochdalek) Diaphragm Hernias ... 38
    Morgagni Hernia ... 38
    Bochdalek Hernia ... 40

14. VATS Evacuation of Hemothorax ... 43
    Essential Operative Steps ... 43
    Potential Complications and Pitfalls ... 43
    Template Dictation ... 43

15. VATS Pericardial Window ... 46
    Essential Operative Steps ... 46
    Potential Complications and Pitfalls ... 46
    Template Dictation ... 46

16. Chest Wall Tumor Resection and Chest Wall Reconstruction ... 49
    Essential Operative Steps ... 49
    Potential Complications and Pitfalls ... 50
    Template Dictation ... 50

17. Pancoast Tumor ... 54

Essential Operative Steps	54
Potential Complications and Pitfalls	54
Template Dictation	55

18. Tracheostomy — **58**
- Essential Operative Steps — 58
- Potential Complications and Pitfalls — 58
- Template Dictation — 59

19. Tracheal Resection and Reconstruction — **61**
- Essential Operative Steps — 61
- Potential Complications and Pitfalls — 61
- Template Dictation — 61

20. Esophageal Stent Placement — **64**
- Essential Operative Steps — 64
- Potential Complications and Pitfalls — 64
- Template Dictation — 64

21. Laparoscopic Nissen Fundoplication — **66**
- Essential Operative Steps — 66
- Potential Complications and Pitfalls — 67
- Template Dictation — 67

22. Laparoscopic Paraesophageal Hernia Repair — **70**
- Essential Operative Steps — 70
- Potential Complications and Pitfalls — 71
- Template Dictation — 71

23. Transhiatal Esophagectomy — **76**
- Essential Operative Steps — 76
- Potential Complications and Pitfalls — 76
- Template Dictation — 77

24. Open Modified Mckeown Esophagectomy — **81**
- Essential Operative Steps — 81
- Potential Complications and Pitfalls — 82
- Template Dictation — 83

25. Open Ivor-Lewis Esophagectomy — **89**
- Essential Operative Steps — 89
- Potential Complications and Pitfalls — 90
- Template Dictation — 91

I. General Thoracic Surgery

26. Minimally Invasive Ivor-Lewis Esophagectomy	**96**
Essential Operative Steps	96
Potential Complications and Pitfalls	98
Template Dictation	98
27. Lung Volume Reduction Surgery	**104**
Essential Operative Steps	104
Potential Complications and Pitfalls	104
Template Dictation	104
28. VATS Wedge Resection	**106**
Essential Operative Steps	106
Potential Complications and Pitfalls	106
Template Dictation	107
29. VATS Sympathectomy	**109**
Essential Operative Steps	109
Potential Complications and Pitfalls	109
Template Dictation	110
30. VATS Thymectomy	**112**
Essential Operative Steps	112
Potential Complications and Pitfalls	112
Template Dictation	113
31. Transcervical Thymectomy	**115**
Essential Operative Steps	115
Potential Complications and Pitfalls	116
Template Dictation	117
32. Trans-Sternal Thymectomy	**119**
Essential Operative Steps	119
Potential Complications and Pitfalls	119
Template Dictation	119
33. Open Lobectomies	**122**
Right Upper Lobectomy	122
Right Middle Lobectomy	125
Right Lower Lobectomy	127
Left Upper Lobectomy	129
Left Lower Lobectomy	132
34. Segmentectomy	**135**

Essential Operative Steps	135
Potential Complications and Pitfalls	135
Template Dictation	136
35. Carinal Pneumonectomy	**143**
Essential Operative Steps	143
Potential Complications and Pitfalls	144
Template Dictation	144
36. Extrapleural Pneumonectomy for Mesothelioma	**149**
Essential Operative Steps	149
Potential Complications and Pitfalls	150
Template Dictation	151
37. Lung Procurement	**154**
Essential Operative Steps	154
Potential Complications and Pitfalls	154
Template Dictation	156
38. Lung Transplantation	**161**
Essential Operative Steps	161
Potential Complications and Pitfalls	161
Template Dictation	163
39. Bronchial and Arterial Sleeve Resection	**167**
Essential Operative Steps	167
Potential Complications and Pitfalls	167
Template Dictation	168

II. ADULT CARDIAC SURGERY   173

1. Aortic Root Replacement for Ascending Aortic Aneurysm	**174**
Essential Operative Steps	174
Potential Complications and Pitfalls	175
Template Dictation	175
2. Aortic Root Replacement (Endocarditis)	**178**
Essential Operative Steps	178
Potential Complications and Pitfalls	178
Template Dictation	178
3. Total Arch/Hemiarch Replacement with DHCA – Dissection	**181**

Essential Operative Steps	181
Potential Complications and Pitfalls	183
Template Dictation	183

4. Elephant Trunk Part 1 — 187
- Essential Operative Steps — 187
- Potential Complications and Pitfalls — 187
- Template Dictation — 188

5. Elephant Trunk Part 2 — 191
- Essential Operative Steps — 191
- Potential Complications and Pitfalls — 191
- Template Dictation — 192

6. Endovascular Management of Acute Type B Dissection — 194
- Essential Operative Steps — 194
- Potential Complications and Pitfalls — 194
- Template Dictation — 194

7. Aortic Valve Replacement for Aortic Insufficiency or Aortic Stenosis — 197
- Essential Operative Steps — 197
- Potential Complications and Pitfalls — 197
- Template Dictation — 198

8. Aortic Valve Replacement with Aortic Root Enlargement — 200
- Essential Operative Steps — 200
- Potential Complications and Pitfalls — 201
- Template Dictation — 202

9. Biatrial Cox-Maze Ablation for Atrial Fibrillation — 206
- Essential Operative Steps — 206
- Potential Complications and Pitfalls — 206
- Template Dictation — 207

10. Coronary Artery Bypass Grafting With Cardiopulmonary Bypass — 210
- Essential Operative Steps — 210
- Potential Complications and Pitfalls — 210
- Template Dictation — 211

11. Coronary Artery Bypass Grafting With Mammary and Vein Grafts - Off Pump — 214
- Essential Operative Steps — 214
- Potential Complications and Pitfalls — 214

Template Dictation   215

12. Coronary Artery Bypass Grafting + Mitral Valve Repair Vs Replacement
    218
    Essential Operative Steps   218
    Potential Complications and Pitfalls   219
    Template Dictation   220

13. Coronary Artery Bypass Grafting With Aortic Valve Replacement   **223**
    Essential Operative Steps   223
    Potential Complications and Pitfalls   224
    Template Dictation   224

14. Devega Tricuspid Valve Repair   **227**
    Essential Operative Steps   227
    Potential Complications and Pitfalls   228
    Template Dictation   228

15. Donor Heart Procurement   **230**
    Essential Operative Steps   230
    Potential Complications and Pitfalls   231
    Template Dictation   231

16. Hemiarch Replacement with DHCA – Aneurysm   **233**
    Essential Operative Steps   233
    Potential Complications and Pitfalls   234
    Template Dictation   234

17. Aortic Root Replacement with Homograft For Aortic Root Abscess (Native And Or Prior Bentall)   **237**
    Essential Operative Steps   237
    Potential Complications and Pitfalls   238
    Template Dictation   240

18. Unexpected Intraoperative Complications   **244**
    Massive Air Embolism   244
    Intraoperative Aortic Dissection   247

19. LVAD – Heartware   **251**
    Essential Operative Steps   251
    Potential Complications and Pitfalls   251
    Template Dictation   252

20. LVAD – Heart Mate II — 254
- Essential Operative Steps — 254
- Potential Complications and Pitfalls — 254
- Template Dictation — 255

21. Minimally Invasive Directed Coronary Artery Bypass — 257
- Essential Operative Steps — 257
- Potential Complications and Pitfalls — 257
- Template Dictation — 257

22. Aortic Valve Surgery with Upper Hemisternotomy Approach — 260
- Essential Operative Steps — 260
- Potential Complications and Pitfalls — 260
- Template Dictation — 261

23. Mitral Valve Replacement — 264
- Essential Operative Steps — 264
- Potential Complications and Pitfalls — 265
- Template Dictation — 265

24. Minimally Invasive Mitral Surgery — 268
- Essential Operative Steps — 268
- Potential Complications and Pitfalls — 269
- Template Dictation — 269

25. Mitral Valve Repair for Bileaflet Prolapse — 273
- Essential Operative Steps — 273
- Potential Complications and Pitfalls — 274
- Template Dictation — 275

26. Orthotopic Heart Transplantation — 277
- Essential Operative Steps — 277
- Potential Complications and Pitfalls — 277
- Template Dictation — 278

27. Thoracoabdominal Aneurysm Repair — 281
- Essential Operative Steps — 281
- Potenital Complications and Pitfalls — 281
- Template Dication — 282

28. Permanent Pacemaker Insertion — 285
- Essential Operative Steps — 285
- Potential Complications and Pitfalls — 285

Template Dictation	286

29. Repair of Post-Infarction Ventricular Septal Defect   288
     Essential Operative Steps   288
     Potential Complications and Pitfalls   288
     Template Dictation   289

30. Repair of Post-Infarction Ventricular Aneurysm (Dor Endoventricular Circular Patch Plasty (EVCPP))   292
     Essential Operative Steps   292
     Potential Complications and Pitfalls   293
     Template Dictation   293

31. Pulmonary Embolectomy   297
     Essential Operative Steps   297
     Potential Complications and Pitfalls   297
     Template Dictation   298

32. Redo Sternotomy and Difficult Sternal Closure   301
     Essential Operative Steps   301
     Potential Complications and Pitfalls   303
     Template Dictation   305

33. Resection of Atrial Myxoma   308
     Essential Operative Steps   308
     Potential Complications and Pitfalls   308
     Template Dictation   309

34. Septal Myectomy   311
     Essential Operative Steps   311
     Potential Complications and Pitfalls   311
     Template Dictation   311

35. Endovascular Repair of Descending Thoracic Aortic Aneurysm (Tevar)   314
     Essential Operative Steps   314
     Potential Complications and Pitfalls   315
     Template Dictation   315

36. Total Arch Replacement with Deep Hypothermic Circulatory Arrest For Aneurysm   318
     Essential Operative Steps   318
     Potential Complications and Pitfalls   320

Template Dictation   320

37. Total Artificial Heart   324
    Essential Operative Steps   324
    Potential Complications and Pitfalls   324
    Template Dictation   325

38. Transcatheter Aortic Valve Implantation (TAVI): (Transfemoral-Transapical Approach)   327
    Essential Operative Steps   327
    Potential Complications and Pitfalls   328
    Template Dictation   328

39. Valve Sparing Root Replacement   330
    Essential Operative Steps   330
    Potential Complications and Pitfalls   330
    Template Dictation   331

III. CONGENITAL CARDIAC SURGERY   337

1. Repair of Atrial Septal Defect- Secundum Atrial Septal Defect   338
    Essential Operative Steps   338
    Potential Complications and Pitfalls   339
    Template Dictation   339

2. Ventricular Septal Defect: Perimembranous   342
    Essential Operative Steps   342
    Potential Complications and Pitfalls   343
    Template Dictation   344

3. Partial AV Canal Repair   347
    Essential Operative Steps   347
    Potential Complications and Pitfalls   348
    Template Dictation   349

4. Complete Atrioventricular Canal Repair   352
    Essential Operative Steps   352
    Potential Complications and Pitfalls   353
    Template Dictation   354

5. Repair of Partial Anomalous Pulmonary Venous Return   357
    Essential Operative Steps   357

Potential Complications and Pitfalls	357
Template Dictation	358

6. Supra-Cardiac Total Anomalous Pulmonary Venous Return (TAPVR) — 361
Essential Operative Steps	361
Potential Complications and Pitfalls	362
Template Dictation	363

7. Total Anomalous Pulmonary Venous Return (TAPVR) - Cardiac Type — 366
Essential Operative Steps	366
Potential Complications and Pitfalls	366
Template Dictation	366

8. Infra-Cardiac Total Anomalous Pulmonary Venous Return (TAPVR) — 369
Essential Operative Steps	369
Potential Complications and Pitfalls	370
Template Dictation	371

9. Patent Ductus Arteriosus Ligation — 376
Essential Operative Steps	376
Potential Complications and Pitfalls	376
Template Dictation	376

10. Aortic Coarctation Repair with Extended End-to-End Anastomosis — 379
Essential Operative Steps	379
Potential Complications and Pitfalls	380
Template Dictation	381

11. Division of Vascular Ring — 384
Essential Operative Steps	384
Potential Complications and Pitfalls	384
Template Dictation	384

12. Pulmonary Artery Banding — 387
Essential Operative Steps	387
Potential Complications and Pitfalls	387
Template Dictation	388

13. Modified Blalock-Taussig Shunt (Using Interposition Gore-Tex Tube Graft) — 390
Essential Operative Steps	390
Potential Complications and Pitfalls	391
Template Dictation	392

14. Norwood Procedure — 395
- Essential Operative Steps — 395
- Potential Complications and Pitfalls — 396
- Template Dictation — 396

15. Bidirectional Glenn Procedure — 400
- Essential Operative Steps — 400
- Potential Complications and Pitfalls — 401
- Template Dictation — 402

16. Completion Lateral Tunnel Fontan — 405
- Essential Operative Steps — 405
- Potential Complications and Pitfalls — 406
- Template Dictation — 406

17. Extra-Cardiac (Non-Fenestrated) Completion Fontan Procedure — 409
- Essential Operative Steps — 409
- Potential Complications and Pitfalls — 410
- Template Dictation — 411

18. Repair of Supravalvular Aortic Stenosis — 414
- Essential Operative Steps — 414
- Potential Complications and Pitfalls — 415
- Template Dictation — 415

19. Ross Procedure for the Correction of Congenital Aortic Stenosis — 417
- Essential Operative Steps — 417
- Potential Complications and Pitfalls — 418
- Template Dictation — 418

20. Repair Of Obstructive Hypertrophic Cardiomyopathy: (Septal Myomectomy) — 422
- Essential Operative Steps — 422
- Potential Complications and Pitfalls — 422
- Template Dictation — 423

21. Arterial Switch Procedure — 425
- Essential Operative Steps — 425
- Potential Complications and Pitfalls — 426
- Template Dictation — 427

22. Tetralogy of Fallot: Transventricular Repair — 430
- Essential Operative Steps — 430

Potential Complications and Pitfalls 431
Template Dictation 431

23. Tetralogy of Fallot Repair - Infundibular Sparing (Transatrial Repair) 434
Essential Operative Steps 434
Potential Complications and Pitfalls 435
Template Dictation 436

24. Pulmonary Valve Replacement and Reconstruction of Right Ventricle Outflow Tract 441
Essential Operative Steps 441
Potential Complications and Pitfalls 442
Template Dictation 443

25. Repair of Truncus Arteriousus (TA) 446
Essential Operative Steps 446
Potential Complications and Pitfalls 447
Template Dictation 448

26. Cone Repair for Ebstein Malformation 451
Essential Operative Steps 451
Potential Complications and Pitfalls 452
Template Dictation 452

27. Pediatric Lung Transplantation: Bilateral Sequential Lung Transplantation 455
Essential Operative Steps 455
Potential Complications and Pitfalls 456
Template Dictation 457

28. Pediatric Heart Transplantation 461
Essential Operative Steps 461
Potential Complications and Pitfalls 462
Template Dictation 462

I. General Thoracic Surgery

1. Flexible Bronchoscopy

Bharat Pancholy MD, and William H Warren MD

Rush University Medical Center, Chicago IL

Essential Operative Steps

Flexible bronchoscopy in a non-intubated patient

1. Monitoring = continuous pulse oximetry, non-invasive blood pressure monitoring, electrocardiographic monitoring.
2. IV access – peripheral or central IV access.
3. Apply supplemental oxygen either via nasal cannula or non-rebreather mask.
4. Sedation for comfort and cooperation:
5. Intravenous opiates (analgesic and antitussive)
6. Benzodiazepines (anxiolysis and antegrade amnesia)
7. Topical anesthetic – spraying hypopharynx with 1% or 2% lidocaine using atomizer
8. If inserting through nares –ask patient to plug one nare and inhale through other nostril. Then reverse. Whichever nare appears to be able to ventilate better, plan to introduce bronchoscopy through that nare. Place cotton tip applicator through the nare with lidocaine gel to anesthetize. Leave cotton tip applicator in place for 1 minute and then remove.
9. Introduce bronchoscope through the nose or mouth
10. Once true vocal cords visualized, inject 5 ml of 4% lidocaine – this will anesthetize the larynx and allow for easier advancement of the bronchoscope.
11. Visualization and inspection of the larynx, and vocal cords.
12. Assess vocal cord mobility
13. All lobar and segmental bronchi must be examined.
14. Tracheobronchial tree remote from the area in question is assessed first.
15. Bronchus leading to the known area of disease is examined.
16. Perform bronchoscopic procedure as indicated – biopsy, brushing, bronchoalveolar lavage, transbronchial needle aspiration.
17. Remove bronchoscope at termination of procedure

Flexible bronchoscopy in an intubated patient

1. Apply swivel adapter to endotracheal tube
2. Maintain ventilation through side arm of adapter
3. Bronchoscope is passed through tight fitting diaphragm on the adapter
4. Perform bronchoscopy and any associated procedures
5. Remove bronchoscopy, remove adapter.

Potential Complications and Pitfalls

1. Hypoxemia

2. Hypercapnia pre procedure/during/post procedure
3. Respiratory depression
4. Aspiration
5. Analgesic in elderly and debilitated patients should be minimized
6. Liver failure patients should not receive any benzodiazepines
7. Bleeding (risk is increased in following)
8. Increased with PT >40% of normal
9. Platelet count < 50,000
10. Uremia
11. Pulmonary hypertension
12. Pneumothorax after patient undergoing transbronchial biopsy
13. Bronchospasm
14. Increase in patients with asthma and severe chronic obstructive disease
15. Laryngospasm
16. Usually because of inadequate anesthetic to vocal cords and tracheobronchial tree.
17. Sepsis (usually after BAL)
18. Do not perform in patients with bilateral vocal cord paralysis
19. Can lead to edema resulting in life-threatening airway obstruction

Template Dictation

Preoperative Diagnosis: [INDICATION – e.g. severe/change in cough, hemoptysis, diffuse lung disease, bacteriologic sampling, lung abscess, aspiration)

Postoperative Diagnosis: Same

Procedure(s) Performed: Flexible bronchoscopy (with associated procedures)

Attending Surgeon: [BLANK]

Secondary Surgeon: [BLANK]

Assistants: [BLANK]

Anesthesia: [BLANK]

Indication(s) for Procedure: [AGE] year old [GENDER] with [DURATION] history of [COMPLAINT] –e.g. worsening cough and unresolving pneumonia]. Chest xray and sputum culture reveals [FINDINGS – collapse of lobe with gram stain with gram negative rods.].

Description of Procedure: The flexible bronchoscopy tower and bronchoscope was brought to the patient's room on [DATE]. The patient's identity and planned procedure were verified, and a time out was performed. Monitors and supplemental oxygen were applied. We proceeded to anesthetize the patient topically. The flexible bronchoscope was inserted [TRANSORALLY/TRANSNASALLY]. The vocal cords were visualized and bilateral movement was noted [or abnormal movement on the (left/right) side

was noted]. 1% lidocaine was injected through the bronchoscopy port anesthetizing the larynx. The tracheobronchial tree remote from the area of interest was assessed first. All lobes and segments were clearly visualized. Pathologic findings included **[FINDINGS, e.g. bronchial irritation, edema, etc). The bronchoscope was then moved to the area of concern. Findings of (e.g. large purulent mucous with edema) was identified in (area of tracheobronchial tree)].** (Further diagnostic procedures performed as indicated and described). Specimens removed included **[X, e.g bronchoalveolar lavage].** The bronchoscope was successfully removed without complication. Patient's hemodynamics continued to be **[X, e.g. stable]** at the end of procedure. The patient remained in a monitored bed post procedure.

Dr. **[BLANK]** was present and scrubbed for **[BLANK]** elements of this procedure.

2. Rigid Bronchoscopy

Cameron T. Stock, MD and Douglas J. Mathisen, MD

Massachusetts General Hospital, Boston, MA

Essential Operative Steps

1. Induction of anesthesia is initiated when all equipment and team members are present
2. The patient's neck is extended and a teeth guard is placed on the upper incisors
3. The bronchoscope is used to lift the epiglottis revealing the vocal cords
4. The bronchoscope is rotated 90 degrees while passing through the cords to minimize trauma
5. The bronchoscope is connected to the ventilator
6. The bronchoscope is advanced under direct vision to the area of interest
7. Serial dilations should proceed with gentle pressure and small incremental increases in the diameter of the bronchoscope. A gentle corkscrew action under direct vision is best.

Potential Complications and Pitfalls

1. Failure to clearly visualize the epiglottis and vocal cords by being posterior and under the larynx
2. Creation of a mucosal flap with the tip of the bronchoscope by advancing forcefully or without clearly visualizing the tracheal lumen
3. Perforation of the tracheal lumen by using excessive force or by not being in the axis of trachea when dilating a stenotic segment
4. Inadequate ventilation leading to CO_2 retention, acidosis and potential for arrhythmias

Template Dictation

Preoperative Diagnosis: Tracheal stenosis, tracheal malignancy

Postoperative Diagnosis: Same

Procedure(s) Performed: Rigid bronchoscopy, dilation of tracheal stenosis, dilation of endobronchial tumor

Attending Surgeon: [BLANK]

Secondary Surgeon: [BLANK]

Assistants: [BLANK]

Anesthesia: [BLANK]

Indication(s) for Procedure: [AGE] year old [GENDER] with known [tracheal tumor, tracheal stenosis, newly diagnosed asthma] who presented with increasing dyspnea and audible stridor. The patient was noted to be hypoxic with an increased work of breathing. Humidified facemask oxygen was administered, and the patient's symptoms stabilized. The patient was observed in the ICU while waiting for the operating room to open. The patient was brought expeditiously to the operating room for evaluation.

Description of Procedure: The patient was taken to the operating room on [DATE]. The patient was identified with two unique identifiers and the correct procedure was confirmed. The patient was placed supine on the operating table. After all necessary equipment and all members of the surgical team were confirmed present, general anesthesia was administered. Rigid bronchoscopes of sizes ranging from 3.5 mm to 9 mm and Jackson-Pilling esophageal bougies were available in the operating room. After the patient was preoxygenated with mask ventilation, the #7 rigid bronchoscope was passed into the patient's mouth and the glottis was clearly visualized. Care was taken not to lever the scope off the patient's incisors. The epiglottis was retracted anteriorly using the tip of the bronchoscope revealing the vocal cords. Both cords were noted to be moving symmetrically and no glottic edema was noted. The bronchoscope was passed through the cords by rotating the scope 90 degrees to enter the trachea parallel to the cords. The scope was cleared of secretions. The visualized tracheal mucosa was noted to be free from inflammation. We discussed with the anesthesiologist paralyzing the patient or using deep inhalation anesthesia. It was decided to proceed with our preferred method of spontaneous ventilation under deep inhalation anesthesia as the patient was adequately ventilating.

[Choose One:]

If obstructing tumor: We observed a near obstructing endobronchial tumor at the takeoff of the right mainstem bronchus. The #7 rigid bronchoscope was able to pass distal to the lesion along the membranous wall revealing a normal appearing bronchus intermedius that was not involved with tumor. The lesion was initially biopsied with a cupped biopsy forceps to check for consistency and avascularity. Next, using the beveled tip of the bronchoscope and advancing slowly with a constant rotary motion, the center of the tumor was cored out. After several passes with the bronchoscope in this manner, we were left with a patent bronchial lumen. Bleeding was controlled with direct pressure applied by the bronchoscope, and tumor fragments were removed with the suction catheter. At the conclusion of the procedure the bronchoscope was able to easily pass through the right main bronchus into the bronchus intermedius.

If benign stenosis: At 3 cm distal to the vocal cords, we observed a tight tracheal stenosis consistent with the patient's known post-intubation stenosis. The tracheal lumen appeared to narrow to a diameter of 2-3mm, and the surrounding tracheal mucosa appeared injected and inflamed. Secretions were cleared with a long suction catheter. Serial dilations of the stricture were initiated using the Jackson-Pilling esophageal bougies beginning with the smallest and progressively increasing their size. Next the #7 bronchoscope was withdrawn, and the 3.5 mm bronchoscope was advanced to the lesion. Using firm but gentle pressure and slight rotation of the bronchoscope, the scope was advanced past the stenotic segment. Care was taken not to exert excessive force so as to avoid perforating the membranous trachea proximal to the lesion. The bronchoscope was immediately connected to the ventilator and the patient was bag ventilated to facilitate clearance of CO_2. The 4 mm bronchoscope was next used to traverse the lesion. We incrementally increased the size of the bronchoscope until the 8 mm bronchoscope was able to pass easily through the area of previous stenosis. Small tissue fragments were carefully removed using the biopsy forceps and suctioning. Areas of bleeding were tamponaded using the bronchoscope and topical dilute epinephrine was also used to control oozing from the tracheal lumen. At this point no further dilations were thought to be necessary. At the conclusion of the procedure, the patient was well oxygenated and hemodynamically stable. All instrument, sponge, and needle counts were confirmed to be correct. The bronchoscope was withdrawn. The patient was awoken from anesthesia and brought to the recovery room in stable condition. In anticipation of some swelling following our dilation, Decadron 10 mg IV then 4 mg IV every 6 hours for 24 hours was ordered for the patient. A chest x-ray was ordered.

Dr. [BLANK] was present and scrubbed for [BLANK] elements of this procedure.

3. Esophagogastroduodonoscopy

Timothy J Pirolli, MD and Ahmad Y. Sheikh, MD

Stanford University Hospital and Clinics, Stanford, California

Essential Operative Steps

1. Lines and Monitoring
2. General endotracheal anesthesia with single-lumen endotracheal tube or monitored anesthesia care
3. Checking all equipment to ensure the video monitor, insufflation and saline infusion ports are working adequately.
4. Insert gastroscope into esophageal inlet (direct laryngosopy may be used to facilitate insertion of scope)
5. Advance gastroscope with insufflation and examine the esophagus. Assess for mucosal changes. Document location of z-line (gastroesophageal junction) and diaphragmatic pinch to assess for a hiatal hernia.
6. Advance gastroscope with insufflation and examine the gastric mucosa
7. Retroflex gastroscope to examine the cardia. Endoscopically grade (i.e., Hill classification) of the gastroesophageal valve.
8. Advanced gastroscope with insufflation to examine the pylorus and duodenum.
9. Take biopsies as needed
10. Retract gastroscope with desufflation under direct vision
11. Extubate patient and transfer to PACU

Potential Complications and Pitfalls

1. Oropharyngeal trauma
2. Difficulty positioning gastroscope down the esophagus due to anatomical anomalies or strictures. A pediatric gastroscope and or gentle dilatation may be helpful
3. Bleeding
4. Esophageal or gastric perforation
5. Failure to desufflate the gastrointestinal lumen

Template Dictation

Preoperative Diagnosis: [INDICATION - e.g. Dysphagia, GERD]

Postoperative Diagnosis: Same

Procedure(s) Performed: Esophagogastroduodenoscopy.

Attending Surgeon: [BLANK]

Secondary Surgeon: [BLANK]

Assistants: [BLANK]

Anesthesia: [BLANK]

Indication(s) for Procedure: [AGE] year old [GENDER] with [DURATION] history of [COMPLAINT – e.g. increasing dysphagia and reflux]. After the risks and benefits were describe to the patient, he/she signed informed consent and proceeded to the operating room for an esophagogastroduodenoscopy

Description of Procedure: The patient was taken to the operating room on [DATE]. The patient's identity and planned procedure verified with a surgical timeout, and the patient was placed on the operating room table in the supine position. General anesthesia with a single-lumen endotracheal tube was obtained. The flexible adult gastroscope was inserted into the posterior oropharynx and posterior to the left arytenoid, into the esophageal inlet. Insufflation was gently used to expand the lumen. The cricopharyngeus was located at [DISTANCE] from the incisors. The cervical and thoracic esophagus were inspected and normal mucosa was observed. There were no strictures, esophagitis, erosions, ulcers, petechiae, or other abnormalities. The gastroesophageal junction was located at [DISTANCE] from the incisors. There was no evidence of Barrett's esophagus, hiatal hernia or other abnormalities. **[Insert abnormal findings]** We then entered the stomach. The gastroscope was retroflexed to examine the cardia, which was normal. A Hill class [X] valve was noted. The remainder of the stomach was examined and appeared normal. The gastroscope was then advanced to the pylorus, which was widely patent. The scope was inserted through the pylorus without difficulty, and the first, second and third portions of the duodenum were inspected and found to be normal, without evidence of ulcer disease. The duodenum and stomach were evacuated free of air and debris and the scope withdrawn into the distal esophagus. There was no evidence of perforation or mucosal irregularity. We then removed the gastroscope without difficulty.

All instrument, sponge and needle counts were confirmed to be correct x 2 at the end of the operation. The patient was extubated and subsequently transferred to the post-anesthesia care unit in stable condition.

Dr. **[BLANK]** was present and scrubbed for **[BLANK]** elements of this procedure.

4. Mediastinoscopy

Nicholas Baker, MD and Ryan Levy, MD

University of Pittsburgh Medical Center, Pittsburgh, PA.

Essential Operative Steps:

1. Right radial arterial line
2. General endotracheal anesthesia
3. Prep and drape entire neck and chest in the event an emergent median sternotomy is required
4. Transverse skin incision one fingerbreadth above sternal notch
5. Divide platysma transversely and strap muscles longitudinally in midline
6. Palpate for high innominate artery
7. Incise pretracheal fascia and enter with mediastinoscope
8. Blunt finger dissection to develop the pretracheal plane to the level of the carina, staying on the trachea during the dissection
9. Insert mediastinoscope with tip angled toward airway
10. Identify carina and level 7 lymph nodes
11. Identify left tracheobronchial angle and level 4L nodes
12. Identify right tracheobronchial angle and level 4R nodes
13. Biopsy superficially with care not to injure deep structures.
14. Check for hemostasis
15. Approximate strap muscles, platysma, and skin

Potential Complications and Pitfalls:

1. Review preoperative CT for calcified lymph node targets, high innominate artery and aberrant anatomy
2. Place patient with head at top of bed with full neck extension
3. Eye protection for the patient
4. Monitor arterial line to identify excess pressure on innominate artery
5. Palpate for high innominate artery.
6. Mediastinoscope must be under pretracheal fascia
7. Keep tip of mediastinoscope angled toward airway when advancing in to chest
8. Stay on the trachea and mainstem bronchi
9. Biopsy superficially only visible nodes
10. Structures at risk for injury when biopsying level 7 nodes: esophagus, deep main pulmonary artery, anterior pericardium, left atrium
11. Structures at risk for injury when biopsying level 4L nodes: lateral aorta and left recurrent laryngeal nerve (NO CAUTERY due to the risk of nerve injury)
12. Structures at risk for injury when biopsying level 4R nodes: lateral azygos, pleura, right pulmonary artery
13. Control bleeding with pressure the pretracheal space (DO NOT REMOVE MEDIASTINOSCOPE WHEN YOU ENCOUNTER

BLEEDING). Pack the pretracheal plane, keep calm, assess the situation and assure you have adequate IV access and help. A Sternal saw should be kept in the room at all times during this operation so that it may be immediately available in an emergency.

Template Dictation

Preoperative Diagnosis: [INDICATION – e.g. Lung cancer, lung nodule, mediastinal lymphadenopathy]

Postoperative Diagnosis: Same

Procedure(s) Performed: Video assisted mediastinoscopy

Attending Surgeon: [BLANK]

Secondary Surgeon: [BLANK]

Assistants: [BLANK]

Anesthesia: [BLANK]

Indication(s) for Procedure: [AGE] year old [GENDER] with [DURATION] history of [Complaint – e.g. lung mass, nodule, or mediastinal lymphadenopathy].

Description of Procedure: The patient was taken to the operative suite on [DATE]. The patient's identity and planned procedure verified and the patient was placed supine of the operating table. Following an uneventful induction of general anesthesia, the patient was intubated with a single lumen endotracheal tube without incident. A right radial arterial line was placed. The patient's arms were tucked, a shoulder roll was placed, and the neck was extended as much as safely possible. Eye protection goggles were placed on the patient. The patient's neck and entire chest was prepped and draped in a sterile standard fashion.

The skin was marked one finger breadth above the sternal notch. A transverse two centimeter skin incision was made and electrocautery was used to incise the platysma in a transverse fashion. The strap muscles were divided in the midline in a longitudinal fashion. The trachea was identified, pretracheal fascia was sharply incised with Metzenbaum scissors and the pretracheal space was developed using blunt finger dissection.

Next the mediastinoscope was placed into the pretracheal space just above the trachea and advanced into the mediastinum. Blunt dissect with a mediastinoscope sucker with intermittent touch cautery was, used to dissect along the anterior trachea down to the level of the carina. The right and left main stem bronchus were identified. Blunt dissection with suction and touch electrocautery was used to identify level 7 lymph nodes. Cup biopsy forceps were used to superficially biopsy visible level 7 nodes. Next, the left tracheobronchial angle was identified. Blunt dissection without using electrocautery was used to dissect level 4L lymph nodes. Cup biopsy forceps were used to superficially biopsy visible level 4L nodes. Next, right tracheobronchial angle was identified. Blunt dissection with suction and touch electrocautery was used to dissect level 4R lymph nodes. Cup biopsy forceps were used to superficially biopsy visible level 4R nodes.

Hemostasis was obtained with careful electrocautery and pressure from packing a sponge into the wound. The sponge was removed and hemostasis was acceptable. The mediastinoscope was removed. The strap muscles were approximated with #2-0 absorbable stitch, the platysma was approximated with a #2-0 absorbable stitch, and the skin was approximated with a #4-0 absorbable stitch. Benzoin, steri-strips, and dry sterile dressing were applied.

All instrument, sponge, and needle counts were confirmed to be correct x 2 at the end of the operation. The patient was extubated in the operating room and subsequently transferred to the post anesthesia care unit in stable condition.

Dr. [**BLANK**] was present and scrubbed for [**BLANK**] elements of this procedure.

5. Chamberlain Procedure

Geoffrey T. Lam, MD, and Jessica S. Donington, MD

NYU School of Medicine, New York, NY

Essential Operative Steps

1. Lines and monitoring
2. General endotracheal anesthesia: double-lumen tube preferable but not essential
3. Bronchoscopy: to confirm double-lumen tube placement
4. Transverse mediastinotomy in second left intercostal space
5. Preservation of internal mammary artery
6. Biopsy
7. Evacuation of pleural air if pleural space entered
8. Closure of incision

Potential Complications and Pitfalls

1. Injury to internal mammary artery or vein
2. Injury to aorta or pulmonary artery
3. Pneumothorax
4. Injury to phrenic nerve
5. Injury to recurrent laryngeal nerve

Template Dictation

Preoperative Diagnosis: [INDICATION – e.g. mediastinal lymphadenopathy, anterior mediastinal mass]

Postoperative Diagnosis: Same

Procedure(s) Performed: Chamberlain procedure with biopsy, fiberoptic bronchoscopy

Attending Surgeon: [BLANK]

Secondary Surgeon: [BLANK]

Assistants: [BLANK]

Anesthesia: [BLANK]

Fluids: [BLANK]

EBL: [BLANK]

Specimens: [BLANK]

Drains: [BLANK]

Indication(s) for Procedure: [AGE] year old [GENDER] with [MEDIASTINAL LYMPHADENOPATHY]. Preoperative imaging revealed [FINDINGS].

Description of Procedure: Informed consent for surgery was obtained from the patient, including a discussion of risks, benefits and alternatives, and the form was documented in the chart. The patient was taken to the operating room on [DATE] and placed on the operating room table in the supine position. Anesthesia inserted appropriate intravascular access and hemodynamic monitoring lines. Preoperative IV antibiotics were administered. A time out was observed to identify the correct patient, procedure and anatomic location. General endotracheal anesthesia through a double-lumen tube was then induced. Bronchoscopy was performed, which confirmed proper placement of the endotracheal tube. The patient was left in the supine position with the neck extended and the arms tucked. A Bair Hugger was applied and all pressure points were padded. The left lung was isolated [IF SINGLE LUNG VENTILATION USED]. The neck and chest were prepped and draped in sterile fashion.

A 3 cm transverse incision was made in the second intercostal space to the left of the sternum. The pectoralis muscle was divided in the direction of its fibers, thereby exposing the chest wall. The intercostal fibers were divided from the superior aspect of the third rib, taking care not to injury the internal mammary artery. The mediastinal space was entered. Exposure was obtained by retracting the internal mammary artery medially, and by dissecting the mediastinal pleural free from the posterior sternum and retracting it laterally. The aortopulmonary window was digitally palpated and examined for enlarged lymph nodes. Lymph nodes were sampled from station 5 and 6 [DIRECTLY/USING THE MEDIASTINOSCOPE] and were passed off the field. The vagus and phrenic nerves were seen along the aortic arch and preserved. Hemostasis was achieved by direct pressure. Because the pleural space was entered, a small red rubber catheter was placed into left pleural space. The incision was closed in layers. The pectoralis fascia was closed using a running 0 Vicryl suture. The patient's back was then raised, and the left lung was re-inflated with the end of the red rubber catheter submerged under saline. When the bubbling ceased, the catheter was removed. The subcutaneous layer was closed using 2-0 Vicryl, and the skin was closed using a running 3-0 Monocryl subcuticular stitch. Sterile dry dressings were applied.

The patient tolerated the procedure well. The patient was extubated in the operating room and transferred in stable condition to the recovery room. At the end of the case, the sponge, needle and instrument counts were correct x2.

Dr. [BLANK] was present and scrubbed for [BLANK] elements of this procedure.

6. Diagnositic Thoracoscopy

Nicholas Engstrom, MD and Brandon Tieu, MD

Oregon Health and Sciences Center, Portland, Oregon

Essential Operative Steps

1. Lines and Monitoring
2. Single lumen endotracheal intubation
3. Flexible Bronchoscopy
4. Dual lumen endotracheal exchange
5. Positioning (lateral decubitus)
   a. Axillary roll
   b. Bean bag
   c. Elevated arm support
   d. Bed Flexion
6. Camera port 7th intercostal space, mid-axillary line
7. Working port in 5th intercostal space, anterior axillary line
8. Parietal pleural visualization
9. Mediastinal pleural visualization
   a. Anterior
   b. Posterior
10. Diaphragm visualization
11. Inspection of the fissures
12. Palpation of the Lung
13. Biopsy
14. Assess hemostasis
15. Intercostal nerve blocks
16. Chest tube placement
17. Assess lung re-inflation

Potential Complications and Pitfalls

1. Chest entrance injuries
   a. Lung
   b. Diaphragm
   c. Heart (left sided approach)
2. Biopsy site bleeding
3. Post op air-leak
4. Insufficient visualization

Template Dictation

Preoperative Diagnosis:

Postoperative Diagnosis:

Procedure(s) Performed: Diagnostic Thoracoscopy

I. General Thoracic Surgery

Attending Surgeon: [BLANK]

Secondary Surgeon: [BLANK]

Assistants: [BLANK]

Anesthesia: [BLANK]

Indication(s) for Procedure: Patient is a **(AGE)** year old **(GENDER)** with **(DURATION)** history of **(COMPLAINTS)**. He/she was evaluated with **(TESTS)** and found to have **(FINDINGS)**. A formal discussion regarding diagnostic thoracoscopy was held with the patient including but not limited to the following risks: **(RISKS)**. The patient agrees to proceed.

Description of Procedure: After obtaining informed consent, the patient was identified in the preoperative holding area, taken to the operating room, and placed in the supine position on the operating room table. All appropriate monitoring devices were placed. Following an uneventful induction of general anesthesia, the patient was intubated using a single lumen endotracheal tube. A timeout was conducted. Flexible bronchoscopy was performed. A complete examination of the lower trachea, bilateral mainstem and lobar bronchi, and segmental bronchi was performed. No blood, pus, or endobronchial lesions were noted. The patient has normal endobronchial anatomy.

The single lumen endotracheal tube was exchanged for a dual lumen endotracheal tube. The patient was then turned to the **(SIDE)** lateral decubitus position. An axillary roll was placed. The arms were secured in an elevated arm support with a padded arm board. Site identification was rechecked, and the patient was prepped and draped in sterile fashion. Anatomical landmarks were identified, and the camera port was created in the 7th intercostal space in the anterior axillary line. The thoracoscope was then introduced, and the chest wall was inspected. A second working **(SIZE)** incision was made in the **(INTERSPACE)** interspace **(LOCATION)**. There was no pleural effusion. The anterior and posterior mediastinal pleura were visualized. The parietal pleura was inspected. No abnormalities were noted. The lung was then retracted to the anterior working incision to allow digital palpation. The fissures were then investigated visually and by palpation. The thoracoscope was changed to the working incision to allow thorough investigation of the diaphragm. Biopsies were taken from **(SITES OF BIOPSY)** and the specimen(s) were sent for frozen section. Frozen sections demonstrated the presence of **(FINDINGS)**. Hemostasis at the biopsy and port sites was assured. Multilevel intercostal nerve blocks were performed using **(LOCAL ANESTHETIC)** from one rib space above the most cranial port site to one rib space below the most caudal port. A 28 French single chest tube was placed through the camera port and secured to the skin using 0 silk suture. Double lung ventilation was initiated and the **(SIDE)** lung fully inflated under direct vision. All sponge and instruments counts were correct. The anterior working incision was closed using 2-0 vicryl for musculofascial closure, 3-0 vicryl for deep dermal, and 4-0 vicryl for subcuticular closure. Sterile dressings were applied. The patient was extubated in the OR and transferred to the PACU in stable condition.

Dr. **[BLANK]** was present and scrubbed for **[BLANK]** elements of this procedure.

7. Tunneled Catheter Placement

Elena M. Ziarnik, MD and Otis Rickman, DO

Vanderbilt University Medical Center, Nashville, TN

Essential Operative Steps

1. Patient positioned in lateral decubitus, 30 degrees. Effusion side up.
2. Ultrasound guidance to evaluate the location of effusion, lung and diaphragm
3. Mark point of entry (approximately 4th-5th intercostal space at the mid-axillary line).
4. Mark exit site (at the costal margin in the midclavicular line)
5. Prep and drape, centering on the entry and exit site marks
6. Infiltrate skin and subcutaneous tissue with 5cc 1% lidocaine
7. Infiltrate exit site and planned tunnel with 10cc 1% lidocaine
8. Access fluid with the introducer needle (placed through the catheter) while applying suction with syringe
9. Remove needle and syringe, place guidewire through catheter, remove catheter
10. Make incisions for entry and exit sites with #11-blade. Exit site should be just big enough to tightly fit tunneling device. Access site should be large enough to accommodate catheter and peel-away trochar
11. Using tunneling device, create a tunnel from catheter exit incision to access incision
12. Position the catheter cuff just deep to the exit site
13. Sequentially dilate pleural tract over the guidewire, and insert the large bore peel-away trochar via Seldinger technique
14. Insert tunneled pleural catheter through trochar and peel away. Have patient hum to minimize air entry into pleural space.
15. Connect to drainage device to ensure catheter is not kinked
16. Secure catheter at exit site with #2-0 silk
17. Close access site with #2-0 silk horizontal mattress
18. Drain fluid as needed, can connect to low wall suction using provided adapter for initial drainage
19. Disconnect from drainage and secure to patients side with padded dressing.

Potential Complications and Pitfalls

1. Lung injury
2. Pneumothoarx
3. Bleeding, intercostal artery laceration
4. Positioning the catheter below the diaphragm
5. Pain with too aggressive initial drainage
6. Poorly positioned exit site (posteriorly or on a rib), which can increase patient discomfort

Template Dictation

Preoperative Diagnosis: [INDICATION – e.g. Malignant pleural effusion]

Postoperative Diagnosis: Same

Procedure(s) Performed: Indwelling tunneled pleural catheter placement, US guidance for catheter placement

Attending Surgeon: [BLANK]

Secondary Surgeon: [BLANK]

Assistants: [BLANK]

Anesthesia: [BLANK]

Indication(s) for Procedure: [AGE] year old [GENDER] with [DURATION] history of [COMPLAINT – e.g. increasing shortness of breath]. Pre-procedure CXR reveals [SIDE] pleural effusion. [Recurrent after thoracentesis, known malignancy, trapped lung}

Description of Procedure: The patient was positioned in lateral decubitus position with the head of bed at 30 degrees with the [AFFECTED] side up. Pleural fluid was identified on the [AFFECTED] side using ultrasound. The access site at the 5th intercostal space in the midaxillary line, and exit site just below the [AFFECTED SIDE] costal margin were marked. The chest was prepped and draped in the usual sterile fashion. The tunnel and exit site were anesthetized with 10 cc of 1% lidocaine, and the access site to pleural space was anesthetized with an additional 5 cc 1% lidocaine. Appropriate choice of the access site was confirmed by free flow of pleural fluid upon aspiration with a finder needle. The pleural space was accessed with a small-bore catheter over a needle. After confirming access into the pleural space by free flow of pleural fluid, the needle was removed, and catheter was left in the pleural space. The wire was advanced into the pleural space through the catheter. Stab incisions were made at the planned exit and access sites with an #11-blade scalpel. Using the tunneling device, the catheter was tunneled through subcutaneous tissue. The cuff was positioned about 5 cm from exit incision. A tapered dilator and peel away sheath trochar were advanced over the wire and advanced into the pleural space. The inner dilator and wire were removed, and the tunneled catheter was fed into the pleural space without resistance. The peel away trochar was pulled apart while advancing and holding pressure on the catheter until the trochar was removed and the catheter was completely in the pleural space. There was no kinking of the catheter. Pleural fluid was easily drained from the catheter. The access site was closed with a #2-0 silk horizontal mattress suture, and the catheter was secured at exit site with a #2-0 silk suture in a Roman sandal fashion. The catheter was capped after cleaning it with alcohol. Skin at the exit site was prepped. Foam padding and a bio-occlusive dressing were applied.

Dr. [**BLANK**] was present and scrubbed for [**BLANK**] elements of this procedure.

8. Open Thoracostomy (Eloesser Flap and Clagett Window)

Jacob Moremen, MD and Thomas Birdas, MD

Division of Cardiothoracic Surgery, Indiana University School of Medicine, Indianapolis, Indiana

Essential Operative Steps

1. Lines and monitoring
2. General endotracheal anesthesia
3. Two lung ventilation (unless empyema not drained and potential for lung reexpansion)
4. Lateral decubitus positioning
5. Skin incisions vary (must include most dependent portion of chest, may include prior incisions and tube thoracostomy site if possible)
6. Clagett window: Lateral 6-8 cm thoracotomy and extended in a "Y" fashion laterally and medially; or elliptical incision may be used
7. Eloesser flap: uses U-shaped incision
8. Raise skin flaps
9. Clagett: 2-3 cm circumferentially
10. Eloesser: Single long flap (area inside the U-curve)
11. Removal of 1-3 ribs (ensure large access to most dependent portion of pleural space)
12. Complete debridement of necrotic tissue and irrigation of space
13. Marsupialize space with heavy absorbable suture
14. Clagett: sew edges of flaps to thickened parietal pleura circumferentially
15. Eloesser: sew large skin flap into base of opened area
16. Ensure adequate hemostasis
17. Pack with sterile moist gauze

Potential Complications and Pitfalls

1. Large window is key
2. Inadequate thoracostomy can result in premature closure of skin before deep space granulation
3. Incision too cephalad may not completely drain basilar space
4. May require single lung ventilation if empyema not fully drained preoperatively
5. Used in patients too frail or with inadequate tissue for muscle flap thoracoplasty or as part of staged repair of bronchopleural fistula
6. Inadequate drainage of infection, debridement of necrotic tissue
7. Chronic *apical* space problems are better managed with extrapleural thoracoplasty

Template Dictation

Preoperative Diagnosis: Chronic basilar space infection [ADDITIONAL SPECIFICS – e.g. bronchopleural fistula, tuberculosis]

Postoperative Diagnosis: Same

Procedure(s) Performed: Open thoracostomy [Clagett window or Eloesser flap]

Attending Surgeon: [BLANK]

Secondary Surgeon: [BLANK]

Assistants: [BLANK]

Anesthesia: [BLANK]

Indication(s) for Procedure: [AGE] year old [GENDER] with [DURATION] history of basilar pleural space infection following [ORIGINAL PROCEDURE/DIAGNOSIS] and failed conservative therapy with antibiotics and tube thoracostomy. Prior decortication did not successfully obliterate space and is here today for open drainage and thoracostomy.

Description of procedure: The patient was taken to the operating room on [DATE]. The patient's identity and planned procedure verified, and the patient was placed on the operating room table in the supine position. Appropriate intravenous antibiotics and subcutaneous heparin were administered prior to the induction of anesthesia. General anesthesia was induced, and the patient was intubated with a double lumen endotracheal tube. Position of the tube was verified via flexible bronchoscopy and was found to be adequate. The patient was then placed in the [SIDE] lateral decubitus position. The tube thoracostomy was removed, and the entire chest prepped and draped in sterile fashion. An 8 cm posterolateral thoracotomy incision was made over the most dependent portion of the right pleural space. Cautery dissection was carried down through muscle layers, and the pleural space was entered on the superior aspect of the rib. A finochietto rib retractor was inserted.

The skin incision was extended in a Y-shaped fashion [or ELIPTICALLY] for better exposure of the ribs. A 2 to 3 cm skin flap was raised circumferentially. The [NUMBER] ribs were identified for resection to optimally expose the basilar space. A 6-8 cm length of each rib was exposed and freed from the surrounding tissue attachments circumferentially with Doyen dissector. A bone cutter was used to divide each rib laterally and medially, and the [NUMBER] ribs were resected. The neurovascular bundles were suture ligated proximally and distally and Intervening tissue resected and discarded.

With the space fully exposed, a sample of the empyema fluid was sent for culture. All necrotic, infected debris was decorticated from the lung and chest wall. A sample of the empyema rind was sent for culture. The chest was irrigated with two liters of warm antibiotic-containing saline. Hemostasis was achieved. Skin flaps were sutured with 0 Prolene suture in interrupted fashion to the thickened parietal pleura circumferentially. The wound was packed with several rolls of moist gauze and a large dry dressing applied over the defect.

All instrument, sponge and needle counts were confirmed to be correct x 2 at the end of the operation. The patient was subsequently transferred to the postoperative surgical intensive care unit in critical condition.

Dr. [BLANK] was present and scrubbed for [BLANK] elements of this procedure.

9. Pleural Biopsy (Open/Thoracoscopic)

David Graham, MD, and Kemp Kernstine, MD, PhD

University of Texas-Southwestern, Dallas, Texas

Essential Operative Steps

1. Lines and Monitoring
2. General endotracheal anesthesia
3. Single lung ventilation with bronchial blocker or dual-lumen endobronchial tube
4. Lateral decubitus position
5. Mark potential thoracotomy incision (generally resection of 7th rib via S-shaped incision)
6. Ask anesthesia to deflate lung on the operating side
7. Open Technique
    a. Review preoperative imaging and mark an area along the thoracotomy line where there appears to be significant thickened pleural tumor
    b. Make a limited 1-4 cm incision depending on thickness of soft tissue from the skin to chest wall
    c. Divide latissimus dorsi, dissect onto chest wall
    d. Dissect above rib dividing intercostal muscles and identify the hard, white pleural mass
    e. (A mediastinoscope can be used to facilitate exposure)
    f. Sharply resect (scalpel or biopsy forceps) a 1 cm square piece of pleura for improved histology and microbiology studies
    g. If more tissue needed, obtain more biopsies along the chest wall near the incision site
    h. Place saline into the wound and have anesthesia give a Valsalva maneuver up to 30 mmHg. If no bubbling, close wound in layers. If bubbling, place a Blake drain and close wound in layers.
8. Thoracoscopic Technique
    a. According to the chest computed tomogram findings and the topographical anatomy of the chest wall, use 25-guage sounding needle to locate effusion; send fluid for cytology/culture
    b. Make a skin incision and insert a 5 or 12 mm trocar into this location
    c. Place the 5 mm 30-degree thoracoscope into the trocar to confirm chest entry and to inspect pleura
    d. Insufflate with 5-10 mmHg CO_2 as needed to help with visualization
    e. Aspirate fluid and send to pathology for culture/cytology/gram stain
    f. Use mediastinal biopsy forceps or thoracoscopic biopsy forceps within the same port to remove tissue
    g. An additional port may be required (along the previously placed thoracotomy incision) if single port/incisional access inadequate

    h. Obtain hemostasis with hook electrocautery as needed
    i. Place chest tube (Blake or Argyle) through port site and secure using Nylon or Ethibond suture

Potential Complications and Pitfalls

1. Certain tumors especially mesothelioma has a propensity to seed and subsequently grow in surgical sites; therefore, keep all biopsy incisions within the planned line of thoracotomy incision.
2. NEVER biopsy the visceral pleura without using a stapling device; this will cause a persistent air leak and delay treatment
3. If additional tissue is needed, do not resect more pleural rind on the lung (Pitfall #2, obtain more tissue along chest wall)
4. Take care not to dissect too deeply into chest wall when taking parietal pleural biopsies as meddlesome bleeding can occur
5. If definitive procedure planned in the near future, chest tube placement without pleurodesis is appropriate; however, if delay is anticipated, then palliation of the effusion can be performed. If the lung fully expands, intraoperative talc or Betadine pleurodesis is an option. If the lung is entrapped, a tunneled, valved pleural catheter for external intermittent drainage would be best for palliation.

Template Dictation

Preoperative Diagnosis: [INDICATION – e.g. Recurrent bloody pleural effusions, Pleural thickening, Pleural neoplasm]

Postoperative Diagnosis: Same

Procedure(s) Performed: Open pleural biopsy

Attending Surgeon: [BLANK]

Secondary Surgeon: [BLANK]

Assistants: [BLANK]

Anesthesia: [BLANK]

Indication(s) for Procedure: [AGE] year old [GENDER] with [DURATION] history of [COMPLAINT – e.g. increasingly dyspnea and recurrent bloody pleural effusions, preoperative imaging shows concern for pleural thickening and prior attempts for percutaneous biopsy and cytology have been negative. Thoracic surgery was consulted for open surgical biopsy.

Description of Procedure: The patient was taken to the operating room on [DATE]. The patient's identity and planned procedure verified, and the patient was placed on the operating room table in the supine position. General anesthesia was obtained and a dual-lumen endobronchial tube was then placed. The patient was positioned in the lateral decubitus position. We then proceeded to prep and drape the chest in sterile fashion. An Ioban dressing was placed. A time out was performed.

A posterolateral thoracotomy incision was marked at approximately the level of the 6th intercostal space. A 2 cm incision was made using a #15 blade along this marking in the posterior axillary line. The dissection was carried down through the latissimus dorsi and onto the chest wall using electrocautery. The intercostal muscles were divided on the superior border of the rib. A white firm mass was encountered. Sharp resection of this mass was performed and sent to pathology for examination. Saline was placed into the wound and anesthesia provided a Valsalva maneuver at 30 mmHg. No air leak was noted. The wound was closed in layers using Vicryl suture followed by a subcuticular monofilament suture. Tegaderm was placed as the sterile dressing.

All instrument, sponge and needle counts were confirmed to be correct x 2 at the end of the operation. The patient was subsequently transferred to the postoperative cardiac surgical intensive care unit in critical condition.

Dr. [BLANK] was present and scrubbed for [BLANK] elements of this procedure.

10. Pleurectomy and Decortication

Abby White, DO and Scott J. Swanson, MD

Brigham and Women's Hospital, Boston, Massachusetts

Essential Operative Steps

1. Lines and monitoring
   a. Arterial catheter
   b. Central Venous Catheter
   c. Naso-gastric tube help avoid esophageal injury
2. General endotracheal anesthesia via dual lumen endotracheal tube.
3. Bronchoscopy
4. Posterolateral thoracotomy, through latissimus dorsi and sparing serratus anterior muscles
5. Sixth rib resection
6. Blunt and cautery dissection between endothoracic fascia and parietal pleura starting at the vicinity of entry and proceeding laterally, anteriorly and posteriorly before reaching the apex.
7. Careful attention must be drawn to avoiding injury to the subclavian vessels, phrenic and vagal nerves, superior vena cava, azygous vein, esophagus and the internal mammary vessels.
8. Packing with lap pads for hemostasis along raw surface areas to minimize blood loss
9. Mobilization of the pleura from the mediastinum, taking care to avoid injury to the phrenic and recurrent laryngeal nerves.
10. Inferior dissection of the pleural off of the diaphragm
11. Mobilization toward the diaphragmatic sulcus, starting from the posterior costophrenic angle and moving anteriorly.
12. Avoid entry into the peritoneum where possible, though this is particularly difficult when dissecting around the central tendon. Entry is repaired as soon as it is seen. We prefer to use running 2-0 Vicryl.
13. Dissection is carried to the posterior pericardium, which is removed en bloc if no planes between tumor and pericardium can be safely identified.
14. Once dissection is complete to the hilum, the parietal pleura is entered and the visceral decortication undertaken.
15. Dissection in the fissures is undertaken with caution, using inflation and deflation of the lung for hemostasis and identification of tissue planes between pleura and parenchyma respectively.
16. Systematic interlobar, hilar and mediastinal lymphadenectomy is done routinely
17. Hemostasis is obtained, often with the help of an Argon beam electrocaogulator to control raw surface area bleeding at the chest wall.
18. The chest is irrigated with multiple liters of normal saline and water.
19. In carefully selected patients, intraoperative heated chemotherapy (IOHC) is delivered. We use weight-based dosing of cisplatin and gemcitabine.

We use a 60-minute chemotherapy run; shorter runs are utilized for patients with borderline renal function.
20. If pericardial resection is required to achieve a complete resection, we reconstruct the pericardium with fenestrated PTFE (0.1mm) to prevent cardiac herniation and epicarditis. The patch is fenestrated to prevent tamponade from accumulation of pericardial fluid or blood
21. If the tumor extension involves the diaphragmatic muscle, with the diaphragm is reconstructed with PTFE (2 mm). Two pieces of 20 x 30 DualMesh are stapled together to create a loose patch that decreases tension, reduces the incidence of patch dehiscence and herniation of abdominal organs into the chest. We secure the diaphragmatic patch circumferentially, using both interrupted 2-0 Prolene and the ProTack device.
22. Three chest tubes are placed, one anteriorly and directed towards the apex, one posteriorly and directed towards the apex, and one right-angled chest tube along the diaphragm. Wide drainage is necessary to control air leaks and to allow complete re-expansion of the lung.
23. The thoracotomy incision is closed in standard fashion.

Potential Complications and Pitfalls

1. Be prepared to manage significant blood loss and maintain closed loop communication with the anesthesia team regarding this. We have typed and cross-matched blood available and in the operating room throughout the duration of the procedure.
2. Injury to the subclavian vessels can occur at the apices bilaterally.
3. On the right, the superior vena cava and azygous vein are at risk with dissection of the mediastinal pleural in this area.
4. On the left, the plane between tumor and adventitia of the aorta, intercostal vessels, and the esophagus should be sought judiciously.
5. Vocal cord injury should be treated with prompt injection medicalization to prevent aspiration in the early postoperative period.
6. A tight pericardial patch can predispose to positional hemodynamic compromise and cardiac tamponade.
7. A tight diaphragmatic patch around the IVC can result in impaired cardiac filling
8. When delivering IOHC, careful attention must be paid pre-, intra- and post-operatively to adequate fluid resuscitation to avoid potential renal toxicity from cisplatin

Template Dictation

Preoperative Diagnosis: [**Indication** – eg. [EPITHELIOD/BIPHASIC] Malignant Mesothelioma of the [LEFT/RIGHT]]

Postoperative Diagnosis: Same (Add invasion of relevant structures)

Procedure(s) Preformed: Bronchoscopy, [RIGHT/LEFT] pleurectomy and decortication, +/- diaphragmatic resection and reconstruction, +/- pericardial resection and reconstruction, +/- Intraoperative Heated Chemotherapy (IOHC), and mediastinal lymph node dissection

Attending Surgeon: [BLANK]

Secondary Surgeon: [BLANK]

Assistants: [BLANK]

Anesthesia: [BLANK]

Indication(s) for Procedure

Description of Procedure: The patient was brought to the operating room on [**DATE**]. Name, birthdate and nature of the procedure were verified. After an uneventful induction of general anesthesia, the patient was intubated with a single-lumen endotracheal tube without incident. Flexible bronchoscopy was performed. There were minimal secretions. No endoluminal abnormalities or anatomic variations were noted.

Single-lumen endotracheal tube was exchanged to a [**RIGHT/LEFT**]-sided double lumen endotracheal tube and the patient was repositioned in the [**RIGHT/LEFT**] lateral decubitus position and was prepped and draped in the usual sterile fashion. A [**RIGHT/LEFT**] posterolateral thoracotomy was performed, transecting the latissimus muscle. The serratus anterior muscle was preserved and retracted anteriorly. The sixth interspace was entered, and 15 cm of the rib was excised. Standard rib and scapular retractors were placed. The extrapleural dissection proceeded circumferentially around the thoracotomy. Starting posteriorly and inferiorly, we were able to define the extrapleural plane down to the base of the diaphragm and then superiorly to the apex, taking care to identify and protect the subclavian vessels, aorta and esophagus. We then performed a radical visceral pleurectomy and decorticated the tumor off the fissure and all lobes to the level of the hilar reflection. All gross disease was resected. Because the diaphragm was involved, it had to be avulsed circumferentially.

Argon beam coagulation was used for tumorolysis and hemostasis along the entire lung surface into the fissures and chest wall. A chemical scrub was performed with 3 cycles of hydrogen peroxide in 1 liter of water followed by 1 liter of saline. The chest was then pulse lavaged. Intracavitary heated chemotherapy was then performed with cisplatin and gemcitabine for 60 minutes. The abdominal peritoneum was inspected and any defects repaired primarily with running #2-0 Vicryl. The chest was evacuated; all chemotherapy fluid was recovered. The chest was irrigated and checked for hemostasis. A Gore-Tex 1 mm **[2mm on Left]** Dualmesh patch was fashioned to reconstruct the diaphragm and secured to chest wall with #2-0 Prolene sutures around the chest wall thru the 8th interspace and thru the tip of the 5th rib anteriorly. The patch was secured posteriorly using a laparoscopic tacking device. The rest of the patch was secured to the anterior chest wall and to the pericardium with interrupted #0-Prolene sutures.

After ensuring hemostasis, three **[RIGHT/LEFT]**-sided chest tubes were placed as follows: a 28 French anterior angled chest tube over the dome of the diaphragm into the costophrenic sulcus, a 28 French straight anterior, and a 28 French straight posterior to the apex along the gutter. Number 2 Vicryl pericostal sutures were placed, and the lung was allowed to re-inflate completely. The incision was closed in layers with Vicryl sutures. One previous port site excised completely down to chest wall. The double lumen endotracheal tube was then exchanged to a single-lumen tube. Toilet bronchoscopy showed moderate amount of secretions that were suctioned to clear. The patient was taken to the ICU intubated in stable condition. All note, sponge, needle, and instrument counts were correct at the end of the operation.

Dr. **[BLANK]** was present and scrubbed for **[BLANK]** elements of this procedure.

11. Pleural Decortication (Open/Thoracoscopic)

David Graham, MD, and Kemp Kernstine, MD, PhD

University of Texas-Southwestern, Dallas, Texas

Essential Operative Steps

1. Lines and Monitoring
2. General endotracheal anesthesia
3. Single lung ventilation with bronchial blocker or dual-lumen endobronchial tube
4. Bronchoscopy to evaluate for bronchial obstruction
5. Lateral decubitus position
6. Mark posterolateral thoracotomy incision (2 fingerbreadths below scapular tip in an S-shaped fashion. Planned incision in the 5th intercostal space)
7. Ask anesthesia to deflate lung on the operating side immediately prior to entering the pleural space
8. Open Technique
    a. Posterolateral thoracotomy. Divide the latissimus dorsi; spare the serratus anterior.
    b. Divide the intercostal muscles above the 6th or 7th rib (5th or 6th intercostal space) and enter pleural cavity taking care to avoid injury to the lung
    c. Drain fluid and send to pathology for cytology/gram stain/culture- aerobic, anaerobic, mycobacterial and fungal
    d. Place rib spreader (Tuffier or Finochietto)
    e. Mobilize lung by detaching pleural adhesions and divide inferior pulmonary ligament
    f. Remove gelatinous/fibrinous deposits and blood clots (if present)
    g. Decorticate chest wall and diaphragm
    h. Sharply incise visceral pleural rind
    i. Carefully develop plane between the lung and the visceral pleural rind, and circumferentially decorticate the visceral pleural peel, thereby freeing the entire lung and allowing it to fully expand. Traction is applied to the peel (Tonsil/Pean clamp) with counter-traction applied to the lung (peanut Kitner, sponge stick). In addition, maintaining lung inflation (and even a Valsalva maneuver) is helpful to develop the dissection plane.
    j. Resect necrotic tissues (if necessary)
    k. Send pleural rind from each lobe to pathology (to rule out malignancy) and to microbiology (for mycobacterial and fungal stains and aerobic, anaerobic, mycobacterial and fungal cultures)
    l. Irrigate hemithorax with sterile saline or water (antibiotic containing saline or water can be used but there is no evidence to support its use)

    m. Widely drain the pleural space with e large bore anterior and posterior chest tubes and secure to skin. Though there is no strong evidence to support it, many surgeons place small bore infusion catheters to infuse saline or antibiotic solution to keep the large drains clear.
    n. Place pericostal sutures for rib reapproximation (#2 Vicryl) in a fashion to avoid intercostal bundle entrapment
    o. Close wound in layers: serratus fascia, latissimus dorsi fascia, deep dermal tissues, and subcuticular layer.
    p. Injection of bupivacaine with epinephrine in the intercostal areas 2-3 interspaces above and below the intercostal space entered and around each of the drains placed. Paravertebral, extra-pleural and intra-incisional catheters may be placed to provide continuous and intermittent infusion of bupivacaine.

9. Thoracoscopic Technique
    a. Enter chest cavity via anterior incision approximately 2 cm below and lateral to the nipple, approximately the 5th intercostal space or in a fashion as directed by the preoperatively performed contrast-enhanced chest computed tomogram (CT). In pleural spaces that appear complex on the CT, we often place a 5 mm port first as there is less parenchyma damage if the thoracoscope is incorrectly placed. It can be enlarged to a 12 mm scope as necessary.
    b. Insert the 5 mm 30-degree thoracoscope into the trocar to confirm chest entry and to inspect pleura for adhesions
    c. Insufflate with 5-10 mmHg CO_2 as needed to help with visualization and assist in the dissection
    d. Place 1-3 additional thoracoports: 5 or 12 mm port in the mid-axillary line just above the diaphragm (approximately the 7th intercostal space) and one posteriorly. In the more complex pleural spaces as determined by direct visualization and the CT, thoracoports may be placed in areas to provide the greatest opportunity for visualization and decortication.
    e. Mobilize lung by detaching pleural adhesions and divide inferior pulmonary ligament, as with the open technique
    f. Using a 5 or 10 mm suction-irrigator system, drain fluid collections and send to pathology for cytology/gram stain/culture; a curved ring forceps may be required to remove gelatinous fibrous deposits and blood clots, if present.
    g. Sharply incise into pleural rind using endoshears or electrocautery
    h. Carefully develop plane between the lung and the rind. Decorticate the visceral pleura, releasing the lung in its entirety. Traction is applied to the peel (thoracoscopic tissue grasper or a Forrester clamp) with counter-traction applied to the lung (thoracoscopic Kitner). Spinning the grasper on the peel can aid in pleural stripping. In addition, to help better define the plane, maintaining lung inflation and even a Valsalva maneuver can help provide traction; this can be

challenging thoracoscopically due to the small working space.
i. Continue diligently until all affected surfaces are released and lung re-expansion is unhindered. Use intermittent lung inflation to check adequacy of decortication and reexpansion.
j. Send rind to pathology to rule out malignancy and to pathology for culture
k. Irrigate hemithorax with saline or water.
l. Place large bore anterior and posterior chest tubes through port sites, using posterior port as a viewing port, and secure to skin.
m. Intercostal block with bupivicaine
n. Close remaining thoracoport sites in a subcuticular fashion using absorbable suture

Potential Complications and Pitfalls

1. Try not to violate the lung parenchyma; this will cause an air leak and bleeding; although these small air leaks are typically well tolerated and will resolve in time
2. The thoracoscopic approach may be time consuming and result in only a partial decortication; failure to progress may warrant open thoracotomy
3. If technically impossible (marked lung injury, failure to develop correct plane), incisions into the visceral pleura either parallel or checkerboard may help allow the lung to expand.
4. Difficult areas to decorticate include the fissures and diaphragmatic surface. Diligence and patience is required.
5. Overnight mechanical ventilation with PEEP of 8 to 10 mmHg is helpful to facilitate lung expansion and to tamponade bleeding
6. Make sure the lung remains fully expanded. Widely drain the pleural space, and keep chest tubes on suction for at least 48 hours. Incomplete expansion (of all or a portion of the lung) can lead to pleural space complications
7. Inadequate pain control for either surgical approach induces splinting and failure to produce adequate cough and clearance of secretions.
8. A portion of rib may need to be removed to facilitate open or thoracoscopic decortication in the case of fibrothorax or limited exposure.

Template Dictation

Preoperative Diagnosis: [INDICATION – e.g. Parapneumonic empyema, Empyema thoracis, Chronic pleural effusion, Entrapped lung, Fibrothorax]

Postoperative Diagnosis: Same

Procedure(s) Performed: Open thoracotomy with full lung decortication

Attending Surgeon: [BLANK]

Secondary Surgeon: [BLANK]

Assistants: [BLANK]

Anesthesia: [BLANK]

Indication(s) for Procedure: [AGE] year old [GENDER] with [DURATION] history of [COMPLAINT] – e.g. recent history of pneumonia, increasingly dyspnea, fever, leukocytosis, preoperative imaging shows multi-loculated pleural fluid collections. Thoracic surgery was consulted for decortication.

Description of Procedure: The patient was taken to the operating room on [DATE]. The patient's identity and planned procedure were verified. The patient was placed on the operating room table in the supine position. General anesthesia was obtained and a dual-lumen endobronchial tube was then placed. Flexible bronchoscopy was performed. The left and right mainstem bronchi, lobar bronchi and segmental bronchial orifices were examined. There were endoluminal masses, bloody secretions, purulent secretions or other endoluminal abnormalities. The patient was positioned in the lateral decubitus position. We then proceeded to prep and drape the chest in sterile fashion. Ioban dressing was placed. A time out was performed.

A posterolateral thoracotomy incision was made using a #10 blade scalpel staying 2cm below the scapular tip. Dissection was carried down through the latissimus dorsi and onto the chest wall using electrocautery, sparing the serratus anterior. The dissection continued into the fifth interspace, dividing the intercostal muscles superior to the sixth rib. The operating lung side was deflated by anesthesia. The pleura was incised where cloudy fluid was encountered. This was sent for culture, gram stain, and cytology. After extensive pleural division both anteriorly and posteriorly, a Finochietto rib spreader was placed. Adhesions were noted from the lung to the chest wall and were divided using electrocautery. The inferior pulmonary ligament was divided. Copious amounts of gelatinous fibrous debris were removed. The chest wall and diaphragm were decorticated. The rind on the lower lobe including the visceral pleura was incised with a scalpel until the underlying parenchyma was encountered. Careful dissection using traction/counter-traction ensued until the peel was fully removed from the entire lung. A peanut dissector aided this process. Small rents in the lung were created during the visceral pleural decortication. Overall, there was minimal parenchymal injury. Intermittent lung ventilation guided the decortication until full release of the lung was achieved. The peel was sent to pathology to rule out malignancy and to microbiology for culture. The chest was irrigated with antibiotic containing saline. Hemostasis was assured. Anterior and posterior 32 Fr chest tubes were placed and secured to the skin using 0 Nylon suture. Pericostal #2 Vicryl sutures were used to re-approximate the ribs. Rib blocks were performed 2 ribs above and 2 ribs below the thoracotomy space with 0.25% Marcaine. The wound was closed in layers using Vicryl suture followed by a subcuticular monofilament suture.

Tegaderm was placed as the sterile dressing.

All instrument, sponge and needle counts were confirmed to be correct x 2 at the end of the operation. The patient was left intubated and subsequently transferred to the postoperative cardiac surgical intensive care unit in guarded condition.

Dr. **[BLANK]** was present and scrubbed for **[BLANK]** elements of this procedure.

12. Open Transthoracic Diaphragm Plication

Jennifer L. Sullivan, MD and Ryan Levy, MD

University of Pittsburgh Medical Center, Pittsburgh, PA

Essential Operative Steps

1. Lines and Monitoring
2. General endotracheal anesthesia
3. Double lumen endotracheal tube or bronchial blocker for lung isolation
4. Lateral decubitus position
5. Thoracotomy incision
6. Identify attenuated portion of diaphragm
7. Pledgeted horizontal mattress sutures
8. Tight repair so diaphragm now in position of maximum end-inspiration
9. Assess hemostasis
10. Chest tube placement
11. Thoracotomy closure

Potential Complications and Pitfalls

1. Not enough sutures or loose re-approximation can lead to recurrence.
2. Too much tension can cause dehiscence
3. Injury to underlying abdominal viscera with bleeding or sepsis
4. High thoracotomy can make it difficult to place sutures adequately
5. Avoid phrenic nerve branches on the diaphragm

Template Dictation

Preoperative Diagnosis: [INDICATION – e.g. diaphragm paralysis)

Postoperative Diagnosis: Same

Procedure(s) Performed: [RIGHT, LEFT] thoracotomy, diaphragm plication

Attending Surgeon: [BLANK]

Secondary Surgeon: [BLANK]

Assistants: [BLANK]

Anesthesia: [BLANK]

Indication(s) for Procedure: [AGE] year old [GENDER] with [DURATION] history of [COMPLAINT –e.g. DOE, orthopnea] and [CAUSE – e.g previous surgery, history of trauma, cancer, central line placement]. A Chest CT/CXR revealed [FINDINGS – e.g. elevated hemidiaphragm, pleural pathology]. A SNIFF test was performed showing paradoxical motion of the affected hemidiaphragm, confirming diaphragm paralysis.

Description of Procedure: The patient was taken to the operating room on **[DATE]**. The patient's identity and planned procedure were verified, and the patient was placed on the operating room table in the supine position. General anesthesia was induced, and the patient was intubated with a double lumen endotracheal tube. Appropriate placement of the tube was verified via bronchoscopy. The patient was placed in the **[LEFT, RIGHT]** lateral decubitus position, taking care to pad all pressure points. The chest was then prepped and draped in a sterile fashion.

A low posterolateral thoracotomy incision was made using a 10-blade scalpel and electrocautery was used to dissect the muscle to enter the 8th intercostal space. A 1 cm segment of the rib was shingled posteriorly and then a Finochietto retractor was used to spread the ribs. Examination of the pleural cavity showed good lung isolation and no pleural effusions or lesions.

The elevated, attenuated area of the diaphragm was identified and grasped with a Babcock clamp to elevate the muscle from the underlying abdominal viscera. Starting on the posterior surface of the diaphragm, a pledgeted #0 Ethibond suture was placed in a horizontal mattress fashion, going lateral to medial, taking wide bites of the muscle. Several rows of these sutures were placed, each about 2 cm apart, going from the posterior to the anterior surface of the diaphragm. The sutures were then tightened, gathering the diaphragm tissue into several pleats, and the knots secured. The diaphragm was then re-examined, showing appropriate at the base of the thorax and the muscle was seen to be taut and drum-like.

Adequate hemostasis was observed. A 24 Fr Blake drain was placed into the diaphragmatic recess and a 28 Fr chest tube was placed along the posterior pleural cavity up to the apex. The tubes were brought out through separate skin incisions in the anterior axillary line and secured to the skin with 0-silk suture. The lung was then re-inflated under direct visualization.

Four interrupted pericostal #1 Vicryl sutures were used to re-approximate the ribs. The underlying musculofascial layers were then closed with #0 Vicryl suture in a running fashion. The deep dermal layer was then closed with #2-0 Vicryl suture in s running fashion. The skin was re-approximated with #4-0 Monocryl in running fashion. The incision was covered with sterile dressings.

All instrument, sponge and needle counts were confirmed to be correct at the end of the operation. The patient tolerated the procedure well, with no apparent intraoperative complications. The patient was subsequently transferred to the cardiothoracic surgical intensive care unit in stable condition.

Dr. **[BLANK]** was present and scrubbed for **[BLANK]** elements of this procedure.

13. Repair of Anterior Restrosternal (Morgagni) and Posterolateral (Bochdalek) Diaphragm Hernias

Abby White, DO and Scott J. Swanson, MD

Brigham and Women's Hospital, Boston, Massachusetts

Morgagni Hernia

Essential Operative Steps

Typically not identified or repaired until adulthood, hernias through the Foramen of Morgagni result from failure of fusion of the septum transversum with the sternum and anterior chest wall or muscular agenesis at the retrosternal position of the diaphragm. This type of hernia rarely causes pulmonary hypoplasia or compromise in the neonatal period.

1. Lines and monitoring
   a. Arterial catheter can be useful in the setting of acute obstruction and/or suspected strangulation
   b. Naso-gastric tubes (NGT) can be useful for prevention of aspiration and decompression of obstruction, especially when the hernia sac contains stomach or proximal small bowel Caution placing NGT if volvulus is suspected.
2. General endotracheal anesthesia via dual lumen endotracheal tube.
3. Supine positioning, with arms tucked.
4. Safe peritoneal entry for laparoscopy
   a. Decision for initial port placement based on surgeon experience, hernia contents and patient-related factors such as prior surgery, anticipated adhesions, body habitus, etc.
   b. Typical port sites:
      i. Two 11mm epigastric ports, one for a 10mm camera and one working port
      ii. Two or three 5mm working ports for retraction and exposure, typically at the right and left lateral costal margins, and a 5mm Nathanson liver retractor (or other self-retaining liver retractor) where anatomy dictates.
5. Reverse Trendelenberg positioning facilitates reduction of hernia contents and allows stomach and omentum to fall away from the hiatus.
6. Reduction of hernia sac and contents
   a. Careful lysis of adhesions and dissection of the hernia sac using available energy sources (LigaSure, Harmonic Scalpel, electrocautery)
   b. Atraumatic hand-over-hand reduction of the hernia sac and contents, minimizing the amount of tissue grasping with retractors.
   c. Assessment of viability of herniated structures. ie. bowel viability
   d. Resection and removal of hernia sac.

7. Primary repair with non-absorbable sutures (small, amenable defects)
   a. Accomplished when there is an anterior cuff of muscle
   b. Leave fascia on diaphragm muscle where possible
   c. Interrupted simple or horizontal mattress sutures with braided non-absorbable suture
   d. +/- Gore-Tex or Teflon pledgets
8. Tension-free repair with prosthetic mesh (Gore-Tex or bioasborbable)
   a. Secured circumferentially with interrupted 0-Ethibond suture.
   b. When there is no anterior muscle cuff, the diaphragm can be fixated to anterior chest wall interspaces (between costal cartilages) or to the rectus muscle or both. This is easily accomplished with a Carter-Thomason guide and suture passer.
9. Hemostasis and closure

Potential Complications and Pitfalls

1. As with all hernias, elective repair is associated with the greatest success rate. Patients presenting with acute obstruction and/or strangulation require careful monitoring, appropriate fluid resuscitation and careful monitoring postoperatively for infection in either pleural space, the mediastinum or the peritoneum.
2. Unique to Morgagni hernias, the internal mammary vessels should be considered when dissecting the hernia at the anterior surface, and when fixating mesh to the anterior chest wall.
3. Care should be taken when dissecting hernia sac from the pleura or pericardium. Rarely does a clinically significant pneumothorax develop, but heightened awareness and consideration should given when direct entry into the pleural space is seen intraoperatively. Most pneumothoraces can be safely observed.

Template Dictation

Preoperative Diagnosis: [Indication – [INCARCERATED/STRANGULATED] Morgagni Diaphragmatic Hernia containing [STOMACH/SMALL BOWEL/COLON/STOMACH/SPLEEN, OMENTUM, ETC]

Postoperative Diagnosis: Same

Procedure Preformed: Diagnostic laparoscopy, repair of diaphragmatic hernia with mesh

Attending Surgeon: [BLANK]

Secondary Surgeon: [BLANK]

Assistants: [BLANK]

Anesthesia: [BLANK]

Indication(s) for Procedure: This is a [BLANK] year-old [SEX] with a history of [SYMPTOMS] who was found to have a [SIZE] anterior diaphragmatic hernia containing [CONTENTS]. Repair was indicated to prevent strangulation. (Typically not indicated for shortness of breath, however, compression of lung from mass effect can be mentioned here).

Description of Procedure: The patient was brought to the operating room on [DATE]. Name, birthdate and nature of the procedure were verified. After an uneventful induction of general anesthesia, the patient was intubated with a single-lumen endotracheal tube without incident. The patient was positioned supine with both arms tucked and the abdomen prepped and draped in usual sterile fashion.

Safe peritoneal entry was accomplished via a small stab incision in the left upper quadrant with Veress needle introduction and insufflation of the abdomen with carbon dioxide to a pressure of 15 mmHg. Two 11 mm incisions were made just to the left and right of midline, halfway between the xiphoid process and umbilicus in the epigastrum and trocars inserted. A 10mm camera was used and laparoscopy confirmed the presence of a [BLANK x BLANK cm] anterior diaphragmatic hernia containing [CONTENTS]. Two additional, right and left lateral 5 mm ports were placed under direct visualization, 2 cm beneath the costal margins.

The hernia sac and its contents were carefully reduced in a hand-over-hand technique, minimizing tissue grasping and tension where possible. The Ligasure device was used to lyse adhesions and free the hernia sac from associated attachments. The fascia overlying diaphragmatic muscle was left intact. The hernia sac was excised and removed. To avoid undue tension, an acellular dermis patch was placed in an underlay fashion and secured using a combination of interrupted nonabsorbable monofilament suture and titanium tacks placed with an automatic device.

The 11 mm port sites were closed with absorbable braided suture. Hemostasis was verified and all port sites were inspected. The carbon dioxide was evacuated and the skin at the port sites closed with absorbable suture. All sponge, needle and instrument counts were correct.

Dr. **[BLANK]** was present and scrubbed for **[BLANK]** elements of this procedure.

Bochdalek Hernia

Essential Operative Steps

Typically identified in the prenatal period, the classic Bochdalek hernia is a 2-4cm, left-sided posterolateral defect in the diaphragm through which the abdominal contents have migrated, more commonly without the development of a hernia sac. Compression of the lung from herniated contents results in pulmonary hypoplasia and/or pulmonary hypertension, the physiology of which is often the more devastating factor to neonates. Surgical repair is secondary to physiologic cardiopulmonary stabilization

1. Lines and monitoring
   a. As dictated by neonatal physiology.
2. General endotracheal anesthesia
3. Left subcostal incision for the more-common left-sided defects.
4. Retractors in the left upper quadrant facilitate visualization of the hernia and contents
5. Careful reduction of abdominal contents, typically using a dry sponge stick
6. Diaphragmatic remnant defect identified and assessed
7. At the posterior recess, the diaphragm can be mobilized from the posterior peritoneum just caudal to the left kidney, allowing for less tension on the repair.
8. Repair of the defect with simple, interrupted, nonabsorbable sutures
   a. In repairs without a posterior cuff of diaphragm, a prosthetic patch, such as GORE-TEX can be used.
   b. Where there is no diaphragm in the posterior location, sutures can be placed around the 11th or 12th rib. The prosthetic mesh may need to be removed if chest wall development is hindered by the fixed mesh on the side of the repair.
9. Once the defect has been repaired, inspect the abdominal contents for rotational anomalies and replace then in a normal anatomic position prior to closure.
10. Closure and hemostasis
    a. Occasionally, an external silo is needed for a mal-developed abdominal cavity
    b. A chest tube is left only for those patients on ECMO as surveillance for bleeding.

Potential Complications and Pitfalls

1. Timing of the operation should be considered in conjunction with a multi-disciplinary pediatric team.
2. Caution when reducing the contents of the hernia, as the left lobe of the liver and spleen are frequently involved and are easily avulsed in neonates.
3. Follow-up data using bioprosthesis closure of the diaphragm showed earlier hernia recurrence as well as a higher incidence of multiple recurrences.
4. Patients are at increased lifetime risk of small bowel obstruction from volvulus or hernia recurrence and parent education is a must.
5. Yearly AP chest radiographs can be performed to detect asymptomatic recurrence.

Template Dictation

Preoperative Diagnosis: Left posterolateral diaphragmatic hernia

Postoperative Diagnosis: Same

Procedure Preformed: Repair of Diaphragmatic Hernia [+/- MESH]

Attending Surgeon: [BLANK]

Secondary Surgeon: [BLANK]

Assistants: [BLANK]

Anesthesia: [BLANK]

Indication(s) for Procedure: This is a [BLANK] year-old [SEX] with a [SIDED] congenital diaphragmatic hernia. Following adequate cardiopulmonary stabilization and cooperative care in a multi-disciplinary fashion, the decision was made to proceed with operative repair.

Description of Procedure: The patient was brought to the operating room on [DATE]. Name, birthdate and nature of the procedure were verified. After an uneventful induction of general anesthesia, the patient was intubated with a single-lumen endotracheal tube without incident. The abdomen was prepped and draped in usual sterile fashion.

A left-sided subcostal incision was made and the muscle fibers split for peritoneal entry. The peritoneum was grasped, elevated and sharply entered.

A body wall retractor was placed and the peritoneal cavity was explored. The diaphragmatic defect was identified. A sponge stick was used to reduce the abdominal contents into the abdomen. A **[SIZE]** cm defect remained. The hernia sac was excised. A transverse incision was made in the posterior peritoneum to reduce tension on the repair and allow for mobilization of the posterior diaphragm.

The diaphragm was repaired with simple, interrupted, #2-0 Ethibond sutures. Following closure of the diaphragm, the abdominal contents were inspected for rotational anomalies and were oriented in usual anatomic position prior to closure. Hemostasis was verified. The anterior and posterior rectus sheath were reapproximated with running #2-0 PDS suture and the wound closed in layers. All sponge, needle and instruments counts were correct.

Dr. **[BLANK]** was present and scrubbed for **[BLANK]** elements of this procedure.

14. VATS Evacuation of Hemothorax

Carlo O. Martinez, MD and Daniel T. DeArmond, MD

University of Texas Health Science Center, San Antonio, TX

Essential Operative Steps

1. Lines and Monitoring
2. General endotracheal anesthesia with double-lumen endotracheal tube
3. Bronchoscopy
4. Repositioning in lateral decubitus positioning, leaned back slightly to allow access to the anterior intercostal spaces and positioned with the hip over the central break to allow for further opening of the intercostal spaces
5. Place first incision at sixth intercostal space in the midclavicular line
6. Thoracoscope is inserted to assess lung parenchyma, adhesions, and site for second incision
7. Second incision is placed low, at the eight intercostal space in the posterior axillary line
8. Evacuate the retained hemothorax
9. Place chest tube at the lowest incision
10. Ensure lung re-expands completely
11. Close incisions
12. Extubate

Potential Complications and Pitfalls

1. The hemothorax should be completely evacuated or chronic pleural effusions (from the oncotic effects of blood), fibrothorax, lung entrapment or empyema may unsue.
2. An organized, chronic hemothorax may require a thoracotomy for complete decortication to allow the lung to fully expand.
3. Avoid inadvertent parenchymal injury.

Template Dictation

Preoperative Diagnosis: [INDICATION – e.g. hemothorax from chest wall trauma]

Postoperative Diagnosis: Same

Procedure(s) Performed: Video Assisted Thoracoscopic Surgery **(DETAILS – e.g. Diagnostic, with Decortication, with Pleurodesis)**

Attending Surgeon: [BLANK]

Secondary Surgeon: [BLANK]

Assistants: [BLANK]

Anesthesia: [BLANK]

Indication(s) for Procedure: [AGE] year old [GENDER] with [DURATION] history of [COMPLAINT] –e.g. trauma]. Initial chest tube thoracostomy insufficient in evacuating hemothorax. Imaging demonstrates retained hemothorax with increasing WBC, compressive atelectasis, etc.]

Description of Procedure:

General: The patient was identified in the holding area. The procedure, benefits, risks, and alternatives were discussed with the patient and [his/her] family including the risks of, recurrence, infection, injury to surrounding structures, and prolonged airleak. The patient verbalized understanding of information provided and agreed to proceed. The informed consent form was signed and placed in the chart.

The patient was taken to the operating room on [DATE]. A Time Out was performed verifying the correct patient, correct procedure, and correct side. Pertinent imaging was available. Perioperative IV antibiotics were administered. The patient was placed on the operating room table in the supine position. Following the induction of general anesthesia, a double-lumen endotracheal tube was placed.

Bronchoscopy: Flexible bronchoscopy was performed. The bronchoscope was inserted through each of the lumens of double-lumen endotracheal tube in order to verify proper positioning. A complete examination was performed. There was no blood, mass, foreign object or other abnormalities. Excess secretions were suctioned out of the airways. The scope was withdrawn.

VATS with Hemothorax Evacuation: The patient was then repositioned in the [left/right] lateral decubitus with [right/left] side up. [His/Her] hips were positioned over the central break to allow flexion and opening of the intercostal spaces. The patient was prepped and draped in standard surgical fashion. An incision was made in the sixth intercostal space along the midclavicular line and directed posteriorly. Entry into the thoracic cavity was uncomplicated and digital inspection revealed no pleural adhesions. The scope was inserted and some retained hemothorax was noted. The [left/right] lung demonstrated [good/fair/poor] isolation and was [completely/partially/poorly] deflated. The second incision at the eighth intercostal space at the posterior axillary line was performed and entry into the thoracic cavity was performed under direct visualization. The thoracoscope was then inserted in the lower incision to obtain a wide view of the thoracic cavity. The retained hemothorax was evacuated with suction through the anterior incision. The thoracic cavity was inspected for areas of active bleeding and hemostasis was obtained. A [28-french] chest tube was inserted through the lower incision, directed apically and posteriorly, and secured with a suture. The [left/right] lung was reinflated completely under direct visualization and double lung ventilation was re-established. The scope was removed.

Closure: The incisions were closed in layers with a #2-O Vicryl deep dermal layer and #3-O Monocryl for subcuticular closure. The incisions were cleaned and dried and Dermabound was applied. A sterile dressing was applied to the chest tube.

All instrument, sponge and needle counts were correct at the end of the operation. The patient was extubated and taken to PACU in satisfactory condition.

Dr. [BLANK] was present and scrubbed for [BLANK] elements of this procedure.

15. VATS Pericardial Window

Jennifer L. Sullivan, MD and Ryan M. Levy, MD

University of Pittsburgh, Pittsburgh, PA

Essential Operative Steps

1. Lines and Monitoring (arterial line)
2. General endotracheal anesthesia
3. Double lumen endotracheal tube or bronchial blocker for lung isolation
4. Lateral decubitus position.
5. Identify phrenic nerve
6. Tent pericardium away from heart
7. Creation of window
8. Assess hemostasis
9. Pericardial drain and chest tube placement
10. Port site closure

Potential Complications and Pitfalls

1. Identify and avoid injury to phrenic nerve
2. Injury to heart, especially if pericardium is adherent to heart
3. Too small of a window will scar closed with recurrence of effusion
4. Herniation of heart with too large of a window
5. Bleeding from pericardial edges
6. Be prepared for patient to become unstable after anesthesia induction from tamponade physiology
7. VATS approach not appropriate for unstable patient who can not tolerate lung isolation – perform subxiphoid approach
8. Failure to recognize a loculated effusion on preoperative echocardiography.

Template Dictation

Preoperative Diagnosis: [INDICATION – e.g. pericardial effusion)

Postoperative Diagnosis: Same

Procedure(s) Performed: [LEFT, RIGHT] VATS pericardial window

Attending Surgeon: [BLANK]

Secondary Surgeon: [BLANK]

Assistants: [BLANK]

Anesthesia: [BLANK]

Indication(s) for Procedure: [AGE] year old [GENDER] with [DURATION]

history of [**COMPLAINT** –e.g. increasing SOB, chest discomfort]. Preoperative echocardiography revealed [**FINDINGS** - e.g. size, signs of tamponade]. A Chest CT revealed [**FINDINGS** – e.g. location, presence of loculation, evidence of pleural pathology].

Description of Procedure: The patient was taken to the operating room on [**DATE**]. The patient's identity and planned procedure were verified, and the patient was placed on the operating room table in the supine position. Appropriate preoperative prophylactic antibiotics were administered. General anesthesia was induced and the patient was intubated with a double lumen endotracheal tube. The patient was placed in the [**LEFT, RIGHT**] lateral decubitus position. The chest was then prepped and draped in a sterile fashion.

A 15-blade scalpel was used to make the camera port at the 8th intercostal space in the posterior axillary line. A 10 mm 30 degree thoracoscope was inserted through the port. Adequate lung isolation was confirmed and the pleural cavity was examined for effusions and lesions. [**FINDINGS**]. A 10 mm incision working port was placed at the 5th intercostal space in the mid-axillary line. A 5 mm port was placed in the anterior axillary line in the 6th intercostal space.

The distended pericardium was visualized. The phrenic nerve was identified running along the pericardium and care was taken to avoid contact with the nerve throughout the case. A long Allis clamp was used to grasp the pericardium to tent the tissue away from the underlying heart. An endoshear was used to create an initial opening in the pericardium about 1 cm anterior to the phrenic nerve. A [**SEROUS/BLOODY**] effusion was observed coming from the pericardial space. The Allis clamp was used to provide traction on the free edge of the pericardium. The pericardium was further incised with the harmonic scalpel, creating about 3 cm square defect in the pericardium. Several other areas of small fenestration were created as well to ensure adequate decompression into the pleural space. The pericardial tissue was sent to pathology as a permanent specimen for further evaluation.

After completion of the window, the pericardial space was then gently probed with the Yankauer sucker to break any fibrinous septa and ensure complete drainage of the effusion. Adequate hemostasis was observed. A 24 Fr Blake drain was placed through the window into the pericardial space and brought out through a separate incision in the skin. A 28 Fr chest tube was inserted along the posterior pleural cavity with the tip at the apex and brought out through the initial camera port incision. The tubes were secured to the skin with #0 silk suture. The lung was then re-inflated under direct visualization.

The fascia was then closed with #0 Vicryl suture and the deep dermal layer was then closed with #2-0 Vicryl suture. The skin was re-approximated with #4-0

Monocryl in running fashion. The incisions were covered with sterile dressings.

All instrument, sponge and needle counts were confirmed to be correct at the end of the operation. The patient tolerated the procedure well, with no apparent intraoperative complications. The patient was subsequently transferred to the cardiothoracic surgical intensive care unit in stable condition.

Dr. [BLANK], the attending, was present and scrubbed for [BLANK] elements of this procedure.

16. Chest Wall Tumor Resection and Chest Wall Reconstruction

George Makdisi, MD, K. Robert Shen, MD

Mayo Clinic, Rochester, MN

Note: there are a variety of resection locations and reconstruction options, to limit the size of the chapter, we describe the most common locations (anterior/lateral chest wall and sternal resection); with skeleton reconstruction (mesh, cadaveric rib grafts and plates) followed by rotational muscle flap (latissimus dorsi) as well as pectoralis muscle flap advancement for sternal resection. Other resections and reconstructions follow same principles.

Essential Operative Steps

1. A combined multidisciplinary approach planning with the anesthesia, plastics and thoracic surgery
2. Preoperative biopsy either percutaneous or incisional is often beneficial to make definitive diagnosis. This will determine how much surgical margin will be necessary
3. Lines and Monitoring
4. General endotracheal anesthesia with double-lumen endotracheal tube
5. Include the biopsy site in your incision
6. Identify, defined and assess the extent of resection
7. Assess for local invasion and resectability
8. Get frozen section to assure negative margins, if positive resect more
9. Resection, assess the size of the defect
10. Reconstruct the bony defect
11. Cover material used to reconstruct bony defect with vascularized soft tissue
12. Good hemostasis and good drainage of any skin flaps to avoid development of seroma
13. Close monitoring to the flap necrosis/ might need early débridements

Reconstruction Options

1. Management of chest wall defect :
    a. Not needed if small defect <5 cm or those located posteriorly underneath the scapula above the fourth rib.
    b. Mesh: Should be thick at least 2 mm: Polypropylene, Marlex, composite Marlex methyl methacrylate, PTFE, biologic mesh.
    c. Mesh and plates.
    d. Mesh and artificial ribs (i.e., titanium rib plates with cadaveric rib graft).
2. Management of chest wall soft tissue defect:
    a. Primary closure.
    b. Muscle advancement: pectoralis major

c. Rotational muscle/musculocutaneous flap: latissimus dorsi, serratus anterior, rectus abdominis, external oblique muscle.
   d. Omental transposition flap with split-thickness skin grafting immediately or 48 hours later.

Potential Complications and Pitfalls

1. A combined multidisciplinary approach with plastic and reconstruction surgeons, thoracic surgeons, anesthesia and critical care specialists affords the best functional results after chest wall resection.
2. Three principles of surgical resection should be maintained 1). Resect all devitalized tissue 2). If a large chest wall resection if performed, the rigid chest wall should be restored to preserve chest wall mechanics and prevent a flail chest. 3). Healthy soft tissue coverage to obliterate pleural dead space, protect the viscera and great vessels, and prevent infection.
3. Location, size, depth, presence of an infection, prior radiation therapy, recurrence of residual cancer, patient performance status, patient comorbidities, immunosuppression, and prognosis are important factors in planning resections and reconstructions.
4. Surgical margins of 4 cm are desirable, for most malignant chest wall tumors. This is influenced by tumor location, pathology, location of tumor recurrence and reconstruction possibilities. For lower grade malignant chest wall tumors or benign tumors, surgical margins of 2cm may be sufficient. For metastatic tumors negative margins are adequate.
5. Reconstruction of the bony chest wall is not necessary and primary soft tissue closure can be performed for small defects <5 cm or those located posteriorly underneath the scapula above the fourth rib.
6. Adequate pain control, early mobility, physical therapy and aggressive pulmonary hygiene are very important factors in postoperative period.
7. Careful hemostasis should be performed to avoid hematomas.
8. Careful monitoring of flap ischemia and necrosis.
9. Complete resection with wide margins >4cm in the first operation is the most important factor in patient survival and recurrence rate as the frozen section is often unreliable in assessing the extent of involvement of the ribs.

Template Dictation

Preoperative Diagnosis: [INDICATION – e.g. primary bone tumors benign/malignant, primary soft tissue tumors, metastatic and recurrent breast cancer, chronic infection...]

Postoperative Diagnosis: [Same]

Procedure(s) Performed: Chest wall resection with [BLANK] reconstruction

Attending Surgeon: [BLANK]

Secondary Surgeon: [BLANK]

Assistants: [BLANK]

Anesthesia: General endotracheal anesthesia, Thoracic epidural

Indication(s) for Procedure: [Mr/ Mrs.] [BLANK] is a [age] year-old [gender] who presented with progressive enlarged mass [or infection] in the [location] chest wall. Workup included [CXR, CT, PET], a core needle biopsy had been performed, and the findings are consistent with a [pathology]. [Mr/ Mrs.] [BLANK] is brought now for surgical resection in conjunction with plastics surgery

Description of Procedure: The patient was brought to the operating room and had a thoracic epidural catheter placed by the Anesthesia Team. The patient was then placed supine on the operating table and underwent an uneventful induction of general endotracheal anesthesia. A double-lumen endotracheal tube was placed. We positioned the patient in the [RIGHT/LEFT] lateral decubitus position. The [RIGHT/LEFT]-sided chest wall and [RIGHT/LEFT] arm were sterilely prepped and draped.

A curvilinear incision was made, centered over the mass in the [RIGHT/LEFT] anterior portion of the chest in order to encompass the prior needle biopsy site. Dissection was carried down through the subcutaneous tissue to the pectoralis major muscle fascia. We then raised soft tissue flaps superiorly and inferiorly as well as medially and laterally. We were able to then mark out a planned 4-cm wide resection encompassing most of the pectoralis major muscle as well as the pectoralis minor muscle, and en bloc resection of the anterior portions of ribs [RIB NUMBERS] was performed. Dissection through the muscle was performed using Bovie electrocautery. Once the medial extent of the planned rid resection was reached, the ribs were scored with Bovie cautery to mark the resection border and the periosteum then stripped with a periosteal elevator. The medial portions of the ribs were sectioned with a microsagittal saw, and the neurovascular bundles then clamped, ligated with 2-0 silk ligatures, and divided. The lateral portions of the ribs were then divided in a similar fashion. The specimen was then removed from the field after marking sutures were placed for orientation, and all our gross surgical margins were clear. Frozen section showed [FINDINGS]. The final diagnosis is held over for permanent section. The mass was quite mobile on the chest wall and did not grossly appear to involve any of the underlying ribs. We then carefully palpated the [RIGHT/LEFT] lung and examined the pleura. No tumoral invasion or masses were noted. We then placed a [SIZE] AlloDerm biologic mesh to fill in the chest wall defect. The mesh was attached to the ribs medially and laterally with mattress style No. 1 Polypropylene sutures, and then superiorly and inferiorly it was secured by suturing it around ribs [RIB NUMBERS], also with No. 1 Polypropylene. We then reconstructed the bony chest wall defect using titanium rib plates to replace the resected ribs [RIB NUMBERS]. The rib plates were bent to the appropriate curvature and then secured to the medial and lateral portions of the ribs using three appropriately sized bicortical locking screws on each side of the rib.

On rib **[RIB NUMBERS]** we also interposed a cadaveric rib graft, which was secured to the rib plate also using four interlocking appropriately sized bicortical screws. In addition, on rib plates **[RIB NUMBERS]** fibular cadaveric bone grafts were secured to the plate to bridge the bony rib defect.

Rotational Latissimus Dorsi Muscle Flap Reconstruction Dictation

Patient was brought to the operating room. A thoracic epidural catheter was placed by the Anesthesia Team. Following an uneventful induction of general endotracheal anesthesia, the patient was intubated with a double-lumen endotracheal tube. We subsequently positioned the patient in the **[RIGHT/LEFT]** lateral decubitus position. The **[RIGHT/LEFT]**-sided chest wall and **[RIGHT/LEFT]** arm were sterilely prepped and draped.

We proceeded with to harvest the latissimus dorsi as a pedicled muscle flap. We marked a curvilinear incision extending from the **[RIGHT/LEFT]** posterior axillary line towards the spine at the mid thoracic region. This was opened sharply, and then Bovie electrocautery was used to dissect the skin and fat into and through the dorsal thoracic fascia from the underlying latissimus muscle. For the large vessels, surgical clips were used to maintain hemostasis. We then identified the borders of the latissimus anteriorly and superiorly. These were dissected free from the underlying serratus anterior muscle. Once the correct plane had been identified, the latissimus muscle was divided just lateral to the midline and then inferiorly above the posterior iliac crest. Dissection was then continued distal to proximal elevating the latissimus muscle from the underlying serratus, trapezius, and rhomboids. As we elevated the flap towards the axilla, the thoracodorsal bundle was identified. Care was taken to protect it from injury. After elevation of the entire muscle and vascular pedicle along the posterior surface of the latissimus dorsi, we buried the elevated muscle in a subcutaneous pocket that was created while harvesting the latissimus muscle. Two 10 flat JP drains positioned in the cavity, brought out through separate stab incisions in the axilla, and secured to the skin using 2-0 nylon suture. The curvilinear incision was closed using 0 Polypropylene in an interrupted fashion for the fascial layer, a running 3-0 Monocryl for the deep dermal layer, and a 4-0 Monocryl subcuticular suture for the skin closure. Wound was dressed with 1-inch Steri-Strips. The patient tolerated the procedure well. There were no intraoperative complications. All needle, sponge, and instrument counts were correct after two counts

Dr. **[BLANK]** was present and scrubbed for **[BLANK]** elements of this procedure.

Sternal Resection and Reconstruction

Patient was brought to the operating room. A thoracic epidural catheter was placed by the Anesthesia Team. Following an uneventful induction of general endotracheal anesthesia, the patient was intubated with a double-lumen endotracheal tube. A roll between the scapulae, and the chest and the abdomen were prepared and draped. We began by making a vertical curvilinear incision centered over the mass *[a transverse incision underneath the breast folds can be used for the lesions in the lower sternum and chest especially in females]* starting at the level of the manubriosternal joint and extending inferiorly to the xiphisternum. An elliptical segment of skin incorporating the biopsy scar was excised. The subcutaneous tissues were then dissected and divided using Bovie electrocautery. The pectoral muscles were dissected off as flaps from the costal cartilages on both sides. The lesion was identified, and the necessary extent of resection was assessed. After dissection of the xiphisternum and dissecting up to the costal cartilages, the internal mammary arteries were identified, ligated and divided on [ONE/BOTH] sides with 2-0 silk suture. The medial portioned of ribs [RIB NUMBERS] were scored with Bovie cautery and the periosteum of these ribs was stripped with a periosteal elevator. After the neurovascular bundles were clamped and divided and ligated with 2-0 silk ligatures, the medial portion of the ribs [RIB NUMBERS] and costal cartilages were divided with a microsagital saw giving an adequate tumour clearance of approximately 4 cm. The sternum is then divided with the sternal saw and scissors. The specimen was then removed from the field. We did mark the specimen for orientation, and all our surgical margins were grossly clear. Frozen section showed [FINDINGS]. The final diagnosis is held over for permanent section.

After assuring hemostasis, we assessed and measured the defect. The resection resulted in a defect of [SIZE] in the anterior chest wall exposing the pericardium and [RIGHT/LEFT] lung. A 28 french straight chest tube was inserted into the [RIGHT/LEFT] pleural space. The sternum and chest wall were reconstructed with Alloderm. The mesh was attached to the ribs medially and laterally with mattress style #1 Polypropylene sutures. Superiorly and inferiorly, it was secured by suturing it around ribs [RIB NUMBERS] with #1 Polypropylene. Once the mesh was in place the pectoral muscles were reattached to the costal cartilages and the prosthesis. Two #10 Jackson-Pratt drains were positioned over the neosternum, brought out through separate stab incisions, and secured in place using 2-0 nylon suture. The pectoral muscles and presternal fascia are sutured together using #0 Vicryl suture in the midline to cover the mesh. After securing hemostasis, the subcutaneous layer was approximated with continuous absorbable suture using #1 Vicryl suture. The skin was closed using a running 4-0 Monocryl subcuticular suture. The patient tolerated the procedure well. No intraoperative complications. All needle, sponge, and instrument counts were correct on two occasions

Dr. [BLANK] was present and scrubbed for [BLANK] elements of this procedure.

17. Pancoast Tumor

R. Taylor Ripley, MD, Valerie W. Rusch, MD

Memorial Sloan-Kettering Cancer Center, New York, NY

Essential Operative Steps

1. Neoadjuvant chemoradiotherapy.
2. Insertion of double lumen endotracheal tube.
3. Lateral decubitus position with slight anterior rotation.
4. Exploratory thoracotomy through standard posterolateral incision.
5. Assessment for metastasis, resectability, and extent of chest wall resection.
6. Removal of Finochietto chest retractor and placement of Rultract internal mammary artery retractor to elevate tip of scapula.
7. Periscapular incision with division of latissimus dorsi and trapezius muscles and detachment of the serratus anterior muscle.
8. Detachment of scalene muscles and elevation of paraspinous muscles to expose first rib and transverse processes.
9. Chest wall resection starting anteriorly with 3-4 cm margin and sending anterior piece for pathological analysis as specimen margins (permanent sections).
10. Posterior division of involved ribs also submitted for pathological analysis.
11. Dissection along superior border of first rib.
12. Exposure of subclavian artery and vein and brachial plexus
13. Determination of nerve root involvement with liberal use of frozen section analysis.
14. Possible T1 nerve root resection.
15. Involvement of a neurosurgeon for completion of spine resection.
16. Mediastinal lymph node dissection of subcarinal and either right level 4 or left levels 5 and 6 lymph nodes.
17. Right or left upper lobectomy with en bloc removal of lobe and chest wall.
18. Closure of thoracotomy with chest tube placement.
19. Reconstruction of chest wall, usually with PTFE patch to support tip of scapula.
20. Closure of wound.
21. Reintubation with single lumen endotracheal tube.
22. Toilet bronchoscopy.

Potential Complications and Pitfalls

1. Proceeding without neoadjuvant chemoradiotherapy.
2. Withholding surgery in patients with radiologically stable disease (persistent mass does not predict pathological response).
3. Pulmonary resection of less than a lobectomy.

4. Bulky N2 disease.
5. Inadequate chest wall margin, especially along spine.
6. Not involving spinal surgeon for posterior spinal resection.
7. Resection of brachial plexus roots other than T1.
8. Failure to ligate nerve root leading to CSF leak and pneumocephalus.
9. Inadequate post-operative pain control and pulmonary toilet.

Template Dictation

Pre-Operative Diagnosis:
1. Right (or Left) Superior Sulcus Non-Small Cell Lung Cancer (Pancoast Tumor).
2. Status Post Induction Chemoradiotherapy.

Post-Operative Diagnosis: Same

Procedure(s) Performed:
1. Right (or Left) Thoracotomy.
2. Right (or Left) Upper Lobectomy.
3. En Bloc Chest Wall Resection (Ribs I – X).
4. Chest Wall Reconstruction with PTFE (if needed).
5. Mediastinal Lymph Node Dissection.
6. Flexible Bronchoscopy.

Attending Surgeon: [BLANK]

Secondary Surgeon: [BLANK]

Assistants: [BLANK]

Anesthesia: [BLANK]

Indication(s) for Procedure [Age] year old [Gender] was diagnosed with a locally advanced non-small cell lung carcinoma of the right superior sulcus (Pancoast tumor). [Additional statements: The tumor involved adjacent vertebral bodies; therefore it was classified as T4. The tumor involved the T1 nerve root, therefore it was classified as T3.] This patient underwent induction chemoradiotherapy with a good clinical response [Additional statement: with decrease in pain and/or a reduction in the SUV on the PET scan] and is being taken to the operating room for resection of the residual primary tumor.

Description of Procedure: Following induction of satisfactory level of general anesthesia and insertion of a double-lumen endotracheal tube, the patient was rotated into the **[left/right]** lateral decubitus position. The patient was rotated slightly anteriorly to improve the exposure to the posterior chest wall. The **[right/left]** chest was prepped and draped in the usual sterile manner. We started with an exploratory thoracotomy as a standard posterolateral incision into the fifth intercostal space. The Finochietto chest retractor was inserted. The chest was explored to determine that the patient did not have metastatic disease, had a potentially resectable tumor, and the extent of a chest wall resection.

The Finochietto chest retractor was then removed. The Rultract internal mammary artery retractor was used to elevate the tip of the scapula. The incision was extended posteriorly to the base of the neck and anteriorly around the anterior border of the scapula to the mid-axillary line, thereby making the incision periscapular in extent. The serratus anterior muscle was completely detached from the chest wall and the latissimus dorsi and trapezius were divided which provided full exposure to the upper portion of the chest wall. The scalene muscles were detached from the first and second ribs. The paraspinous muscles were elevated to the spinous processes to expose the costovertebral junction and the transverse processes.

The resection was started with the anterior portion of the chest wall. The [RIB NUMBERS, e.g., first through fifth] ribs were divided with at least 3-4 cm margin. A small piece of each of the ribs anteriorly was sent for permanent analysis. A portion of the posterior 5th rib was resected to facilitate anterior mobility. Next, the posterior resection was completed by resecting the entire posterolateral aspect of the first, second, third, and fourth ribs. Small portions of the ribs posteriorly were submitted for routine pathology.

After the anterior portion of the first rib had been divided at the costochondral junction, dissection along the superior border of the first rib was performed down to the insertion on the spine to join the posterior dissection. The chest wall was retracted inferiorly to display the subclavian artery and vein and the brachial plexus. [Additional statement: During the completion of dissection along the brachial plexus, multiple frozen sections were obtained. The patient did [OR DID NOT] have residual microscopic disease along the C8 nerve root. The tumor surrounded the T1 nerve root therefore it was resected. No area of gross residual disease remained. Posteriorly, the paraspinous muscles were retracted to expose the transverse processes. At this point, the neurosurgeon came to the operating room to complete the posterior aspect of this dissection along the spine.

The upper lobectomy and mediastinal lymph node dissections were completed next. An en bloc resection of the subcarinal and paratracheal (or AP window) lymph nodes was performed and submitted for frozen section analysis. The upper lobe bronchus was dissected free, ligated with a TA-30 4.8 mm stapler and then transected distally. The branches of the pulmonary artery to the upper lobe were dissected free, ligated, and divided with the Endo-GIA vascular stapler. The superior pulmonary vein branches were ligated with the Endo-GIA vascular stapler. The fissure was divided with Endo-GIA stapler to complete the resection.

Finally, the chest was closed and reconstructed. Intercostal nerve blocks were performed with 0.5% Marcaine. Two 28 French chest tubes were inserted via separate inferior stab wounds and placed anteriorly and posteriorly in the pleural space. The thoracotomy incision was then closed by reapproximating the fifth and sixth ribs with #2 Vicryl pericostal sutures. The chest wall defect was repaired with 2 mm thickness Gore-Tex patch, which was secured in place with #0 Prolene sutures. The sutures approximated the paraspinous muscles to the patch posteriorly and to the intercostals and chest wall muscles anteriorly. The entire incision was closed in layers with #0 Vicryl to the chest wall muscles, #2-0 Vicryl to the subcutaneous tissues, and #3-0 subcutaneous Monocryl for the skin closure. Dressings were applied.

The patient was returned to supine position and reintubated with a single lumen endotracheal tube. Toilet bronchoscopy was performed. The patient was awoken from general anesthesia, extubated, and transferred to the recovery room.

Dr. [BLANK] was present and scrubbed for [BLANK] elements of this procedure.

18. Tracheostomy

Lara Schaheen, MD, and Jonathan D'Cunha, MD, PhD

University of Pittsburgh Medical Center, Pittsburgh, PA

Essential Operative Steps

1. Lines and Pulse Ox Monitoring
2. General endotracheal anesthesia
3. Time out and administer pre-operative antibiotics according to institutional standards
4. Pre-oxygenate with FiO_2 at 100%
5. Neck hyperextension and shoulder roll placement
6. Perform flexible bronchoscopy for pulmonary toilet and evaluate anatomy
7. Arms tucked
8. Sterile prep and drape of the neck and entire chest including lateral aspect in case chest tube needed
9. Palpate cricoid and thyroid cartilages
10. Midline transverse incision one finger breadth above the sternal notch
11. Dissect in midline to the trachea
12. Retract the strap muscles laterally and thyroid isthmus superiorly
13. Palpate the tracheal rings
14. Insert tracheostomy hook if needed to elevate the trachea anteriorly by retracting superiorly.
15. Decrease FiO_2 to room air to avoid airway fire (from cautery if required)
16. Have the anesthesiologist deflate the endotracheal tube balloon
17. Make a vertical incision between the second and third tracheal rings
18. Dilate the trachea with a tracheal spreader
19. Withdraw endotracheal tube under vision to just above the tracheotomy
20. Insert tracheostomy tube (typically #8 Shiley).
21. Connect tracheostomy tube to ventilatory circuit. Inflate tracheostomy balloon. Confirm placement with end-tidal CO2.
22. Confirm placement with flexible bronchoscopy via tracheostomy tube and clear any residual secretions
23. Secure tracheostomy with tracheal sutures x 4 (#2-0 Prolene).
24. Place tracheostomy ties.
25. Perform flexible bronchoscopy via endotracheal tube to ensure good position of tracheostomy and no upper airway bleeding.
26. Remove endotracheal tube.
27. Order chest x-ray post operatively.

Potential Complications and Pitfalls

1. Caution with hyperextension of the neck with history of cervical spine injury or fusion.

2. Overextension of the neck should be avoided. It narrows the airway and can lead to placement of the tracheostomy too low (near the carina and innominate artery).
3. Have several sizes of tracheostomy tubes available. Including a tracheostomy tube that is the same size as the endotracheal tube and one size smaller in event that placement is difficult.
4. Have reintubation supplies at the ready
5. Stay midline during dissection
6. If difficulty ventilating consider the potential for a pneumothorax
7. Bronchoscopy after placement should ensure that there is no membranous tracheal tear
8. Bleeding must be evaluated carefully
9. Tracheostomy malposition must be inspected for via the tracheostomy tube and via the endotracheal tube
10. Pre-oxygenate patient with 100% FiO2 to avoid hypoxia during tracheostomy placement.
11. Decrease FiO2 to room air prior to making a tracheotomy to avoid an airway fire.

Template Dictation

Preoperative Diagnosis: [INDICATION – e.g. Respiratory Failure, need for prolonged airway management, inability to manage airway secretions, airway obstruction at or above the level of the larynx,]
Postoperative Diagnosis: Same
Procedure(s) Performed: Tracheostomy, Flexible Bronchoscopy **(DETAILS – e.g. type and size of tracheostomy placed)**

Attending Surgeon: [BLANK]

Secondary Surgeon: [BLANK]

Assistants: [BLANK]

Anesthesia: [BLANK]

Indication(s) for Procedure: [AGE] year old [GENDER] with [DURATION] history of [COMPLAINT – e.g. respiratory failure, need for prolonged airway management, inability to manage airway secretions, airway obstruction at or above the level of the larynx].

Description of Procedure: The patient was identified in the pre-operative holding area and taken to the operating room on [DATE]. The patient's identity and planned procedure verified, and the patient was placed on the operating room table in the supine position. General anesthesia was obtained. A shoulder role was placed to assist in neck hyperextension. The neck and anterior chest were then prepped and draped in sterile fashion. A time out was performed prior to beginning the procedure. The patient was pre-oxiginated with 100% FiO2. The trachea, cricoid cartilage, thyroid cartilage and sternal notch were palpated. A 4 cm midline transverse incision was made one fingerbreadth above the suprasternal notch. The incision was carried down through the subcutaneous tissues using cautery. The platysma was divided with cautery. The strap muscles were identified, divided in the midline, and retracted laterally. The thyroid gland was retracted superiorly, and dissection continued down to the level of the pretracheal fascia. Hemostasis was maintained. The second tracheal ring was identified. A tracheostomy hook was placed between the first and second tracheal rings and the tracheal was retracted superiorly. The FiO2 was decreased to room air. Anesthesia was instructed to deflate the endotracheal tube balloon prior to incising the trachea. Using an #11 blade scalpel, a vertical incision was made in the trachea between the 2nd and 3rd tracheal rings. The endotracheal tube was withdrawn so that its tip was immediately proximal to the tracheostomy site. A #___8 tracheostomy tube was successfully inserted and advanced into the trachea. The tracheostomy balloon was inflated and the tracheostomy was connected to the ventilatory circuit. Placement was confirmed by return of end tidal C02. Oxygen saturations were excellent. A flexible bronchoscope was placed through the tracheostomy tube to confirm appropriate placement under direct vision. The tracheostomy tube was secured in place using a #2-0 Prolene sutures in each of the four quadrants. A soft tracheostomy tie was placed around the patient's neck leaving two fingerbreadths space beneath the tape. Bronchoscopy was performed through the endotracheal and tracheostomy tubes to ensure hemostasis and for pulmonary toilet. There were no immediate complications. Counts were correct x 2 at the end of the case. The patient tolerated the procedure well. A post-operative chest xray was ordered. The attending surgeon was scrubbed and present for the critical portion of the procedure. The patient was subsequently transferred to intensive care unit in stable condition.

Dr. **[BLANK]** was present and scrubbed for **[BLANK]** elements of this procedure.

19. Tracheal Resection and Reconstruction

Cameron T. Stock, MD and Douglas J. Mathisen, MD

Massachusetts General Hospital, Boston, MA

Essential Operative Steps

1. Careful radiologic evaluation
2. General endotracheal anesthesia
3. Preoperative bronchoscopic evaluation of the trachea by the operating surgeon
4. Dilation of the stenotic tracheal segment to secure the airway for resection or palliation until resection can be safely performed
5. Careful dissection of the trachea from surrounding structures staying immediately on the tracheal surface to avoid injury to the recurrent laryngeal nerve
6. Cross field ventilation
7. Placement of traction sutures in the midlateral position on the proximal and distal tracheal ends to gauge tension on the anastomosis and to take tension off the anastomosis when tying the anastomotic sutures.
8. Placement of interrupted absorbable sutures in an organized and systematic fashion for the anastomosis
9. Coverage of the anastomosis with a pedicled muscle flap
10. Neck drainage / placement of a guardian stitch

Potential Complications and Pitfalls

1. Poor preoperative patient selection
2. Injury to the recurrent laryngeal nerve by electrocautery or sharp dissection
3. Excessive tension on the anastomosis when tying
4. Compromise of the tracheal blood supply by excessive dissection
5. Injury to the brachiocephalic artery during dissection inferiorly
6. Postoperative wound infection
7. Air leak/subcutaneous air
8. Anastomotic separation/dehiscence

Template Dictation

Preoperative Diagnosis: Tracheal stenosis, tracheal malignancy

Postoperative Diagnosis: Same

Procedure(s) Performed: Tracheal resection and reconstruction, muscle flap coverage of the anastomosis

Attending Surgeon: [BLANK]

Secondary Surgeon: [BLANK]

Assistants: [BLANK]

Anesthesia: [BLANK]

Indication(s) for Procedure: [AGE] year old [GENDER] with [INDICATIONS, e.g., post-intubation tracheal stenosis, tracheal mass, etc.] who presented with increasing dyspnea and audible stridor with exertion. Preoperative imaging showed [CXR and CT findings] and bronchoscopy revealed **[BRONCHOSCOPIC FINDINGS AND PATHOLOGY RESULTS]**. After discussing the risks and benefits of the procedure, the patient provided informed consent for a flexible bronchoscopy, tracheal resection and reconstruction and muscle flap coverage of the anastomosis.

Description of Procedure: The patient was brought to the operating room on [DATE]. The patient was confirmed with two unique identifiers and the correct procedure was verified. The patient was placed supine on the operating table and general anesthesia was administered. After flexible bronchoscopy revealed healed, non-inflamed tracheal mucosa at the area of known stenosis, the patient's neck was extended by insufflating the thyroid bag placed under the patient's shoulders, and the head was supported with blankets. The patient's neck and chest were prepped and draped in the usual fashion. A time out was performed. A low transverse collar incision was made between the cricoid cartilage and the sternal notch. The incision was carried through the dermis and subcutaneous fat to the platysma. The platysma was divided transversely and cutaneous sub-platysmal flaps were raised to the level of the cricoid superiorly and the sternal notch inferiorly. Gelpi retractors were placed at the lateral aspects of the incision for exposure. The midline of the trachea was identified and the overlying sternohyoid and sternothyroid muscles were dissected off the surface of the trachea laterally for a short distance. The cricoid cartilage was identified in the midline and the anterior surface of the trachea was dissected to the thyroid isthmus. The isthmus was divided sharply and the ends were suture ligated. At the level of the sternal notch dissection of the pretracheal fascia was initiated using finger dissection and the anterior surface of the trachea was dissected bluntly down to the carina. This maneuver was employed to allow the distal trachea to slide cephalad with less tension when creating the anastomosis.

Sharp dissection of the affected tracheal segment was performed using scissors and short bursts of electrocautery. Care was taken to stay immediately on the surface of the trachea to avoid injury to the recurrent laryngeal nerve. Circumferential dissection of the trachea was completed only on the affected segment. The trachea was divided between cartilages distal to the tracheal lesion and the trachea was retracted cephalad to facilitate posterior dissection. Care was taken to avoid injury to the esophagus. Ventilation of the distal trachea was performed by intermittent cross field ventilation with sterile tubing and an armored Tovell endotracheal tube. After careful dissection of the tracheal lesion was completed, it was divided sharply on the proximal end of the affected segment and the specimen was passed off the field.

The tracheal ends were inspected and determined to be satisfactory to complete the anastomosis. Full thickness #2-0 Vicryl traction sutures were placed around the cartilage 1.5 cm from the cut tracheal ends on the proximal and distal airway in the midlateral position on both sides of the trachea. Next, the neck was flexed by deflating the thyroid bag and placing 2-3 folded blankets under the patient's head. The proximal and distal traction sutures were grasped on either side of the trachea and by pulling them together it was determined there would not be excessive tension on the completed anastomosis. The anastomosis was performed using interworked #4-0 Vicryl stitches. The first stitch was placed in the posterior membranous trachea at the 6 o'clock position such that the knot would was on the outside of the trachea. The ends were clipped to the drapes cephalad at the 12 o'clock position. Subsequent stitches were placed on the posterior wall of the tracheal to level of the lateral traction sutures and were clipped to the drapes in the caudal position. Each subsequent suture was affixed anterior to the proceeding stitch on the drapes. Sutures were placed approximately 4 mm apart and 2-3 mm from the cut end of the trachea such that all knots would lie on the outside. Cross field ventilation was performed between stitches. Next, stitches were placed from traction suture to traction suture along the anterior wall of the trachea and the ends were clipped to a surgical towel placed cephalad to the incision. After all the anastomotic stitches were placed the proximal and distal traction sutures were then tied to each other, pulling the tracheal ends together. Next the #4-0 Vicryl stitches placed along the anterior wall were tied from traction suture to traction suture. The stitches on the back wall were then tied, first on the left side followed by the right side. The anastomosis was inspected and found to be satisfactory by deflating the cuff on the endotracheal tube, closing the nose and mouth, and giving a breath to 20-40 cm of H_2O pressure.

Next the right sternothyroid muscle was identified and dissected from the sternohyoid muscle. It was divided inferiorly and rotated over the anastomosis and sutured in place over the anastomotic suture line using interrupted #4-0 Vicryl sutures in a mattress fashion. The sternohyoid muscles were closed in the midline using interrupted sutures. A #10 flat Jackson-Pratt drain was placed in the neck near the anastomosis and the platysma and skin were closed. All instrument, sponge and needle counts were confirmed to be correct. A heavy #2 Vicryl "guardian" stitch was placed from the chin to the presternal skin to prevent tension on the anastomosis. A sterile dressing was applied to the neck incision. The patient was extubated and brought to the ICU in stable condition.

Dr. [BLANK] was present and scrubbed for [BLANK] elements of this procedure.

20. Esophageal Stent Placement

Thomas Caranasos, MD and Kfir Ben-David, MD

University of Florida, Gainesville, FL

Essential Operative Steps

1. Preoperative imaging to determine pathology (Malignant esophageal stricture, Begin esophageal stricture, Esophageal perforation, Leak following esophageal or gastric surgery, Tracheoesophageal fistula)
2. Appropriate noninvasive monitoring
3. Conscious sedation or general endotracheal anesthesia.
4. Introduction of the scope into the esophagus to the pylorus or duodenum depending on pathology
5. Examination of the stomach and hiatus with retroflexion
6. Examination of the GE junction and esophagus
7. Recognition of pathology
8. Deployment of the stent
9. Examination of appropriate positioning
10. Safe withdrawal of the scope

Potential Complications and Pitfalls

1. Appropriate administration of sedation (avoiding over-sedation, hemodynamic instability, or aspiration)
2. Introduction of the scope within the esophagus
3. Careful advancement of the scope, especially in the face of stricture as to not cause perforation.
4. Appropriate examination of the entire stomach, possibly the duodenum, GE junction, and esophagus for underlying pathology. Biopsy if needed.
5. Management of bleeding with clips or submucosal epinephrine injection
6. Deployment of stent bridging area of pathology
7. Anchoring the stent to prevent stent migration
8. Evaluation of placement of the stent for concern of perforation or mucosal injury
9. Appropriate timing of stent removal to avoid late complications (Perforation, Erosion, Migration, Bleeding)

Template Dictation

Preoperative Diagnosis: Esophageal Perforation

Postoperative Diagnosis: Same

Procedure(s) Performed: EGD, Esophageal Stent Placement

Attending Surgeon: [BLANK]

Secondary Surgeon: [BLANK]

Assistants: [BLANK]

Anesthesia: [BLANK]

Indication(s) for Procedure: [Blank] is a 60 year old male who is post procedure day 2 from EGD for Achalasia. He returned to the hospital with worsening mid-epigastric pain. Oral contrasted CT imaging showed evidence of distal esophageal leak. The risks, benefits, and alternatives to the above procedure were discussed at length with the patient and he agreed to and accepted the risks.

Description of Procedure: The patient was brought to the endoscopy suit. Noninvasive blood pressure and continuous heart rate and pulse oximetry monitoring were utilized throughout the procedure. Versed and fentanyl were used for conscious sedation. The endoscope was introduced through the bite block in the mouth and into the posterior oropharynx. The vocal cords were visualized anteriorly and the scoped passed posterior to the left arytenoid and into the esophagus. Under direct visualization the scope was carefully advanced. The proximal and middle esophagus appeared normal. A [**Finding and description - e.g.** *10 mm mucosal laceration was noted at 38 cm from the incisors. The tear was located on the left anterior-lateral portion of the esophagus. The lesion extended from 38-39 cm from the incisors*]. The GE junction was measured at [**X**] cm from the incisors. The scope is slowly advanced into the stomach and retroflexed to examine the GE junction. No evidence of hiatal hernia or gastric perforation was visualized. The stomach and first portion of the duodenum were examined. No abnormalities were noted. The scope was slowly withdrawn 10 cm proximal to the level of the [**lesion to be stented**]. Under direct endoscopic visualization, a 0.97 mm guide wire was advanced into the stomach. A [**dimensions X by X**] [**brand**] stent was deployed according to the manufacturer's recommendation. The proximal end of the stent was positioned at [**X**] cm from the incisors with the distal end bridging the GE junction and positioned in the stomach. The string at the proximal end of the stent was clipped to the mucosa with two endo-clips to prevent migration. The scope was then passed back into the stomach to confirm appropriate positioning and slowly withdrawn and removed. The bite block was removed and the patient transferred to the endoscopy recovery room in stable condition.

Dr. [**BLANK**] was present and scrubbed for [**BLANK**] elements of this procedure.

21. Laparoscopic Nissen Fundoplication

Luis F. Alberton, MD and Sean Kwon, MD

North Shore Long Island Jewish Health System, New Hyde Park, NY

Essential Operative Steps

1. Lithotomy position or supine with foot rest to allow steep reverse Trendelenburg position
2. Foley catheter
3. Additional peripheral IVs +/- arterial line
4. Gain access to abdominal cavity with Veress needle or open Hassan technique
5. Inspect abdominal cavity and place additional ports
6. Place liver retractor to provide exposure of hiatus
7. Mobilize lesser curvature, divide gastrohepatic ligament
8. Dissect right crus
9. Mobilize greater curvature
10. Dissect left crus
11. Complete anterior portion of mediastinal dissection of the distal esophagus starting on the pericardium anteriorly and then working from pleura to pleura
12. Take down retrogastric and retroesophageal attachments and identify the decussation of the right and left crus
13. Complete the mediastinal dissection in the posterior (periaortic plane) until the distal esophagus has been mobilized circumferentially taking care to spare both vagal trunks
14. Dissect the GEJ fat pad to identify the true GEJ
15. Collis gastroplasty if there is inadequate length of intraabdominal esophagus
16. Place Bougie (i.e., 54 Fr)
17. Grasp fundus along the line of the short gastrics and pass from left to right in the retroesophageal window inside of the vagus nerves
18. Shoe shine technique to assure the absence of rotational torsion
19. Place 2 to 3 sutures to secure the wrap around the esophagus
20. Remove Bougie
21. Close diaphragmatic hiatus
22. Remove liver retractor and ports under direct visualization
23. Close port sites

Special Equipment

1. 5 and/or 10 mm 30 or 45 degree laparoscopes
2. Endoscopic suturing instrument or pledged sutures
3. Self-retaining liver retractor
4. Electrocautery / ultrasonic dissector

Potential Complications and Pitfalls

1. Injury to abdominal viscera or blood vessels while entering the abdominal cavity.
2. Esophageal or gastric perforation
3. Tension pneumothorax
4. Hypotension secondary to CO2 insufflation
5. Injury to replaced left hepatic artery while dissecting gastrohepatic ligament
6. Spleen or splenic vascular injury
7. Bleeding secondary to injury to the short gastrics
8. Wrap or hiatal closure too tight or too loose
9. Injury to vagus nerves
10. When dissecting the GEJ fat pad, always work from right to left
11. Inadequate mobilization of the esophagus and failure to recognized a short esophagus
12. Constructing the wrap around the cardia
13. Denuding the peritoneum off the right or left crus

Template Dictation

Preoperative Diagnosis: [INDICATION – e.g. reflux disease unresponsive to medical therapy]

Postoperative Diagnosis: Same

Procedure(s) Performed: Laparoscopic Nissen Fundoplication and hiatal hernia repair

Attending Surgeon: [BLANK]

Secondary Surgeon: [BLANK]

Assistants: [BLANK]

Anesthesiologist: [BLANK]

Anesthesia: GETA   **IVF:** [BLANK]   **EBL:** [BLANK]   **UO:** [BLANK]

Indication(s) for Procedure: [AGE] year old [GENDER] with [DURATION] history of gastroesophageal reflux disease manifesting as [SYMPTOMS] that has failed to respond to maximal medical therapy. [HIS/HER] preoperative evaluation has included a barium esophagram which revealed [FINDINGS]. Esophageal manometry demonstrated [FINDINGS]. A pH study demonstrated a DeMeester score of [X]. A upper endoscopy was obtained which revealed a [X] cm hiatal hernia and [OTHER FINDINGS, i.e., Barrett's esophagus, esophagitis, etc]. After discussing the risks and benefits of the procedure, the patient provided informed consent for a laparoscopic Nissen fundoplication and hiatal hernia repair.

I. General Thoracic Surgery

Description of Procedure: The patient was taken to the operating room on **[DATE]**. The patient's identity and planned procedure were verified, and the patient was placed on the operating room table in the supine position. Sequential compression devices were placed in both legs for DVT prophylaxis. Following an uneventful induction of general anesthesia, the patient was intubated without incident. A Foley catheter was inserted. **[Patient was placed on lithotomy position]**. The abdomen was then prepped and draped in the usual sterile fashion. The camera and insufflation equipment were connected and checked. A time out was then performed according to hospital policy.

Access to the abdominal cavity was obtained using **[Hassan/Veress needle]** technique. A camera port was placed in the midline supraumbilical area, approximately 15cm from the xiphoid process. Pneumoperitoneum was established with carbon dioxide to a pressure of 15 mmHg, paying close attention to the vital signs and flow and total volume of gas infused. Inspection of abdominal cavity was performed and no abnormalities or injuries were identified. Four additional ports were placed. A 10-mm trocar was placed below the left costal margin, 11 cm away from the xiphoid process. A 5-mm assistant's port was placed a hand's breadth lateral to the 10 mm trocar along the left costal margin. A 5-mm trocar for the liver retractor was inserted just below the right costal margin in the lateral aspect of the right upper quadrant. A self-retaining liver retractor was then used to elevate the left lateral segment of the liver to expose the esophageal hiatus. The retractor is stabilized with a table-mounted mechanical arm. An additional 5-mm trocar was inserted just to the right side of the Falciform ligament and angled toward the hiatus.

Once all the trocars were in place, the gastrohepatic ligament was divided directly over the caudate lobe using **[electrocautery / ultrasonic dissector]**. The dissection was continued towards the base of the right crus. The medial border of the right crus was defined, taking care to preserve its peritoneal lining. We began the lateral mediastinal portion of the dissection, sweeping the pleura laterally. We then divided the peritoneum anteriorly and continued along the medial border of the left crus, taking care to preserve its peritoneal lining. We then completed mobilization of the distal esophagus in the anterior plane, working directly on the pericardium and then working from pleura to pleura, taking care to preserve the anterior vagus nerve.

Attention was then directed to the greater curvature of the stomach. The gastrosplenic ligament was opened with the ultrasonic dissector, and the short gastric vessels were divided to the level of the Angle of His. We then completed our dissection along the medial border of the left crus.

Attention was then redirected to the lesser curvature of the stomach. The stomach was elevated. The retroesophageal and retrogastric attachments were taken down. **[A Penrose drain was passed around the esophagus and used for retraction.]** The distal esophagus was then mobilized posteriorly in the pre-aortic areolar soft tissue plane. The distal esophagus was then circumferentially mobilized. Both vagal trunks were identified and were spared during the dissection. In order to identify the true gastroesophageal junction, we mobilized the GEJ fat pad laterally off the esophagus, sparing both vagal trunks. We noted approximately [x] cm of intraabdominal esophagus. [**Variation: Collis gastroplasty may be performed if a short esophagus (<2 cm of intra-abdominal length) is present**]. The Penrose drain was removed.

The posterior aspect of esophageal hiatus was then closed with interrupted [**SIZE and TYPE;** e.g, non-absorbable, pledged] sutures. The fundus of the stomach was then grasped and passed from left to right in the retroesophageal window between the esophagus and the fat pad. The lines of the short gastrics on either side of the wrap were aligned with one another, thereby forming a 360 degree wrap. A [**SIZE**] Bougie was advanced transorally down the esophagus and into the stomach under direct vision. We performed a "shoeshine maneuver" to assured the absence of rotational torsion. The wrap was then sutured in place using [**TYPE AND NUMBER OF SUTURES**], taking a bite of the fundus on one side, the esophagus, and then the fundus on the other side. The Bougie was removed. An NG tube was placed under and the liver retractor and ports then removed under direct visualization. The abdominal cavity was again inspected and no bleeding or sites of injury were seen. Pneumoperitoneum was then desufflated. The fascial incisions of the 10 mm ports were closed with [**SUTURE**]. Finally the skin was closed with [**SUTURE / GLUE**] and sterile dressings then applied.

All instrument, sponge and needle counts were confirmed to be correct x 2 at the end of the operation. The patient was subsequently transferred to the postanesthesia care unit in satisfactory condition.

Dr. [**BLANK**] was present and scrubbed for [**BLANK**] elements of this procedure.

22. Laparoscopic Paraesophageal Hernia Repair

Andrew B. Nguyen, MD and James D. Luketich, MD

University of Pittsburgh Medical Center, Pittsburgh, PA

Essential Operative Steps

1. Upper endoscopy.
2. Supine position (far right on operating bed), arms out 45 degrees, and foot board placement for steep reverse Trendelenburg.
3. Place 10 mm port via open Hasson technique in the right paramedian line approximately one-third of the way from the xiphoid to the umbilicus.
4. CO_2 insufflation to 15 mmHg.
5. Confirm position within the peritoneal cavity and inspect abdomen with laparoscope.
6. Place additional ports under direct laparoscopic visualization. An 11 mm left paramedian port one hand's breadth to the left initial cutdown port. A 5 mm right and left subcostal port a hand's breadth from the paramedian port sites. A 5 mm port in the lateral right upper quadrant directed along the lower edge of the liver.
7. Insert liver retractor to elevate the left lobe of the liver for exposure of the hiatus.
8. Place patient in steep reverse Trendelenburg position to facilitate visualization of the hiatus.
9. Reduce herniated content gently while avoiding placing traction on the stomach.
10. Evert and incise hernia sac anteriorly.
11. Complete the anterior portion of the dissection, beginning on the pericardium and then working from pleura to pleura.
12. Open the gastrohepatic omentum directly above the caudate lobe
13. Define the medial border of the right crus, while preserving its peritoneal lining.
14. Divide the short gastric vessels.
15. Define the medial border of the left crus, while preserving its peritoneal lining.
16. Medistinal dissection in areolar periaortic soft tissue plane
17. After mobilizing the esophagus circumferentially to the level of the inferior pulmonary veins, excise the hernia sac
18. For a Nissen-Fundoplication
    a. Dissect gastric fat pad off stomach to precisely identify the gastroesophageal junction.
    b. Develop a retroesophageal window between the esophagus and posterior vagus nerve.
    c. Pass a 54-French bougie transorally into the stomach under direct laparoscopic visualization.

      d. *[Perform Collis gastroplasty if more intrabdominal esophageal length is required.]*
      e. Create a "floppy" Nissen wrap.
19. For a gastropexy:
      a. Interrupted u-stitches between the line of the short gastrics and left hemidiaphragm
20. Close hiatus with interrupted sutures approximating crura posteriorly (and anteriorly if necessary).
21. Place NG tube
22. Close

Potential Complications and Pitfalls

1. Avoid upper overinsufflation during upper endoscopy which will increase the difficulty of a laparoscopic repair.
2. Trocar injuries.
3. Injury to esophagus.
4. Injury to stomach.
5. Injury to spleen.
6. Vagal nerve injury. Be cognizant of the location of both nerves during the dissection. Minimize the risk of anterior vagal nerve injury by beginning the dissection anteriorly and dissecting in the areolar soft tissue plane. Dissect the fat pad by working from left to right
7. Inadequate esophageal mobilization or failure to recognize a short esophagus can result in a recurrence. Many patients with giant paraesophageal hernias require gastroplasties
8. A poorly planned gastroplasty can result in undue angulation of the stomach
9. An excessively tight hiatal repair can cause obstructive symptoms. An excessively loose repair can contribute to a recurrence.
10. Hypercapnea from CO_2 insufflation
11. Pneumothorax

Template Dictation

Preoperative Diagnosis: Paraesophageal hernia

Postoperative Diagnosis: Same

Procedure(s) Performed: Laparoscopic paraesophageal hernia repair

Attending Surgeon: [BLANK]

Secondary Surgeon: [BLANK]

Assistants: [BLANK]

Anesthesia: [BLANK]

Indication(s) for Procedure: This is a [AGE]-year-old male/female who presented with [SYMPTOMS AND SIGNS]. The patient was found on [ESOPHAGRAM/UPPER ENDOSCOPY/COMPUTED TOMOGRAPHY SCAN] to have a type [II/III/IV] paraesophageal hernia involving a large portion of the stomach/ +/- OTHER ABDOMINAL STRUCTURES]. The risks and benefits had been discussed with the patient regarding surgical repair. The patient provided informed consent for an upper endoscopy, laparoscopic (possible open) paraesophageal hernia repair, and [NISSEN FUNDOPLICATION/GASTROPEXY], [AND POSSIBLE COLLIS GASTROPLASTY].

Description of procedure: The patient was identified in the preoperative area, taken to the operating room, and placed supine on the operating table. General anesthesia was induced. The patient was intubated with a single-lumen endotracheal tube. [CEFAZOLIN/OTHER ANTIBIOTIC] was given for perioperative antibiotic prophylaxis. A Foley catheter was inserted. Sequential compression devices were placed bilaterally in the lower extremities and a dose of 5000 units of subcutaneous heparin was given for deep venous thrombosis prophylaxis. A proper time-out was conducted.

An upper endoscopy was first performed. A flexible endoscope was inserted transorally and advanced distally into the esophagus. The esophagus appeared [DESCRIBE FEATURES, NORMAL, ESOPHAGITIS, BARRETT'S ESOPHAGUS, ETC]. The gastroesophageal junction was noted at about [LOCATION FROM INCISORS] cm and the crural pinch at [LOCATION FROM INCISORS] cm from the incisors, consistent with a [SIZE] hiatal hernia. The endoscope was advanced into the stomach, which had herniated in the chest. Care was taken to not over insufflate the stomach to avoid gastric and intestinal distention. The scope was advanced through a patent pylorus into the duodenum, which appeared normal. The duodenum, stomach, and esophagus were then desufflated as the endoscope was withdrawn.

The patient is positioned far right on the operating room table in preparation for the subhepatic liver retractor. A foot board was placed for support during steep reverse Trendelenburg positioning. The patient's arms were secured to the arm board, carefully padded, and rotated 45 degrees away from the bed. The patient was then prepped and draped in the usual sterile fashion.

The first port was placed using the open Hasson technique in the right paramedian line approximately one-third of the distance from the xiphoid process to the umbilicus. The skin was incised and the subcutaneous tissue was bluntly dissected with S retractors. The anterior sheath was opened vertically with electrocautery. The S retractors were used to separate the rectus muscles in the direction of the fibers. The posterior sheath was then grasped with tonsils, elevated, and incised. The peritoneal cavity was entered with S retractors and a 12-mm Hassan port was then placed, taken care to avoid dissecting into the falciform ligament. The abdomen was insufflated to 15 mmHg and the 30-degree laparoscope was inserted to confirm position within the peritoneal cavity and inspect the abdomen. The Hasson port was then secured to the skin with Vicryl sutures. Additional ports were then placed under direct laparoscopic visualization. A left paramedian port was placed approximately one hands breadth to the left and slightly lower to the initial cutdown port. Bilateral 5 mm subcostal ports were placed a hand's breadth from the paramedian ports. A 5 mm port was placed in the lateral aspect of the right upper quadrant and in-line with the lower edge of the liver for insertion of the liver retractor. Under direct laparoscopic visualization, the liver retractor was inserted and used to elevate the left lobe of the liver for exposure of the hiatus.

The patient was placed in steep reverse Trendelenburg position to facilitate visualization of the hiatus. The herniated content was then reduced gently. The herniated sac was then grasped near the 12'oclock position and everted. Using the harmonic scalpel, the sac was opened, exposing the areolar plane between the hernia sac and the mediastinum. The sac was sharply and bluntly dissected from the pleura laterally on both sides, the pericardium anteriorly, and the aorta posteriorly with the use of the harmonic scalpel. The anterior and posterior vagus nerves were identified during the mediastinum dissection and preserved.

Attention was then turned to opening the gastrohepatic omentum directly over the caudate lobe. The dissection was continued towards the base of the right crus.

After the division of the gastrohepatic omentum, the esophagus was mobilized first by dissecting out the right crus and taking down the phrenoesophageal ligament, making sure to preserve the peritoneal lining of the right crus. The areolar plane between the esophagus and the right crus was entered. Extensive, circumferential mobilization of the esophagus was then performed high in the mediastinum to the level of the inferior pulmonary veins to help re-establish adequate intraabdominal esophageal length of 2-3 cm. Again, the vagus nerves were identified and preserved. The left crus and base of the crura were also dissected during the mobilization of the esophagus.

Attention was then turned to the mobilization of the fundus and the division of the short gastric vessels. With the traction of gastrosplenic omentum and countertraction of the stomach, the short gastric vessels were ligated with a harmonic scalpel along the upper third of the greater curve of the stomach. Care was taken as the superior pole of the spleen was approached to avoid injury to the spleen. Gastrosplenic attachments were carefully ligated. Retrogastric attachments were also taken down, and a window was created into the lesser sac. Division of the short gastric vessels provided exposure to the left crus and angle of His, which was further dissected to help facilitate retroesophageal mobilization.

To help facilitate precise identification of the gastroesophageal junction, the gastric fat pad was dissected anteriorly off the stomach and distal esophagus, taking care to preserve the anterior vagus nerve. A retroesophageal window was then developed between the esophagus and posterior vagus nerve through which a Nissen fundoplication would be performed.

[**Collis Gastroplasty**] *Despite extensive esophageal mobilization, additional esophageal length was required, which was achieved through laparoscopic wedge Collis gastroplasty. A 54-French bougie was placed transorally into the stomach under direct laparoscopic visualization to allow for safe passage. The stomach was then grasped just proximal to the planned initial staple site. Using a 4.8 mm green load/3.5mm blue load cutting endostapler, serial fires were taken perpendicular to the bougie to divide the stomach toward the bougie. With gentle traction of the partially stapled gastric wedge, additional serial firings of the endostapler were placed parallel to the bougie to complete the creation of the neoesophagus.*

In preparation for a "floppy" Nissen fundoplication, a 54-French bougie is placed transorally into the stomach under direct laparoscopic visualization to allow for safe passage. A grasper was then passed through the retroesophageal window. The fundus was grasped at the level the divided short gastric vessels along the greater curvature and pulled through the window to the right side. A "shoe-shine" maneuver was then performed with the created wrap to ensure adequate mobility without twists or tension. The "floppy" Nissen fundoplication was then secured with two #2-0 Surgidac sutures with the use of the Endo Stitch suturing device. Each stich incorporated full thickness of the stomach and partial thickness of the esophagus, spaced 2 cm apart to prevent slippage of the wrap.

[**Gastropexy**] *Due to concerns for the patient's intraoperative instability/age/co-morbidities/viability of the stomach/preoperative symptoms and esophageal dysmotility, a gastropexy was performed. With an Endo Stitch suturing device, multiple serial interrupted horizontal mattress of #0 Surgidac sutures were placed between the stomach and the anterior abdominal wall over a distance of about 10 cm, spaced 2 cm apart.*

Attention was then turn to performing a tension-free hiatal closure. The bougie was removed and the crura were assessed for adequate tissue integrity and mobility. [*Due to the enlarged hiatus and significant tension with the approximation of the crura, left pneumothorax was induced with a placement of the pigtail catheter in the left pleural space under direct laparoscopic view of the diaphragm. The diaphragm was noted to become relaxed and bulged into the peritoneal cavity. The pigtail catheter was then secured to the skin and placed to drainage after the closure of the hiatus.*] The crura were reapproximated with 2 (or 3) posterior interrupted sutures of #0 Surgidac using the Endo Stich suturing device. [*After approximating the crura posteriorly, the hiatus was re-evaluated and noted to have a patulous anterior space. A single stitched was then placed anteriorly in the upper aspect of crura.*] Care was taken to avoid artificially creating an angulation of the esophagus at the hiatus. At the completion of the hiatal closure, a grasper was easily passed through the hiatus and the closure did not appear tight.

A nasogastric tube was then placed under direct laparoscopic vision to confirm placement in the stomach.

After ensuring adequate hemostasis, the right paramedian port placed via open Hasson technique was removed under direct laparoscopic visualization. The fascial defect was closed with a single #0 Vicryl suture using a Carter-Thomason device. The other ports were removed under direct laparoscopic visualization. The abdomen was desufflated. The camera port was then removed. All skin incisions were closed and sterile dressings were applied.

The patient tolerated the procedure well and was transferred to the postanesthesia care unit in stable condition.

Dr. [BLANK] was present and scrubbed for [BLANK] elements of this procedure.

23. Transhiatal Esophagectomy

Michelle C. Ellis, MD & Jules Lin, MD

University of Michigan, Ann Arbor, MI

Essential Operative Steps

1. Lines and monitoring (arterial line, large bore IV)
2. Consider epidural catheter placement
3. General endotracheal anesthesia
4. Intraoperative esophagoscopy
5. Laparotomy
6. Assess for resectability, conduit choice
7. Gastric mobilization
8. Kocher maneuver
9. Pyloromyotomy/pyloroplasty
10. Placement of feeding jejunostomy
11. Hiatal dissection and lower esophagus mobilization with mediastinal lymphadenectomy
12. Cervical incision and upper esophagus mobilization
13. Transhiatal mobilization of entire esophagus
14. Division of cervical esophagus
15. Packing of the mediastinum and chest tube placement (if needed)
16. Preparation of gastric conduit
17. Gastric conduit pull through and positioning
18. Reapproximation of the diaphragmatic crus
19. Maturation of feeding jejunostomy
20. Abdominal closure
21. Cervical anastomosis
22. Placement of cervical drain and wound closure

Potential Complications and Pitfalls

1. Unrecognized progression of disease
2. Unrecognized replaced left hepatic artery
3. Splenic injury
4. Inadequate/unhealthy conduit (ischemic, traumatized, or narrowed), need for alternate conduit (colon, jejunum)
5. Control of left gastric artery
6. Inadequate duodenal mobilization
7. Inadvertent pyloric mucosal injury
8. Mediastinal bleeding (azygous vein injury)
9. Injury to the membranous trachea
10. Recurrent laryngeal nerve injury
11. Torsion of conduit

12. Tension free cervical anastomosis

Template Dictation

Preoperative diagnosis: [INDICATION – high grade dysplasia, esophageal squamous or adenocarcinoma] [with or without neoadjuvant chemoradiation therapy]

Postoperative diagnosis: same

Procedure(s) Performed:

1. Flexible esophagoscopy
2. Transhiatal esophagectomy
3. Cervical esophagogastric anastomosis
4. Pyloromyotomy
5. Jejunostomy tube placement
6. +/- chest tube placement

Attending Surgeon: [BLANK]

Secondary Surgeon: [BLANK]

Assistants: [BLANK]

Anesthesia: [BLANK]

Estimated blood loss: [BLANK]

Specimens: Esophagus and proximal stomach, proximal esophageal margin

Drains: Nasogastric tube, cervical Penrose drain, jejunostomy tube, +/- chest tube

Indication(s) for Procedure: [AGE] year old [GENDER] with [DURATION] history of [COMPLAINT-dysphagia, reflux]. Preoperative workup reveals [TESTING performed and FINDINGS]. I have discussed with the patient the risks and benefits of a transhiatal esophagectomy including the risks of an anastomotic leak, stricture, damage to surrounding structures including the recurrent laryngeal nerve resulting in hoarseness, the airway, blood vessels, spleen resulting in a splenectomy, thoracic duct resulting in a chylothorax, cancer recurrence, heart attack, stroke, and death. She/He asked appropriate questions and would like to proceed.

Description of Procedure: The patient was taken to the operating room on [DATE]. A time-out was completed verifying correct patient, procedure, site, positioning, and implant(s) or special equipment. After induction of satisfactory general endotracheal anesthesia, the flexible esophagoscope was introduced through the cricopharyngeus sphincter without difficulty. The squamocolumnar epithelial junction was located at **X** cm and the gastroesophageal junction at **X** cm. The tumor extended from **X** cm to **X** cm. There [was **X** cm of/no] extension onto the stomach. The gastroscope was advanced into the stomach and retroflexed.

[FINDINGS ON EXAMINATION OF STOMACH]. The esophagoscope was then removed without difficulty.

The patient was positioned supine with a folded blanket under the shoulders. The head was turned to the right and supported on a head ring. The arms were padded and tucked at the sides. The skin of the neck, chest and abdomen was prepped and draped. A second time-out was completed verifying correct patient, procedure, site, positioning, planned operation and site.

The peritoneal cavity was entered through a supraumbilical midline incision. The triangular ligament of the liver was divided with cautery, and the left lobe of the liver was padded and retracted to the right. An upper hand self-retaining table mounted retractor was inserted. Exploration of the upper abdomen revealed no evidence of metastatic disease and no palpable mass in the stomach. After identifying the course of the right gastroepiploic artery, and beginning at the midpoint of the greater curvature of the stomach, the greater omentum was separated from the stomach to the level of the pylorus between right-angled clamps applied at least 1-2 cm below this vessel using #2-0 silk ties. The left gastroepiploic artery and short gastric vessels were divided between right-angled clamps using #2-0 silk ties. Care was taken to avoid injury to the spleen. The peritoneum overlying the esophageal hiatus was incised. The gastrohepatic omentum was incised, preserving the right gastric artery. The left gastric vein was divided between right angle clamps and ligated with a #2-0 silk. The left gastric artery was dissected, doubly ligated with #2-0 silk and divided.

A generous Kocher maneuver was performed. A 2 cm long pyloromyotomy was carried out, beginning 1.5 cm on the stomach and extending onto the duodenum for 0.5-1 cm. This was performed using the cutting current of a needle tipped electrocautery and a fine tipped mosquito clamp. The duodenal mucosa **[WAS/WAS NOT]** entered during this dissection. [Due to a mucosal injury, a pyloroplasty was performed opening the pylorus longitudinally. The pyloroplasty was closed transversely in 2 layers reapproximating the mucosa with a running #4-0 PDS suture and a second layer of interrupted Lembert #4-0 PDS sutures. The pylorus was marked with silver clips for future radiographic identification.

A #14 French rubber jejunostomy tube was inserted 4-6 inches beyond the ligament of Treitz and was secured in place with two #4-0 Prolene purse-string sutures and then a 4 cm long Witzel maneuver. Attention was then turned to the mobilization of the esophagus. With downward traction on the Penrose drain encircling the esophagogastric junction, the diaphragmatic hiatus was progressively dilated until the hand could be inserted into the posterior mediastinum through the diaphragmatic hiatus. The following findings relative to the esophagus were encountered: [**FINDINGS**: e.g., There were moderate mediastinal adhesions. There was a palpable distal esophageal mass.]. Dissection of the distal 5-10 cm of the esophagus was performed using electrocautery and a long right-angled clamp and then more superiorly keeping the fingers closely applied to the esophagus. Narrow retractors placed into the hiatus allowed visualization, division, and ligation of the lateral attachments of the distal half of the esophagus. Accessible paraesophageal, left gastric, and celiac axis lymph nodes were mobilized for resection with the esophagus and proximal stomach. During the mediastinal dissection, arterial blood pressure was monitored with a radial arterial line to avoid prolonged hypotension due to displacement of the heart. The dissection was carried to the level of the carina. Attention was then turned to the neck.

Through an oblique left cervical incision paralleling the anterior border of the sternocleidomastoid muscle, the platysma muscle was divided. The carotid sheath and its contents were retracted laterally, the trachea and thyroid gland medially, and the prevertebral fascia identified. Care was taken throughout the cervical dissection to avoid direct pressure on the recurrent laryngeal nerve in the tracheoesophageal groove. The cervical esophagus was encircled with a one inch Penrose drain, and with gentle upward traction, blunt mobilization of the upper thoracic esophagus from the superior mediastinum was performed. Working upward from the diaphragmatic hiatus and downward through the cervical incision, mobilization of the esophagus was completed using a combination of finger dissection and dissection with a sponge stick. Blood was evacuated from the mediastinum with a #28 French Argyle Saratoga sump catheter. Once the entire intrathoracic esophagus was free from the mediastinum, the nasogastric tube was withdrawn into the cervical esophagus. The upper esophagus was delivered into the neck wound and divided with a 3.8 mm GIA surgical stapler. The stomach and esophagus were delivered out of the abdominal wound. Narrow retractors were inserted into the diaphragmatic hiatus, and the mediastinum inspected for bleeding. No significant mediastinal bleeding was encountered. Both sides of the mediastinal pleura were inspected for injury. Entry into both pleura [**WAS/WAS NOT**] identified [28F straight chest tubes were placed bilaterally, secured to the skin with #2-0 vicryl, and attached to Pleurovacs].

The esophagus and proximal stomach were then separated from the remaining stomach by applying the 3.8 mm GIA surgical stapler several times along the lesser curvature of the stomach 4-5 cm distal to the esophagogastric junction. The thoracic esophagus and proximal stomach were then removed from the field. The gastric staple suture line was oversewn with a running #4-0 Prolene Lambert suture. The stomach was then gently manipulated through the hiatus and advanced manually upward through the posterior mediastinum until the gastric fundus could be visualized at the base of the neck wound and drawn into the field. The position of the stomach in the neck wound was maintained by packing a small moistened gauze into the thoracic inlet alongside the stomach to prevent it from retracting down into the mediastinum. Care was taken to be certain that the stomach was not twisted within the mediastinum. The abdomen was then inspected for hemostasis. The diaphragmatic hiatus was narrowed to three fingerbreadths with [**X**] interrupted #1 silk sutures and was then loosely tacked to the adjacent stomach with one interrupted #3-0 silk suture. The left lobe of the liver was returned to its normal location and reapproximated to the diaphragm with a #3-0 silk suture.

The jejunostomy tube was brought out through a separate left upper quadrant incision and sutured to the adjacent peritoneum with interrupted #3-0 silk sutures. The tube was secured to the skin with a #2-0 Prolene suture. The abdomen was closed using a running #1 looped PDS suture on the muscle fascia, running #2-0 vicryl on the subcutaneous tissue and a #4-0 monocryl subcuticular suture on the skin.

After closure of the abdomen, the cervical esophagogastric anastomosis was performed. A 1.5 cm anterior gastrotomy was made and the stapled end of the cervical esophagus amputated. A side to side anastomosis between the cervical esophagus and gastric fundus was performed using the 3.8 mm Endo-30 GIA stapler. Two lateral suspension sutures of #4-0 Vicryl were placed between the cervical esophagus and the stomach on either side of the anastomosis. A 16 Fr nasogastric tube guided across the anastomosis and into the intrathoracic stomach. The anterior esophagotomy and gastrotomy were closed in 2 layers with running and then interrupted #4-0 PDS sutures. A silver hemoclip was placed on either side of the anastomosis for future radiographic identification. The neck was irrigated with warm water, and a 1/4 inch Penrose drain was placed next to the anastomosis. Muscle fascia was loosely reapproximated with interrupted #3-0 Vicryl, and the skin edges were reapproximated with a #4-0 monocryl subcuticular suture. Dry sterile dressings were applied to all incisions.

The sponge and needle counts were correct.

A postoperative chest radiograph obtained in the operating room demonstrated [**CORRECT/INCORRECT**] placement of chest tubes with no pneumothorax or effusion.

The patient tolerated the procedure well and left the operating room extubated and in satisfactory condition.

Dr. [**BLANK**] was present and scrubbed for [**BLANK**] elements of this procedure.

24. Open Modified Mckeown Esophagectomy

Zarrish S. Khan, MD and Subroto Paul, MD

New York Presbyterian –Weill Cornell Medical Center

Essential Operative Steps

1. Preoperative workup-staging, neoadjuvant treatment, cardiopulmonary workup.
2. General anesthesia, endotracheal tube, lines and monitoring
3. Flexible Bronchoscopy
4. Esophagogastroduodenoscopy
5. Double lumen endotracheal tube
6. Left lateral decubitus position, right posterolateral thoracotomy.
7. Divide inferior pulmonary ligament, open mediastinal pleura, divide Azygous vein.
8. Dissect esophagus (from the hiatus to the thoracic inlet) en bloc with lymph nodes. Penrose drains looped around the esophagus and knotted. One is tucked in thoracic inlet, and one is tucked in hiatus.
9. Ligate thoracic duct
10. Confirm hemostasis and place chest tube
11. Close thoracotomy in layers
12. Turn patient supine.
13. Midline laparotomy. Look for ascites. Examine and palpate abdominal cavity and liver for metastases.
14. Mobilize left lobe of liver. Place retractors
15. Divide lesser omentum in avascular plane.
16. The transverse colon mobilized from the greater omentum
17. Greater omentum resected, leaving the gastroepiploic arcade.
18. The greater curvature of the stomach grasped protecting the right gastroepiploic arcade. Lesser sac entered. Beginning inferiorly travelling along the greater curvature, tissues and short gastric vessels were divided outside of the right gastroepiploic arcade to completely free greater curvature.
19. Dissect gastroesophageal junction. Previously placed Penrose drain is grasped and used for retraction.
20. Divide left gastric vessels
21. Take down remaining retrogastric attachments
22. Widely Kocherize the duodenum.
23. Pyloromyotomy/pyloroplasty
24. Jejunostomy tube inserted 40 cm distal to ligament of Treitz; Witzle, secured to abdominal fascia, and brought out abdominal wall.
25. Incision along medial aspect of left sternocleidomastoid muscle. Divide omohyoid.

26. Bluntly retract sternocleidomastoid and carotid sheath laterally. Bluntly dissect down to prevertebral fascia, identify and grasp the previously placed Penrose drain at the thoracic inlet.
27. Esophagus is divided at the level of the clavicle and then withdrawn from the abdomen through the esophageal hiatus
28. Construct a 4cm wide gastric conduit based on the line of the short gastric vessels, beginning at level of Crow's foot and extending to Angle of His. Oversew the staple line.
29. Deliver the gastric conduit preserving appropriate orientation (staple line facing patient's right side) through the mediastinum into the cervical incision.
30. End-to-end two layer handsewn anastomosis using interrupted 3-0 Vicryl for the inner layer and 3-0 PDS for the outer layer
31. Nasogastric tube passed distally through the conduit.
32. #10 flat Jackson-Pratt placed into the neck incision,
33. Neck incision closed in layers.
34. Redundancy in the conduit is reduced and conduit is tacked to hiatus to prevent herniation
35. Abdominal fascia and incision closed in layers
36. Exchange double lumen for single lumen endotracheal tube
37. Toilet bronchoscopy and assess airways for thermal injury.

Potential Complications and Pitfalls

Procedure Specific Complications:

1. Anastomotic complications (i.e., leak/dehiscence and strictures)
2. Gastric conduit necrosis
3. Recurrent nerve injury, resulting in aspiration and impaired ability to swallow.
4. Chylothorax from thoracic duct injury
5. Gastric outlet obstruction
6. Tracheobronchial tree injury with or without tracheoesophageal fistula
7. Diaphragmatic herniation of abdominal contents

General Complications of Abdominal and Chest Surgery:

1. Bleeding requiring transfusion and reoperation.
2. Cardiovascular complications including arrhythmias and myocardial infarction
3. Thromboembolic complications including deep venous thrombosis with pulmonary embolism.
4. Respiratory complications including pneumonia, pneumothorax, empyema, and atelectasis.
5. Infectious complications including urinary tract infection and line infections.
6. Wound complications including infection and dehiscence.

7. Gastrointestinal complications including ileus, colitis, perforation, volvulus, and obstruction.

Template Dictation

Preoperative Diagnosis: [Indication stage, location and type of esophageal cancer]

Postoperative Diagnosis: Same.

Procedure(s) Performed:

1. Flexible Bronchoscopy
2. Esophagogastroduodenoscopy and
3. Modified McKeown Esophagectomy and creation of gastric conduit

Attending Surgeon: [BLANK]

Secondary Surgeon: [BLANK]

Assistants: [BLANK]

Anesthesia: [BLANK]

Estimated Blood Loss:

Complications:

Drains: 28 Fr right chest tube, #10 Jackston-Pratt drain, 14 Fr red rubber feeding jejeunostomy tube

Fluids: [CRYSTALLOID, COLLOID, BLOOD PRODUCTS]

Indication(s) for Procedure: The patient is a [AGE] year old [GENDER] with history of [PAST MEDICAL HISTORY] who was found to have esophageal mass during endoscopy as part of workup for [BLANK]. The biopsy of the mass was positive for [ADENOCARCINOMA/SQUAMOUS CELL CARCINOMA], which was subsequently staged as a [TxNxMx] tumor by EUS and PET/CT. The patient had a favorable response to neoadjuvant chemoradiaiton therapy was deemed an appropriate candidate for esophagectomy.

In preparation for surgery, the patient underwent a cardiopulmonary evaluation which included a negative stress test and normal PFTs. He is able to walk 5 city blocks without any symptoms (Exercise capacity). He was advised to undergo the aforementioned procedure. The risks, benefits and alternatives were explained to the patient and family including the risk of pain, infection, bleeding, need for further surgery, pneumothorax, prolonged air leak, damage to surrounding structures, recurrent laryngeal nerve injury, chylous effusion, anastomotic leak, bowel obstruction, empyema, arrhythmia, myocardial infarction, stroke and venous thrombosis with pulmonary embolism, and the potential need for anastomotic dilatation. [HE/SHE] and [HIS/HER] family expressed understanding and agreed to proceed.

Description of Procedure:

BRONCHOSCOPY AND ESOPHAGOGASTRODUODENOSCOPY

After general anesthesia via endotracheal tube was induced, flexible bronchoscopy was carried out through the endotracheal tube. The trachea was normal. The carina was sharp. Examination of the right and left mainstem bronchi and all lobar and segmental bronchi bilaterally down to the level of the subsegments failed to reveal any endobronchial abnormalities such as blood, tumor or frankly purulent secretions. A moderate-to-large amount of mucopurulent secretions was suctioned from the airways bilaterally. The normal anatomy was otherwise present. The flexible bronchoscope was withdrawn.

Next, the adult flexible gastroscope was advanced through the oropharynx, beyond the cricopharyngeus, and into the esophagus. The proximal and mid-thoracic esophagus were normal. Beginning at 38 cm and extending to the gastroesophageal junction (at 40cm), there was a partially obstructing mass. The gastroscope could be advanced through the gastroesophageal junction without difficulty. The endoscope was advanced through the pylorus without difficulty. The first and second portions of the duodenum were normal. The endoscope was then pulled back, and the stomach and esophagus were examined. The gastric antrum and fundus were normal. The incisura was sharp; the stomach distended normally. The gastroscope was retroflexed. There was no hiatal hernia. There was no evidence of tumor invasion onto the cardia. The stomach appeared endoscopically suitable for use as a conduit. The stomach was completely decompressed of air. The gastroscope was pulled back into the esophagus. Proximal to the tumor, the esophagus appeared normal. The gastroscope was then withdrawn. A nasogastric tube was passed by anesthesia into the stomach without difficulty.

Next, the patient's single-lumen endotracheal tube was exchanged for a double lumen endotracheal tube by anesthesia, and appropriate positioning was confirmed by bronchoscopy.

THORACIC DISSECTION

The patient was placed in the left lateral decubitus position, and the right chest was prepped and draped in the usual sterile fashion. The right lung was isolated. We performed a limited serratus-sparing posterolateral thoracotomy and entered the right hemithorax via the fifth intercostal space without incident. The sixth rib was shingled. Palpation of the lung revealed no abnormalities. The inferior pulmonary ligament was divided to the level of the inferior pulmonary vein using electrocautery. A station 9 lymph node was sampled and sent to pathology as a permanent specimen. The lung was retracted anteriorly. The mediastinal pleura anterior to the esophagus was divided between the inferior pulmonary vein and azygous vein. An avascular window was created around the azygous vein, and the vein divided with a endo-GIA vascular load stapler. The pleura was divided posterior to the esophagus between the inferior pulmonary vein and the azygous vein. Just inferior to the level of azygos vein, the esophagus was circumferentially dissected free from the surrounding soft tissues. A Penrose drain was passed around the esophagus and tied to facilitate retraction and further dissection.

We then turned our attention back to the lower thoracic esophagus and completed the anterior portion of the dissection. The periesopheal lymphatics were dissected off the pericardium. The dissection was continued cephalad, dissecting the periesophageal lymphatics off the bronchus intermedius. The subcarinal lymph node packet was removed en bloc with the esophagus. The periesophageal tissues were then dissected off the right mainstem to the level of the azygous vein. We then turned our attention to the posterior dissection plane and took down the periesophageal lymphatics from the level of the esophageal hiatus to the azygous vein. Branch lymphatic vessels and aortoesophageal vessels were divided between clips. The esophagus was completely mobilized circumferentially.

The dissection was continued inferiorly to and below the level of the hemidiaphragm. At the hiatus, the muscle fibers of the crura were identified. Dissection was continued until nearly circumferential intraperitoneal access was achieved. The thoracic duct was ligated with a figure-of-eight #0 Ethibond suture. The previously placed Penrose drain was tucked through the hiatus and into the peritoneal cavity.

A second Penrose drain was passed around the esophagus and tied. We then completed the mobilization of the proximal esophagus. Staying directly on the wall of esophagus, the esophagus was circumferentially mobilized from the surrounding soft tissues to the level of the thoracic inlet. During the dissection, the vagus nerves were divided directly on the esophagus to minimize the risk of recurrent laryngeal nerve injury. The Penrose drain was tucked into the thoracic inlet to facilitate identification of the proper dissection plane from the cervical dissection.

The right hemithorax was copiously irrigated with sterile water followed by sterile saline. After a final check for hemostasis was made, a #28 French chest tube (with extra drainage holes cut into it) was inserted through a small incision in the anterior axillary line at approximately the 7th intercostal space. The chest tube was positioned posteriorly to the apex and secured in place using a #0 silk suture. The right hemithorax was then copiously irrigated with antibiotic irrigation. Number 2 Vicryl pericostal sutures were inserted to reapproximate the ribs. After a final check for hemostasis, the right lung was re-expanded under direct vision. Once complete reinflation was confirmed, the pericostal sutures were secured. The remainder of the incision was closed anatomically in layers. Steri-Strips and sterile dressings were applied.

ABDOMINAL DISSECTION

The patient was then placed in the supine position. The neck was slightly extended, and the head turned towards the right. The neck, chest and entire abdomen were prepped and draped in the usual sterile fashion. A midline incision from the xiphoid to the supraumbilical area was used to gain access atraumatically to the peritoneal cavity. The xiphoid process was resected at the commencement of the laparotomy incision using Mayo scissors.

The abdomen was explored. There was no ascities. There were no liver, peritoneal or omental lesions. There was no celiac adenopathy. The stomach was inspected. There was no evidence of T4 disease.

The Penrose drain was readily identified. The triangular ligament was divided using electrocautery. This allowed insertion of an upper hand retractor. The left lobe of the liver was gently folded on itself, covered with a moist laparotomy pad, and a liver retractor was placed. The lesser omentum was divided in an avascular plane above the caudate lobe of the liver using electrocautery. The peritoneum overlying the gastroesophageal junction was divided and the previously placed Penrose drain was grasped and used for retraction purposes.

The transverse colon was mobilized from the greater omentum using a combination of electrocautery and the ligasure device in an avascular plane. The portion of the greater omentum to the left of midline and extending to the splenic flexure was resected, taking care to leave the gastroepiploic arcade, which was readily palpable, undisturbed. This omentectomy specimen was sent to pathology.

The greater curvature of the stomach was cautiously grasped with a gauze sponge, being certain that the right gastroepiploic arcade was protected at all times. The lesser sac was taken entered, and the short gastrics were taken down all the way to the Angle of His using a Ligasure. The remaining retrogastric and retroesophageal attachments were taken down. The left gastric vessels were left intact. We then completed the caudal dissection along the greater curvature of the stomach. The antropyloric attachments were taken down. The pylorus was identified. The duodenum was widely Kocherized.

Next, a pyloromyotomy **[OR PYLOROPLASTY]** was performed. Electrocautery was used to begin to divide the muscle fibers of the pylorus longitudinally. As the fibers were divided, blunt dissection using a Schnidt clamp was performed to further disrupt the circular fibers of the pylorus. The pyloromyotomy was extended a few centimeters onto the distal antrum. The duodenum was not injured. At the end of the pyloromyotomy, the pylorus was inspected and noted to be widely patent.

Next, the transverse colon was elevated, and the ligament of Treitz was identified. Approximately 40 cm distal to the ligament of Treitz, a freely mobile loop of jejunum was chosen for jejunostomy tube insertion. Concentric pursestring sutures of 3-0 Vicryl were passed through the antimesenteric aspect of the jejunum, and an enterotomy was created in the center of the pursestrings using electrocautery. A #14 French whistle-tip jejunostomy tube was inserted through the jejunotomy and advanced distally into the jejunum. The pursestring sutures were secured. The jejunostomy tube was Witzled at the jejeunostomy entrance site using interrupted 3-0 Vicryl sutures. The jejunostomy tube was brought out through a stab incision in the left abdomen lateral to the umbilicus. The jejunum at the jejunostomy tube site was approximated to the anterior abdominal wall in four quadrants using interrupted 3-0 Vicryl sutures. The jejunostomy tube was sutured at its skin exit site using an #0 Ethibond suture. Antiobstruction stitches were placed 5 cm proximal and 5 cm distal to the jejeunostomy using 3-0 Vicryl sutures. After assuring that it flushed easily, the jejeunostomy was capped.

NECK DISSECTION AND ANASTOMOSIS

An oblique incision was made in the neck paralleling the anterior aspect of the left sternocleidomastoid muscle. The incision was carried down through the subcutaneous tissues. The platysma was divided. The omohyoid was isolated, tied in continuity with #0 Vicryl ties and then divided using electrocautery. The sternocleidomastoid and carotid sheath were retracted laterally, and the thyroid was retracted medially. The middle thyroid vein was divided. The dissection was continued down to the prevertebral fascia. The previously placed Penrose drain at the thoracic inlet was grasped and brought up into the wound. Staying directly on the esophagus, the esophagus was mobilized off the trachea to the level of the cricopharyngeus using bipolar cautery.

An ampule of glucagon was then administered by Anesthesia. Palpation through the esophageal hiatus confirmed dilation to four fingers width. After adequate circulation time of glucagon, the nasogastric tube was withdrawn by anesthesia to just proximal to the neck incision. The esophagus was divided at the level of the clavicle using an endo GIA purple load stapler. A #2 silk suture was passed through the staple line of the distal end of the divided esophagus. The esophagus was then withdrawn from the abdomen, thereby pulling the silk suture through the mediastinum. An Allis clamp was placed on the proximal esophagus to maintain appropriate orientation. The suture in the abdomen was disconnected from the specimen. The left gastric vessels were divided at their takeoff with an endo GIA vascular load stapler. Beginning on the cardia and continuing caudally parallel to the line of the short gastrics, a 3 cm wide gastric conduit was constructed using multiple firings of an endo GIA purple load stapler. At approximately the level of the 3rd arcarde along the lesser curvature, the staple firings were angled towards the lesser curvature. The lesser curvature vessels were divided using an endo GIA vascular load stapler. The esophagogastrectomy specimen was inspected. The margins were grossly negative. The specimen was sent to pathology, and frozen sections confirmed microscopically negative margins for metaplasia, dysplasia, and carcinoma. The entire staple line of the newly created gastric conduit was oversewn using running 3-0 Vicryl sutures. The end of a silk suture passed through the mediastinum into the abdomen was connected to a Foley catheter with 30 mL balloon inflated to approximately 20 mL. An arthroscopy bag was placed around the Foley and tied proximally to the balloon. The bag was cut to an appropriate length. At this point, the gastric conduit was inserted into the arthroscopy bag. Proper orientation was maintained on the gastric conduit. The Foley catheter was placed to suction and the arthroscopy bag sealed down around the gastric conduit. While maintaining continuous suction, the bag was carefully advanced through the mediastinum, thereby atraumatically delivering the gastric conduit in appropriate orientation through the mediastinum and out through the cervical incision. The arthroscopy bag was removed. The conduit appeared pink and healthy.

The staple lines from the remnant esophagus and gastric conduit were resected. An end-to-end two layer handsewn anastomosis was then completed using interrupted 3-0 PDS sutures for the inner (mucosal) layer and 3-0 interrupted Vicryl sutures for the outer (muscular) layer. An 18 French nasogastric tube was advanced through the esophageal conduit prior to completion of the cervical anastomosis and positioned with its tip just proximal to the pyloromyotomy. The cervical anastomosis was completed and allowed to fall into the mediastinum. A #10 flat Jackson-Pratt drain was inserted through a separate stab incision in the neck, positioned posterior to the anastomosis, and secured to the skin using a 3-0 nylon suture. The neck incision was then copiously irrigated. The omohyoid was reapproximated using a figure of 8-0 Vicryl sutures and then the remainder of the incision was closed anatomically in layers. Steri-Strips and sterile dressings were applied.

The redundant portion of the conduit was pulled back into the abdomen. The conduit was tacked to the hiatus using 3-0 silk suture. The abdomen was copiously irrigated with antibiotic-containing saline. After a final check for hemostasis was made, the abdominal incision was closed. The fascia was closed using a running #2 Prolene suture. The subcutaneous tissues were copiously irrigated. The subdermal tissues were closed using a running 2-0 Vicryl suture. The skin was closed using a 4-0 Vicryl subcuticular suture. Steri-Strips and sterile dressings were applied. The double-lumen endotracheal tube was exchanged for a single-lumen endotracheal tube by anesthesia, and completion bronchoscopy was carried out through the endotracheal tube. A moderate to large amount of mucopurulent secretions was again suctioned from the airways bilaterally. There was no evidence of airway injury. The flexible bronchoscope was withdrawn.

Sponge and needle counts were reported as correct. The patient was transported to Thoracic Surgical Intensive Care Unit, intubated and in stable condition

Dr. **[BLANK]** was present and scrubbed for **[BLANK]** elements of this procedure.

25. Open Ivor-Lewis Esophagectomy

Jordy C. Cox, MD, David M. Jablons, MD

University of California San Francisco

Essential Operative Steps

1. Lines, monitoring (+/- epidural analgesia).
2. General endotracheal anesthesia - double lumen endotracheal tube.
3. Prophylactic antibiotics, urinary catheter and SCDs.
4. Upper endoscopy & bronchoscopy. Place nasogastric tube.

Abdominal Phase

5. Upper midline laparotomy
6. Explore abdomen: look for ascites; look for liver, peritoneal or omental implants; feel the primary tumor and feel for surrounding adenopathy.
7. Gastric mobilization
   a. Divide Falciform and left triangular ligaments & retract left lateral segment
   b. Expose right crus- incise pars flaccida overlying caudate lobe
   c. Dissect periesophageal tissue circumferentially.
   d. Encircle with Penrose drain for traction.
   e. Widen esophageal hiatus:
   f. (If required) Ligate and divide the phrenic vein and divide crural fibers vertically towards the central tendon.
   g. Mobilize the distal esophagus in the mediastinum.
   h. Enter the lesser sac and mobilize greater curvature of the stomach. Divide the omentum towards the fundus 1-2 cm lateral to the right gastroepiploic arcade. Stay wide and preserve vascularized omentum to serve as a buttress for the anastomosis.
   i. Divide vasa brevia 1 cm off the stomach.
   j. Divide posterior gastric attachments.
   k. Open gastrohepatic ligament. Retract stomach cephalad and isolate and divide the left gastric vessels. Include all left gastric lymph nodes within the specimen..
8. Kocher maneuver.
9. Pyloroplasty or pyloromyotomy
10. Feeding Weitzel jejunostomy: 16 French catheter placed 40cm distal to the ligament of Treitz
11. Close laparotomy.

Chest Phase

12. Reposition, prep and drape for right thoracotomy. Re-confirm ETT position.
13. Posterolateral thoracotomy: 5th intercostal space.

14. Open mediastinal pleura over the entire length of the thoracic esophagus: from hiatus to 5-10 cm above the azygos vein.
15. Mobilize esophagus circumferentially & encircle with Penrose drain. Control all vessels and lymphatics with clips or energy devices (i.e. Ligasure)
16. Divide azygos vein and preserve supreme intercostal vein.
17. Manually deliver stomach into the chest.
18. Place esophageal traction sutures at proximal margin of resection.
19. Withdraw nasogastric tube. Complete transection of the esophagus and tubularize the gastric conduit (4cm diameter).
20. Systematically sample mediastinal lymph node stations 2R, 4R, 7, 8, 9.
21. Construct a stapled (or alternatively, a hand-sewn) anastomosis at approximately the level of the azygous vein
    a. 25-28 mm EEA stapler
    b. Place the anvil directly into esophagus and secure it with a purse-string suture
    c. Insert the EEA stapler through a gastrotomy. Advance the pin through the posterior wall of the greater curve and engage the anvil.
    d. Complete the anastomosis, remove the EEA and check the anastomotic rings.
    e. Reinforce the anastomosis with additional Lembert sutures.
    f. Send the anastomotic doughnuts for frozen section analysis.
    g. Close the gastrotomy and oversew staple lines with running Prolene.
    h. Advance NG tube through the anastomosis and secure it just below the diaphragm.
    i. Check final margins for metaplasia, dysplasia or carcinoma
22. Cover the anastomosis with omentum, or a pedicled-flap of parietal pleura.
23. Place a chest tube. Add additional holes with a double-action Rongeur to increase drainage capacity.
24. Irrigate and check for hemostasis
25. Multilevel intercostal block
26. Close thoracotomy in layers

Potential Complications and Pitfalls

1. Preoperative considerations:
    a. Pretreatment staging includes a barium contrast study, CT scan, PET scan and upper endoscopy with endoscopic ultrasound.
    b. Consider doing a diagnostic laparoscopy initially to rule out disseminated abdominal disease and evaluate for resectability.
    c. Timing between induction chemo-radiation and surgery should be 4-6 weeks. In general, allow enough time for recovery of the patient's performance status and nutritional markers.

d. Placement of a feeding jejunostomy tube prior to neoadjuvant therapy should be considered in some cases, especially if there is severe dysphagia and/or a history of weight loss.
   e. Repeat PET scan preoperatively to asses for response to induction therapy and evaluate for distant metastatic disease.
   f. Preoperative workup should include pulmonary function testing, echocardiogram and nutritional parameters.
2. Bronchoscopy in the operating room to asses for double lumen ETT positioning and rule out malignant invasion of the airway
3. Upper endoscopy in the operating room to asses for tumor burden, location, extension, associated stricture or Barrett's metaplasia.
4. Technical considerations:
   a. Avoid entering the pericardial space when widening the hiatus.
   b. Wide Kocher maneuver. To assure adequate mobilization, the pylorus should easily reach the level of the caudate lobe to assure that a tension-free intrathoracic anastomosis can be constructed.
   c. Narrow gastric conduits are better for emptying. Wide are better for perfusion. It should be approximately 4cm in diameter.
   d. Take care to avoid thoracic duct injuries when mobilizing the esophagus.
   e. Avoid thermal injuries to the airways when mobilizing the esophagus.
   f. Carefully preserve the orientation of the gastric conduit when hand-delivering it into the chest. The lesser curve staple line should face upwards (towards the thoracotomy)
   g. Dividing the esophagus with a TA stapler allows for a 90-degree angle of transection even high in the chest
   h. Cover anastomosis with omentum, pleura or a portion of redundant stomach.
   i. If gentle ventilation or CPAP of the right lung is required for oxygenation, pack the lung out of the operative field with moist towels.

Template Dictation

Preoperative Diagnosis: [indications] – e.g.GE Junction Adenocarcinoma, High-grade Barrett's dysplasia, distal esophageal stricture.

Postoperative Diagnosis: Same

Procedure(s) Performed: Flexible bronchoscopy, flexible upper endoscopy, Ivor-Lewis esophagogastrectomy, and feeding jejeunostomy tube placement

Attending Surgeon: [BLANK]

Secondary Surgeon: [BLANK]

Assistants: [BLANK]

Anesthesia: General with a double lumen ETT tube.

Fluids:

Estimated Blood Loss:

Drains:

Disposition: To ICU

Complications:

Indication(s) for Procedure: [age] year old [gender] with [duration] history of [chief complaint] (e.g. progressive dysphagia). Upper endoscopy demonstrated a mass at the GE junction. Biopsies confirmed adenocarcinoma. EUS was used for staging. The patient underwent induction chemo-radiation with excellent clinical response. Repeat PET scan confirmed the absence of distant metastatic disease. He presents for possible esophago-gastrectomy.

Description of Procedure: The patient was taken to the operating room on [DATE]. A time out was done, and the patient's identity and planned procedure were verified by the surgical and anesthesia teams.

An epidural catheter was placed prior to induction.

General anesthesia was induced, and the patient was intubated with a double lumen endotracheal tube without difficulty. The position of this tube was confirmed by flexible bronchoscopy.

The patient was placed in a supine position with adequate padding of all bony prominences and received prophylactic antibiotics per protocol. A Foley catheter and a nasogastric tube were placed.

We performed an upper endoscopy that demonstrated [FINDINGS].

The abdomen was prepped and draped in usual sterile fashion. An upper midline incision was performed and carried down through the fascia. The abdomen was entered. A self-retaining retractor was used to achieve adequate exposure.

The abdomen was thoroughly explored and no evidence of macroscopic metastatic disease was found.

The falciform and left triangular ligaments were divided and the left lateral segment of the liver was retracted towards the right upper quadrant

We began mobilization of the stomach and the distal esophagus at the hiatus. The right and left crus were exposed. The distal esophagus was mobilized circumferentially and encircled with a Penrose drain. The hiatus was enlarged and blunt dissection was used to free the distal esophagus.

We then entered the lesser sac and divided the greater omentum, paying close attention to preserving the right gastroepiploic arcade. The short gastric vessels were doubly ligated and divided. All adhesions to the posterior gastric wall were divided sharply.

We directed our attention to the gastro-hepatic ligament, and divided it sharply. The left gastric vessels were identified, triply ligated and divided. There was no evidence of an accessory left hepatic artery. Any noticeable lympahdenopathy was included in the specimen or dissected individually.

A wide Kocher maneuver was done to provide adequate mobilization of the gastric conduit. The stomach and distal esophagus were now free.

Next, we performed a pyloroplasty. The pylorus was identified and elevated. Two traction sutures were placed laterally and a full-thickness longitudinal duodenotomy was done. This was closed transversely in two layers of #3-0 [TYPE] suture. The repair was palpated and felt to be widely patent. A small tongue of omentum was draped over the closure to provide additional buttressing.

We directed our attention to the small bowel. We measured 40cm distal to the ligament of Treitz and identified a portion of jejunum that would accommodate a feeding tube and easily reach the abdominal wall. Two concentric purse-string sutures were placed on the anti-mesenteric border of the bowel and a small enterotomy was made in the center of the pursestring sutures. A 16 French feeding tube was advanced through the enterotomy. A Weitzel tunnel was fashioned with interrupted #3-0 [TYPE] suture. The catheter was brought out through a separate stab incision in the left upper quadrant. The small bowel was tacked to the underside of the abdominal wall and the catheter was secured to the skin with additional sutures.

The abdomen was re-examined. Hemostasis was felt to be adequate and the conduit was clearly viable. The bowel was returned to the abdomen in an anatomical position and the fascia was closed with running [SIZE AND TYPE] suture. The skin was closed after irrigation of the subcutaneous tissues. Sterile dressings were applied.

We now proceeded with the thoracic portion of the procedure. The patient was placed in lateral decubitus and the position of the endotracheal tube was re-confirmed with the bronchoscope. Single lung ventilation was initiated. The chest was prepped and draped.

We made a limited muscle-sparing postero-lateral thoracotomy. The latissimus dorsi was divided sharply for the length of the incision, and the serratus was retracted anteriorly. The chest was entered in the 5th intercostal space. There was minimal rib spreading and no shingling was required.

The right lung was retracted anteriorly. The mediastinal pleura was incised, and the esophagus was dissected free of surrounding structures from the hiatus to just above the azygos vein. The azygous vein was also dissected free and divided with and endo-GIA vascular load stapler.

The stomach was delivered into the chest, paying close attention to maintaining an adequate orientation and avoiding torsion. Two traction sutures were placed laterally on the esophagus, the nasogastric tube was removed and the esophagus was divided proximally with a single firing of a TA stapler.

The gastric conduit was then fashioned with multiple firings of an endo-GIA thick-tissue stapler beginning at a point low on the lesser curve and directed towards the fundus in order to construct a 4 cm tubularized gastric conduit. The specimen was sent to Pathology. Frozen sections demonstrated that the proximal and distal margins were negative for metaplasia, dysplasia and carcinoma.

A systematic lymph node dissection was done in the posterior mediastinum and the peri-esophageal region. Hemostasis was optimized with cautery and surgical clips.

We now performed a [SIZE] mm EEA esophago-gastrostomy. Dr [NAME] scrubbed out at this point to place the Orovil. The anvil was advanced into the proximal esophageal pouch. The stapler was placed in the gastric conduit through a gastrotomy and the anastomosis was completed after adequate coupling of the device. The anastomotic doughnuts were inspected and found to be satisfactory. They were sent for frozen section analysis.

The gastrotomy was closed with additional firings on the endo-GIA stapler and the staple line was oversewn with a running [TYPE] suture.

The anastomosis was inspected and found to be tension-free, widely patent and clearly viable. Additional sutures were placed at the anastomosis to minimize traction injuries and a nasogastric tube was re-inserted under direct vision through the anastomosis and secured just below the diaphragm.

A portion of viable omentum was draped over the anastomosis and the right chest was irrigated with warm saline.

A [SIZE] French chest tube was placed through a separate stab incision and secured to the skin. The right lung was re-inflated under direct vision and a sustained Valsalva ensured adequate recruitment. Intercostal blocks were done with 0.25% bupivacaine.

Pericostal sutures were used to approximate the ribs and the thoracotomy was closed in layers with [SIZE and TYPE] suture. Sterile dressings were applied and the patient was returned to the supine position.

All sponge, needle and instrument counts were confirmed to be correct at the end of the case.

The patient was extubated in the operating room and transferred with physician escort to the cardiac surgical intensive care unit in [type] condition.

Dr. [BLANK] was present and scrubbed for [BLANK] elements of this procedure.

There were no immediate complications. The patient tolerated the procedure well.

26. Minimally Invasive Ivor-Lewis Esophagectomy

David D. Odell, MD, MMSc and James D. Luketich, MD

University of Pittsburgh Medical Center, Pittsburgh, PA

Essential Operative Steps

Laparoscopic Phase
1. Upper endoscopy to assess tumor location and extent of stomach involvement.
2. Supine position (far right on operating bed), arms out 45 degrees, and foot board placement for steep reverse Trendelenburg. Double lumen endotracheal intubation.
3. Place 10 mm port via open Hasson technique in the right paramedian line approximately one-third of the way from the xiphoid to the umbilicus.
4. CO_2 insufflation to 15 mmHg.
5. Confirm position within the peritoneal cavity and inspect abdomen with laparoscope to assess for any injury or evidence of advanced disease.
6. Place additional ports under direct laparoscopic visualization. An 11 mm left paramedian port one hand's breadth to the left initial cutdown port. A 5 mm right and left subcostal port a hand's breadth from the paramedian port sites. A 5 mm port in the lateral right upper quadrant directed along the lower edge of the liver. An 11 mm port in the right lower quadrant.
7. Insert liver retractor to elevate the left lobe of the liver for exposure of the hiatus.
8. Place patient in steep reverse Trendelenburg position to facilitate visualization of the hiatus.
9. Open the gastrohepatic ligament and dissect the right crus.
10. Complete the anterior portion of the dissection, beginning on the pericardium and then working from pleura to pleura.
11. Complete dissection of tissue from the left crus.
12. Divide the short gastric vessels preserving 5-10 mm of fatty tissue along the stomach border.
13. Posterior medistinal dissection in areolar pre-aortic soft tissue plane
14. Isolate and divide the left gastric artery and vein, sweeping all nodal tissue up towards the stomach
15. Complete retrogastric dissection to the level of the pylorus.
16. Divide the gastrocolic omentum in the filmy portion (taking care to avoid the gastroepiploic arcade)
17. Mini-Kocher maneuver to mobilize the 1st and 2nd portions of the duodenum. Mobilization is adequate when the pylorus reaches the caudate lobe.
18. Create a narrow gastric conduit (3-4 cm in width) using serial firings of the Endo-GIA stapling device. Staple line begins at the first branch of the

right gastric artery on the lesser curvature and follows the arc of the greater curvature.
19. Laparoscopically place a feeding jejunostomy (Seldinger technique using a needle jejunostomy kit)
20. Pyloroplasty – full-thickness incision across the pylorus closed transversely in a Heineke-Mickulicz fashion
21. Orient the gastric conduit and suture to the end of the specimen for delivery into the chest during the thoracoscopic phase of the operation.
22. Close the right paramedian cutdown port with a #0 Vicryl suture using a Carter Thompson Suture passing device.

Thoracoscopic Phase
1. Left lateral decubitus position with the arm out and supported at a 90 degree angle and parallel to the floor.
2. Initial 10 mm camera port placed via cutdown through the 9th intercostal space at the level of the posterior axillary line.
3. Additional ports are place under direct vision. A 10 mm surgeon's working port in the 9th intercostal space in the line of the scapular tip. A 5 mm assistant port in the midaxillary line at the 6th interspace. A 5 mm port for the surgeon's left hand at the scapular tip. A 10 mm port for lung retraction in the 4th intercostal space at the posterior axillary line.
4. Complete lung mobilization and lysis of any adhesions.
5. Division of inferior pulmonary ligament
6. Dissection along lateral pericardium.
7. Dissection along posterior border of bronchus intermedius and subcarinal lymphadenectomy.
8. Division of the Azygous vein
9. Dissection along the esophagus above the Azygous to the level of the thoracic inlet
10. Dissection of the posterior aortic plane. Multiple clips are used for hemostasis and to prevent delayed lymphatic leak.
11. Cirumferential mobilization of the esophagus.
12. Conduit is brought into the chest, maintaining proper orientation, and the specimen is divided at or above the level of the Azygous.
13. Minithoracotomy (4 cm) is made in the 6th intercostal space and protected with a wound protector. The specimen is withdrawn and sent to pathology for margins.
14. EEA (usually a #28) anvil is sewn into the cut end of the proximal esophagus with 2 pursestring sutures.
15. The gastric conduit is opened along the staple line. And the EEA stapler inserted. The spike is advanced through the greater curve side once the appropriate length of conduit is determined. The stapler is docked to the anvil and fired. Rings are evaluated for completeness.
16. The excess conduit is resected using an endo-GIA stapler.
17. An NG tube is advanced beyond the anastomosis under direct vision.

18. A 10 French flat Jackson-Pratt drain is positioned behind the anastomosis.
19. A 28 French chest tube is positioned posteriorly toward the apex.
20. A multilevel intercostal nerve block is performed.
21. The thoracotomy incision is closed in layers.
22. The mouth and nasopharynx are irrigated and suctioned free of debris and the double lumen endotracheal tube is exchanged for a single lumen endotracheal tube. A completion bronchoscopy is performed to toilet secretions and assess for airway injury.

Potential Complications and Pitfalls

1. Avoid upper overinsufflation during upper endoscopy which will increase the difficulty of laparoscopic dissection.
2. Extension of tumor onto the stomach, compromising the planned conduit – *requires alternative conduit choice (i.e. colon interposition).*
3. Injury to the gastroepiploic arcade during dissection – *requires alternative conduit choice (i.e. colon interposition).*
4. Tumor involvement of other organs – *requires intraoperative decision regarding resectability en bloc.*
5. Hypercapnea from CO2 insufflation
6. Pneumothorax
7. Failure to achieve adequate lung isolation or inability to tolerate single lung ventilation
8. Loss of proper orientation of the conduit (spiraling) as it is brought into the chest (the staple line should face the lateral chest wall – towards the camera).
9. Anastomotic leak
10. Airway injury (from excessive use of energy adjacent to the airway)
11. Aspiration events during endotracheal tube manipulation

Template Dictation

Preoperative Diagnosis: [esophageal cancer, end-stage achalasia, etc.]

Postoperative Diagnosis: Same

Procedure(s) Performed:

1. Flexible Bronchoscopy.
2. Flexible Esophagogastroscopy with Biopsies.
3. Laparoscopic Thoracoscopy Minimally Invasive Ivor-Lewis Esophagectomy.
4. Laparoscopic Creation of Gastric Tube.
5. Laparoscopic Pyloroplasty.
6. Laparoscopic Insertion Of #10 French Feeding Jejunostomy Tube.
7. Right Video-Assisted Thoracoscopic Immobilization of the Esophagus.
8. Right Vats #28 Eea Esophagogastric Anastomosis.

9. Multilevel Intercostal Nerve Block.
10. Omental Pedicle Flap Covering of the Esophagogastric Anastomosis.

Attending surgeon: [BLANK]

Resident surgeon: [BLANK]

Assistants: [BLANK]

Anesthesia: **General endotracheal through a double lumen endotracheal tube.**

Complications: None.

Estimated Blood Loss: [Blank]

Specimens:
1. Esophageal biopsies at **[Blank]**
2. Esophagogastrectomy
3. EEA rings (final esophageal margin and final gastric margin)

Tubes and Drains:
1. #12 French feeding jejunostomy tube.
2. #28 French chest tube posteriorly directed towards the apex.
3. #10 French Jackson-Pratt drain in the posterior esophageal bed draining the anastomosis.

Indication(s) for Procedure: [*DESCRIBE THE SALIENT DETAILS OF THE INDIVIDUAL PATIENT PRESENTATION AND ANY RELEVANT TREATMENT UNDERTAKEN PRIOR TO SURGERY (FOR EXAMPLE CHEMOTHERAPY AND RADIATION).*] The patient was counseled regarding the risks, benefits, and alternatives to minimally invasive esophagectomy and was agreeable to proceed. An informed consent was signed by the patient.

Description of Procedure: The patient was identified in the preoperative holding area and the operative site marked. The patient was then taken to the operating room by Anesthesia. (S)He was placed supine on the operating room table. Bilateral lower extremity sequential compression devices placed and 5000 units of subcutaneous heparin were administered prior to induction of anesthesia. A Foley catheter was inserted and adequate intravenous access assured. **[Appropriate intravenous antibiotics and dose]** were administered within an hour of the skin incision and re-dosed as needed throughout the operation. The patient was successfully intubated with a double lumen endotracheal tube.

A time-out was observed to identify patient and intended procedure. The flexible bronchoscope was then passed through the endotracheal tube. Complete examination of the airway was performed through the proximal trachea to the carina into the subsegmental airways bilaterally. Endobronchial anatomy was normal, there were no endobronchial lesions. The position of the endotracheal tube was judged to be appropriate. The bronchoscope was then withdrawn. The flexible esophagoscope was passed posterior to the posterior arytenoid and into the esophagus under direct vision. The proximal and mid esophagus were normal in appearance. At approximately [Blank] cm from the incisors tumor seen extending to [Blank]. The stomach distended normally without evidence of linitis plastica. The incisura was sharp. The gastric cardia was free of disease. The proximal portion of the duodenum was visually normal. The stomach was desufflated and the scope withdrawn.

The abdomen was then sterilely prepped and draped in the usual surgical fashion. A Hasson cut-down incision was made 1/3 of the distance between the umbilicus and the xiphoid just to the right of midline. The anterior rectus fascia was scored with Bovie and the posterior sheath grasped between tonsils and sharply incised and the peritoneal cavity entered. A Hasson trocar was then placed and the abdomen insufflated with 15 mmHg of carbon dioxide insufflation. The 10 mm 30 degree laparoscope was inserted and the abdomen visually examined. There was no evidence of injury at the abdominal entry site. Five additional laparoscope port sites were placed. A left subcostal 5 mm port, a left upper quadrant 5/11 port, right subcostal 5 mm port and a right flank 5 mm port and right lower quadrant 5/11 port. All port sites were hemostatic.

Laparoscopic exploration was then performed. There was no evidence of omental, peritoneal or hepatic metastasis noted. The left lateral segment of the liver was elevated with a flexible liver retractor to facilitate exposure of the hiatus. The gastrohepatic ligament was then incised along its filmy portion towards the right crus. The peritoneal lining along the right crus was identified and preserved and the loose areolar plane of the mediastinum entered along the right crus. A circumferential mediastinal mobilization of the intrathoracic esophagus along the lower third was performed from the pericardium anteriorly to the periaortic plane posteriorly and from the right pleura to the left pleura.

Attention was returned to the abdomen, and the phrenoesophageal membrane was divided anteriorly and dissection continued onto the left crus. The peritoneal lining along the left crus was identified and preserved. The upper portion of the gastric cardia and fundus was slowly mobilized with the attachments to the diaphragm being divided. The left gastric artery and vein pedicle were identified and all lymphatic and fatty tissues were swept along this vascular pedicle towards the specimen. Once circumferentially mobilized, the pedicle was divided at its base with a vascular load of the Endo GIA stapler. We next worked along the greater curvature of the stomach, entering the lesser sac. The upper short gastric vessels were divided, meeting the plane of dissection along the left crus. The lesser sac was entered and division of the omentum was continued along the greater curve between the transverse colon and the Right gastroepiploic arcade taking care to preserve the vessel and surrounding tissue. We next mobilized and divided the retrogastric attachments to the superior border of the pancreas down to the level of the pylorus. We then performed an antropyloric mobilization maneuver, and a limited Kocher maneuver, mobilizing the first and second portion of the duodenum.

At this point the pylorus readily reached the base of the caudate lobe. We placed 2 stay sutures in the pylorus, 1 inferiorly and 1 superiorly. We then removed all of the underlying tubes and devices from the esophagus and proceeded to fashion a neurogastric tube. We started this with vascular load along the lesser curvature vascular and fatty tissues just above the takeoff of the right gastric artery. This was done so as to preserve the first few branches of this vessel feeding the antrum of the stomach. After the initial vascular load we then used serial purple loads of the Endo GIA stapler to fashion the 3.5-4 cm neurogastric tube. We preserved the proper orientation of the tube because we made it to prevent any spiraling. We then opened the pylorus longitudinally and with the ultrasonic scalpel and proceeded to close it transversely in a Heineke-Mikulicz fashion so as to fashion our pyloroplasty. The incision was closed with #2-0 Surgidac sutures using the EndoStitch device with a total of 6 sutures being placed. We then checked for hemostasis along the lesser curvature and staple line, which was found to be free of any active bleeding.

The transverse colon was then elevated and the ligament of Treitz identified. The freely mobile loop of jejunum was identified approximately 40 cm distal to the ligament of Treitz. The appropriate site in the left lower abdominal wall was identified for placement of the feeding jejunostomy tube. The jejunum was tacked along its antimesenteric border to the anterior abdominal wall with #2-0 Surgidac EndoStitch and the finder needle inserted, followed by the feeding jejunostomy kit needle. This needle was brought in through the subserosal plane in a Witzel type fashion and then the lumen of the bowel entered. An air insufflation test was performed to confirm the intraluminal placement. Surgidac #2-0 Witzel type stitch was placed and the guidewire passed through the needle distally into the bowel under direct laparoscopic vision. A nick was made in the skin at its wire site with an 11 blade and utilizing a Seldinger technique the dilator sheath complex was centered over the wire and into the bowel lumen under direct laparoscopic vision. The feeding jejunostomy tube, a #12 French, catheter was inserted through the peel away sheath under direct vision and the tube secured with a #2-0 silk suture at the insertion site. The loop of jejunum was then circumferentially tacked to the anterior abdominal wall with a #2-0 Surgidac purse-string suture. We then placed an anti-obstruction suture approximately 3 cm distal again using #2-0 Surgidac Endo Stitch. Intraluminal placement was again confirmed with air insufflation and the tube secured to the skin with 2-0 silk sutures.

We tacked the omental flap previously fashioned at the gastric tube in 2 locations with #2-0 Surgidac Endo Stitches such that our omental pedicle would come up with the tube. We tacked the tube using a mattress type suture to the esophagogastrectomy specimen again with 2-0 Surgidac Endo Stitches. The specimen was then delivered along with the gastric tube and omental flap through the hiatus and pushed superiorly into the chest as able. Hemostasis was again insured and the liver retractor removed under direct vision. The Hasson trocar site was closed with an #0 Vicryl suture on a Carter-Thompson suture passing device. The wounds were irrigated and stapled shut with Band-Aids applied.

The patient was then re-positioned in the lateral decubitus position. The position of the double lumen endotracheal tube was re-confirmed using a pediatric bronchoscope. This was found to be adequate. All pressure points were padded and the axillary roll was placed. The lung was isolated and the right chest sterilely prepped and draped in the usual surgical fashion. An incision was made over the 9th rib in the posterior axillary line and the chest cavity entered above the diaphragm. Additional thoracoscopic ports were placed under direct vision including an infrascapular 5 mm port, 10 mm surgeon's working port over the 10th rib in a line parallel to the scapular tip, and a 5 mm port in the 6th interspace in the mid anterior axillary line along with a 10 mm port in the 4th interspace in the posterior axillary line. All port sites were hemostatic. A thoracoscopic exploration was then performed. There was no pleural pericardial or diaphragm metastasis noted. The inferior pulmonary ligament was mobilized using the ultrasonic scalpel. An #0 Surgidac suture was placed in the diaphragm for retraction purposes and brought out through the right flank and secured to the chest wall with a snap. The esophagus was mobilized with a video-assisted thoracoscopic approach. The anterior pericardial plane was followed along its avascular line. An en bloc subcarinal lymphadenectomy was then performed using a combination of ligature and ultrasonic scalpel. The anatomic strictures, including the right mainstem bronchus, main carina bronchus intermedius, left mainstem bronchus and subcarinal space were all identified and preserved in their entirety. All lymph nodes were swept towards the esophagectomy specimen. The azygos vein was identified, mobilized and divided with a surgical stapler using a single load of the vascular Endo GIA. The vagus nerve was identified and divided at the level of the azygos vein and swept aside so as to avoid traction injury on the recurrent laryngeal nerve.

Above the level of the azygos vein we carried our dissection towards the esophagus and mobilized the esophagus upwards towards the thoracic inlet. In the posterior plane the plane along the esophagus was similarly identified and maintained with all aorto-esophageal vascular and lymphatic branches controlled with clips and divided using ultrasonic scalpel. This technique of dissection was utilized to mobilize the entire length of the esophagus from the diaphragm to the thoracic inlet. We then brought the specimen, along with the attached gastric tube, into the chest taking care to preserve the orientation of the gastric tube. The gastric tube was then tacked to the diaphragm with a #2-0 Surgidac to prevent slippage into the abdomen or a loss of orientation. The posterior dissection was then completed using clips to control aortoesophageal and lymphatic branches.

We next made an access incision through a mini thoracotomy one interspace above our surgeon's working port by dividing the latissimus and intercostal muscles with electrocautery. An Alexis wound retractor was placed and brought into position. Using an endoscopic guidance, we transected the esophagus approximately **[Blank]** cm below the level of the thoracic inlet roughly **[Blank]** cm from the incisors by endoscopy. We removed the specimen and passed it off the table for margins. All frozen section margins were negative. A #28 EEA Anvil was sewn into the cut end of the proximal esophagus with 2 concentric #2-0 Surgidac purse-string sutures. The first was a baseball type stitch and the second a series of horizontal bites. We then opened the conduit along the right side of the staple line using an ultrasonic scalpel and delivered the EEA stapler, #28 size, into the conduit. Preserving the proper orientation, we fashioned the #28 EEA esophagogastric anastomosis. Two complete staple rings were noted subsequent to completion of this anastomosis. These were passed off the table for permanent pathology. The redundant portion of the gastric tube was retracted superiorly with and resected with 2 purple loads of the Endo GIA stapler.

The omental pedicle flap was then secured in place with #2-0 Surgidac Endo Stitches taking care to incorporate the anastomosis in the area of coverage. A #2-0 Surgidac was placed in the diaphragm and attached to the tube along the right crus. A #10 French flat Jackson-Pratt drain was placed in the posterior medistinal bed during the anastomosis. Antibiotic irrigation consisting of 2 liters of water was used to irrigate the chest and was suctioned free. A #28 French chest tube was then posteriorly directed towards the apex and secured at the skin with a #0 silk suture. The JP was secured with 3 independent #2-0 silk sutures. The lung was aerated and seemed to expand well. All port sites were examined for hemostasis and found to be adequate. The mini thoracotomy access incision was closed with #0 Vicryl in a running fashion. All port sites were closed with interrupted #2-0 Polysorb in an inverted subcuticular fashion. The wounds were irrigated and staples were used to close the skin incisions. Sterile dressings were applied. The JP was hooked to bulb suction on the chest tube to 20 cm of water Pleur-Evac suction. The patient was then returned to the supine position and nasopharyngeal/oropharyngeal pulmonary toilet performed. The double lumen endotracheal tube was exchanged for a single lumen tube by Anesthesia under direct vision without the use of a tube changer. A pulmonary toilet bronchoscopy was then performed. There was some evidence of ecchymosis of the level of the carina and the right mainstem bronchus. There was no obvious airway injury noted. There was a moderate amount of secretions, which were toileted free without difficulty.

At the completion of the operation all sponge and needle counts were correct. The patient tolerated the procedure well and was transferred to the Surgical Intensive Care Unit, extubated and in stable condition. There were no immediate complications.

Dr. **[BLANK]** was present and scrubbed for **[BLANK]** elements of this procedure.

27. Lung Volume Reduction Surgery

Desmond M. D'Souza, MD and David P. Mason, MD

Thoracic and Cardiovascular Surgery, Cleveland Clinic, Cleveland, Ohio

Essential Operative Steps

1. Lines and Monitoring.
2. General endotracheal anesthesia
3. Double lumen endotracheal tube
4. Approach: Median sternotomy versus bilateral video-assisted thoracoscopic (VATS)
5. VATS: 3 port incisions
6. Proceed anterior to posterior over the apex of the upper lobe
7. Start in the anterior segment of the upper lobe – above the minor fissure on the right and the lingual on the left
8. Use a buttressed staple fire for the entire resection
9. Gentle handling of the lung is paramount to preventing air leaks; avoid contact with the remnant lung.
10. Extract resected specimen through the large utility port
11. Two well placed chest tubes
12. Check for hemostasis
13. Sternotomy or port site closure
14. Chest tubes to waterseal. Do not connect to suction.

Potential Complications and Pitfalls

1. For open approach: stay midline during sternotomy
2. Staple misfire, buttress failure, or inadvertent lung injury can result in a difficult airleak.

Template Dictation

Preoperative Diagnosis: INDICATION – Emphysema.

Postoperative Diagnosis: Same

Procedure(s) Performed: Bilateral Video assisted thoracoscopic (VATS) Lung Volume Reduction Surgery (LVRS)

Attending Surgeon: [BLANK]

Assistant Surgeon: [BLANK]

Assistants: [BLANK]

Anesthesia: [BLANK]

Indication(s) for Procedure: [AGE] year old [GENDER] with [DURATION] history of [COMPLAINT –e.g. progressive shortness of breath, emphysema with predominant upper lobe disease and low exercise capacity.]

Description of Procedure: The patient was taken to the operating room on [DATE]. The patient's identity, and the planned procedure were confirmed. The patient was placed on the operating room table in a supine position. General anesthesia with a double lumen endo-tracheal tube was obtained. An arterial line and central venous catheter were placed. Proper positioning of the double lumen endotracheal tube was confirmed bronchoscopically, administration of pre-operative antibiotics and DVT prophylaxis were confirmed with the anesthesiologist and operating team.

The patient was repositioned in the left lateral decubitus position. The chest was prepped and draped in the usual sterile fashion. A 2 cm incision was made in the ninth intercostal space in the anterior axillary line. A 30-degree thoracoscope was inserted, and the lung was inspected. Two secondary ports were then placed in the sixth intercostal space in the mid-clavicular line, and the fourth intercostal space in the posterior axillary line.

The thoracoscope was then directed anteriorly with the 30-degree lens pointed superiorly. A ring forceps was used through the posterior port to retract the lung and align the parenchyma of the right upper lobe in the direction of the anterior port. A biological, buttressed purple load stapler was then inserted via the anterior port. Caution was taken while inserting the stapler to avoid inadvertent injury to the friable parenchyma. Multiple staple loads were fired across the apex of the right upper lobe in an anterior to posterior fashion. The thoracoscope was switched to the anterior port, and an endo-catch bag was inserted through the large utility port. The specimen was placed into the endo-catch bag and removed.

The pleural cavity was filled with saline, and the anesthesiologist was asked to ventilate the right lung. The staple line and lung were inspected. There were no air leaks. Multilevel rib blocks with 0.5% marcaine was performed. One 28 French chest tube was placed anteriorly, and one 28 French chest tube was placed posteriorly. The ports were removed, and the port sites were inspected for hemostasis. The lung was re-expanded under direct vision. Prior to closure all instrument, sponge and needle counts were confirmed correct. The port sites were closed using a #2-0 vicryl suture for the fascia and a #4-0 vicryl suture on the skin. The chest tubes are connected to waterseal with no suction.

The patient was then repositioned in the right lateral decubitus position to proceed with the left sided procedure in a similar fashion.

Estimated blood loss was [X] cc. There were no intra-operative adverse events. The patient was extubated in the operating room and subsequently transferred to the postoperative thoracic surgery unit.

Dr. [BLANK] was present and scrubbed for [BLANK] elements of this procedure.

28. VATS Wedge Resection

John R. Spratt, MA, MD and Eitan Podgaetz, MD, MPH

University of Minnesota, Minneapolis, MN

Essential Operative Steps

1. Availability of relevant imaging in OR
2. Operative-side-up lateral decubitus jackknife positioning with reverse Trendelenberg allowing chest wall to be parallel to the floor
3. General endotracheal anesthesia with double lumen endotracheal tube and single-lung ventilation
4. Double lumen tube position must be confirmed by flexible bronchoscopy
5. Surgeon stands on anterior side of patient, assistants posterior
6. Placement of camera port low in the chest (7th-8th intercostal space, midaxillary or anterior axillary line)
7. CO_2 insufflation can be considered to allow better lung collapse
8. First working port in 4-5th intercostal space in anterior axillary line
9. Inspection of lung and hilum with finger/ ring forceps to determine placement of remaining incision(s) if needed
10. Placement of utility thoracotomy (2 – 4 cm) in 4th or 5th intercostal space between anterior border of latissimus dorsi and lateral border of pectoralis major (anterior axillary line)
11. Retraction of soft tissue over utility thoracotomy for easy chest access. [Self-retaining plastic (i.e., Alexis) wound protector]
12. Identification of target lesion and control with ring or Duval forceps proximal to lesion
13. Resection of target lesion with endoscopic stapler
14. Removal of specimen using endoscopic retrieval bag or through wound protector
15. Assess staple line integrity and hemostasis
16. Chest tube placement
17. Port closure

Potential Complications and Pitfalls

1. Incomplete flexion of patient during positioning
   a. May compress intercostal spaces
   b. Ipsilateral hip may limit freedom of thoracoscope
2. Patient intolerance of single-lung ventilation, requiring CPAP or intermittent ventilation of operative-side lung. Can infuse ipsilateral lung with oxygen.
3. Improper endotracheal tube placement leading to hypoxemia or poor lung isolation
4. Failure to appropriately triangulate camera and working incisions around target tissue (good rule of thumb is to leave a hand's breadth between ports)

5. Failure to retract soft tissues over utility thoracotomy may result in lung re-expansion during intrathoracic suctioning. This is especially true in obese patients.
6. Failure to remove sample using retrieval bag may lead to tumor spillage and port site recurrence
7. Avoid crushing the lesion with the ring forceps.

Template Dictation

Date of Service: [DATE]

Preoperative Diagnosis: [INDICATION]

Postoperative Diagnosis: Same

Procedure(s) Performed: [L or R] VATS wedge resection

Attending Surgeon: [BLANK]

Secondary Surgeon: [BLANK]

Assistants: [BLANK]

Anesthesia: [BLANK]

Specimens: [BLANK]

Fluids: [BLANK]

EBL: [BLANK]

Complications: [BLANK]

Drains: [BLANK]

Disposition: [BLANK]

Indication(s) for Procedure: [AGE] year old [GENDER] with a [SIZE] peripheral lung nodule discovered by [IMAGING RESULTS]. The decision was made to perform VATS wedge resection of the lesion for pathologic diagnosis. The risks and benefits of the procedure were described to the patient, who verbalized good understanding, and informed consent was obtained.

Description of Procedure: The patient was taken to the operating room from the preoperative holding area. The patient's identity and planned procedure were verified and the patient was then placed on the operating room table in the supine position. General endotracheal anesthesia was induced, and the patient was intubated with a double lumen endotracheal tube **[OR SINGLE LUMEN ENDOTRACHEAL TUBE AND SUBSEQUENT PLACEMENT OF A BRONCHIAL BLOCKER]**. Tube position was confirmed by flexible bronchoscopy, allowing selective ventilation of the lung on the non-operative side. Once this was completed, the patient was then moved into the

I. General Thoracic Surgery

[NONOPERATIVE SIDE]-lateral decubitus position ensuring his bony prominences were well padded. The upper extremity was not on any undue stretch. The operating table was maximally flexed at the level of the patient's hip. Appropriate endotracheal tube placement was again confirmed with a pediatric bronchoscope. The [SIDE] chest was then prepped widely from the axilla to inferior to the costal margin longitudinally and from the midclavicular line to the tip of the scapula transversely. A surgical time out was performed to identify patient and intended procedure.

The [SIDE] lung was isolated. Rib blocks with [VOLUME AND TYPE OF LOCAL ANESTHESIA] were made prior to each incision. The 8th intercostal space was identified and a 2 cm skin incision was made [LOCATION]. Dissection down to the parietal pleura was performed with electrocautery. The chest was entered sharply and the absence of adjacent adhesions or adherent lung tissue was confirmed by finger palpation. A 10 mm trocar was placed, and the chest cavity was inspected with a 10 mm 30-degree thoracoscope. [FINDINGS]. The chest was then insufflated with CO_2 via the trocar to facilitate lung collapse.

After determining that it was safe to proceed, a second port was placed in the 6th intercostal space in the midaxillary line using the same technique as above. An endoscopic alligator grasper was used to retract the lung and inspect the pleura and the anterior hilum, as well as to identify the lesion. A third and final incision, 3-4 cm in length, was made between the anterior border of the latissimus dorsi and the anterior axillary line at the level of the 4th intercostal space, after instillation of local anesthesia. A small wound protector was placed.

The target lesion was identified at [LOCATION] by visualization and direct finger palpation. The lesion and surrounding lung parenchyma were grasped atraumatically using a Duval clamp. The lesion was elevated and resected with serial firings of a [SIZE, COLOR, STAPLER TYPE] endoscopic stapler. The staple line was noted to be hemostatic. The stapler was removed and a specimen retrieved through the wound protector.

Additional rib blocks were given under direct vision using [VOLUME AND TYPE OF LOCAL ANESTHESIA] and a thoracoscopic aspiration needle. A [SIZE] chest tube was then placed through the camera port, tunneled anteriorly, and directed posteriorly and towards the apex. Chest tube position was confirmed by thoracoscopic visualization. All the ports were removed and the lung was reinflating with Valsalva maneuvers obliterating the pleural space and reversing atelectasis. Each of the ports were closed in layers with absorbable suture.

The sponge, instrument, and needle counts were said to be correct at the conclusion of the procedure. The patient was then extubated without incident and taken to the post-anesthesia care unit in [CONDITION].

Dr. [BLANK] was present and scrubbed for [BLANK] elements of the procedure.

29. VATS Sympathectomy

John R Spratt, MA, MD and Eitan Podgaetz, MD, MPH

University of Minnesota, Minneapolis, MN

Essential Operative Steps

1. Semi-Fowler position with reverse Trendelenburg, arms abducted beyond 90° bilaterally, and entire chest prepped into the field
2. General endotracheal anesthesia with double lumen endotracheal tube and single-lung ventilation
3. Double lumen tube position confirmed by flexible bronchoscopy
4. Surgeon stands on ipsilateral side
5. 1 cm incisions over 5th intercostal space at lateral border of pectoralis major and 4th intercostal space in anterior axillary line with placement of 5 mm trocars in each
6. CO_2 insufflation to facilitate better lung collapse (pressure 6 to 10 mmHg)
7. Inspection of chest cavity and identification of sympathetic chain crossing rib heads posteriorly
8. Meticulous counting of ribs to determine proper level; 2nd rib is most superior rib visible from within pleural cavity, T2 ganglion located between heads of 2nd and 3rd ribs
9. Use hook cautery to dissect parietal pleura above and below isolating the sympathetic chain at the levels desired
    a. T2-T3 transection is best for palmar hyperhidrosis
    b. T3-T4 transection is best for axillary hyperhidrosis
    c. May extend as low as T5 for lower-extremity symptoms
    d. T1-T3 for reflex sympathetic dystrophy
    e. T4-T10 for chronic pancreatic pain
10. Cautery or clips may be used to transect/ clip sympathetic chain. (Clips are believed to be reversible in cases of severe compensatory hyperhidrosis)
11. Lung is re-inflated under direct vision, may use small chest tube through one of the working incisions to evacuate residual gas
12. Removal of chest tube following closure of subcutaneous layer, followed by skin closure
13. Procedure is then repeated on contralateral side
14. Chest radiograph in PACU

Potential Complications and Pitfalls

1. Meticulous identification of proper level of transection is mandatory
    a. Landmarks:
        i. 2nd rib is most superior rib visible from within the chest
        ii. Azygos vein lies at 5th interspace
        iii. Aortic arch reaches 4th interspace

b. Named ganglia located inferior to corresponding rib (e.g. T2 ganglion is located between heads of 2nd and 3rd ribs)
2. Bleeding complications rare, but may result from damage to intercostal vasculature or great vessels, hemothorax from port site bleeding also possible
3. Clinically insignificant postop pneumothoraces are common
4. Horner's syndrome may result from misidentification of level of transection
5. Compensatory sweating of the torso, thighs, and legs may result, can be as severe as original palmar/ axillary hyperhidrosis in some cases
6. Patients must have documented proof of at least two medical treatments (topicals, iontophoresis, Botox, etc.) to be considered for surgical intervention.

Template Dictation

Preoperative Diagnosis: [INDICATION]

Postoperative Diagnosis: Same

Procedure(s) Performed: [L or R] [LEVEL] VATS sympathectomy

Attending Surgeon: [BLANK]

Secondary Surgeon: [BLANK]

Assistants: [BLANK]

Anesthesia: [BLANK]

Specimens: [BLANK]

Fluids: [BLANK]

EBL: [BLANK]

Complications: [BLANK]

Drains: [BLANK]

Disposition: [BLANK]

Indication(s) for Procedure: [AGE] year old [GENDER] with [INDICATION]. The patient has failed maximal medical management of this condition, which included [MEDICAL THERAPY], and the decision was made to perform thoracoscopic sympathectomy. The risks and benefits of the procedure were described to the patient, who verbalized good understanding, and informed consent was obtained.

Description of Procedure: The patient was taken to the operating room from the preoperative holding area. The patient's identity and planned procedure were verified and the patient was then placed on the operating room table in the supine position. General endotracheal anesthesia was induced with the use of [SINGLE LUNG VENTILATION – double lumen endotracheal tube, bronchial blocker, endobronchial intubation, etc.]; tube position was confirmed by flexible bronchoscopy, allowing selective ventilation of the lung on the non-operative side. Once this was completed, the patient was moved into a Semi-Fowler position with both arms abducted beyond 90 degrees. All bony prominences were padded, and it was ensured that the patient's upper extremities were not under undue stretch. The chest was prepped bilaterally from the clavicle to below the costal margin longitudinally and to out to the tip of the scapulae transversely. The patient was draped appropriately and a surgical time out was performed.

The [SIDE] lung was isolated. The fifth intercostal space was identified at the lateral border of the pectoralis muscle. A rib block was performed with [VOLUME AND TYPE OF LOCAL ANESTHESIA], after which a 5mm skin incision was made. Ventilation was held. A 5 mm trocar was placed and the chest was inspected with a 5 mm 30 degree thoracoscope. The lung was noted to be deflated. [FINDINGS]. The chest was then insufflated with CO2 via the trocar to facilitate lung collapse to a pressure of 10 mmHg. After determining that it was safe to proceed, a second 5 mm port was placed in the 4th intercostal space in the anterior axillary line using the same technique described previously.

The second rib was identified high in the chest cavity and this was used as a landmark to identify the location of the [TARGET GANGLIA] ganglia along the visualized sympathetic chain. Hook cautery was used to open the parietal pleura at [LEVELS]. The exposed sympathetic chain was dissected from the parietal pleura. Surgical clips were placed at the proximal and distal level. A 14 French chest tube was then placed through the working trocar; the trocar was then removed over the tube. Suction was applied to the chest tube. The lung was then re-inflated under direct vision and the subcutaneous tissues were then closed after the final trocar and camera were withdrawn. The chest tube was removed under Valsalva maneuver and the skin was closed in a subcuticular fashion with absorbable suture.

[PROCEDURE IS REPEATED ON CONTRALATERAL SIDE]

The sponge, instrument, and needle counts were said to be correct at the conclusion of the procedure. The patient was then awoken from anesthesia, extubated in the OR, and then taken to the PACU in [CONDITION], where a chest radiograph is pending at the time of this dictation.

Dr. [BLANK] was present and scrubbed for [BLANK] elements of the procedure.

30. VATS Thymectomy

Manu S. Sancheti, MD and Allan Pickens, MD

Emory University, Atlanta, GA

Essential Operative Steps

1. Lines and Monitoring
2. General double lumen endotracheal tube anesthesia
3. Partial right lateral decubitus positioning
4. Prep and drape entire chest
5. Single lung ventilation
6. Thoracoscopic guided trocar placement
7. CO_2 insufflation 6 mmHg to 15 mmHg as tolerated
8. Additional left trocars placement
9. Open mediastinal pleura anterior to phrenic nerve
10. Isolate and divide left inferior horn
11. Free thymus from pericardium moving superiorly to thoracic inlet
12. Free thymus anteriorly from sternum along IMA/IMV
13. Enter right pleural space
14. Right trocars placement and move camera/ultrasonic coagulator to right
15. Isolate and divide right inferior horn
16. Free thymus from pericardium moving superior to thoracic inlet
17. Divide attachments to innominate vein
18. Isolate and divide right superior horn
19. Move camera and instruments back to left
20. Divide attachments to innominate vein
21. Isolate and divide left superior horn
22. Place thymus in endoscopic bag and remove
23. Examine specimen
24. Hemostasis
25. Ensure no residual thymic tissue present
26. Place chest tube transmediastinally
27. Observe lung re-expansion
28. Closure

Potential Complications and Pitfalls

1. Improper double lumen endotracheal tube placement
2. Improper positioning and poor padding of pressure points/traction on shoulder or elbow
3. Improper trocar positions
4. Lung injury with initial thoracoscopic guided trocar placement
5. Hemodynamic compromise with insufflation
6. Injury or division of phrenic nerve
7. Bleeding from thymic vessels at horns due to inadequate coagulation or clipping

8. Injury to IMA/IMV
9. Injury to right lung when entering right pleural space
10. Injury to innominate vein or inadequate control of vein branches from innominate vein
11. Poor hemostasis
12. Residual thymic tissue left at end of case
13. Chest tube not placed transmediastinally
14. Poor lung re-expansion

Template Dictation

Preoperative Diagnosis: [INDICATION – e.g Myasthenia Gravis, Thymoma, Thymic cyst, Thymic carcinoma]

Postoperative Diagnosis: Same

Procedure(s) Performed: Thoracoscopic thymectomy

Attending Surgeon: [BLANK]

Secondary Surgeon: [BLANK]

Assistants: [BLANK]

Anesthesia: [BLANK]

Indication(s) for Procedure: [AGE] year old [GENDER] with [DURATION] history of [COMPLAINT –e.g. chest pain, muscle weakness, incidental finding]. Preoperative imaging revealed [RADIOLOGY RESULTS]. Patient was evaluated in Thoracic Surgery Clinic and recommended to undergo thymectomy via bilateral thoracoscopy. Risks/alternatives discussed, questions answered and patient agrees to proceed.

Description of Procedure: The patient was taken to the operating room on [DATE]. The patient's identity and planned procedure verified, and the patient was placed on the operating room table in the supine position. General anesthesia was obtained and the patient was intubated with a double lumen endotracheal tube. Proper position was confirmed with flexible bronchoscopy. A Foley catheter was inserted under sterile conditions. [PREOPERATIVE ANTIBIOTIC AND DOSE] was administered within 1 hour of skin incision. Bilateral lower extremity sequential compression devices were placed for DVT prophylaxis. A warming blanket was placed for intraoperative hypothermia.

The patient was placed in a partial right lateral decubitus position with a bump placed under the patient's left side. The left arm was placed in a sling above the head. All pressure points were padded well and no traction was placed on the shoulder or elbow. Hair removal was performed with clippers. The entire chest was prepped and draped in sterile fashion. The right lung was selectively ventilated. A time out was performed.

LOCAL ANESTHETIC MEDICATION AND DOSE] was used to infiltrate each trocar site prior to incision. A 12 mm incision was made in the 7th intercostal space in the mid-axillary line. A 12 mm thoracoscopic port was placed into the left pleural space under direct thoracoscopic guidance using a 10 mm 30-degree thoracoscope. Upon entrance into the pleural space, insufflation was started up to 15 mmHg as tolerated. Two 5 mm thoracoscopic ports were then placed under direct visualization: one in the left 4th intercostal space at the anterior axillary line and one in the left 6th intercostal space at the anterior axillary line.

The dissection was started by opening the mediastinal pleura with a grasper and ultrasonic coagulator approximately 1-2 cm anterior to the phrenic nerve. This was followed inferior to the diaphragm. The left inferior pole of the thymus gland was freed from its attachments inferiorly. The thymus was then dissected free from the pericardium moving superiorly toward the thoracic inlet. The thymus was then mobilized from the sternum anteromedially along the length of the internal mammary artery/vein. The right pleura was then opened and carried inferiorly. Next, two 5 mm thoracoscopic ports were placed under direct visualization in the right inframammary fold approximately 8 cm apart. The thoracoscope was moved to one of these ports and the ultrasonic coagulator in the other. The thymus was grasped from a left sided port and retracted towards the left. The right inferior horn was isolated and divided. The thymus was then freed from the pericardium moving superiorly toward the thoracic inlet being careful to stay at least 1-2 cm anterior to the phrenic nerve. Superiorly, the thymus was freed from its attachments to the innominate vein using coagulation and clips. The right superior horn was then isolated and divided assisted by inferior retraction of the gland. The camera was then moved back to the left-sided 5 mm port. The left superior horn was then isolated and divided in a similar fashion. A 10 mm endoscopic bag was then placed through the 12 mm port. The thymus gland was extracted in the bag from this port. The gland was examined on the back table and finding include [FINDINGS e.g. mass, cyst, normal, etc]. The specimen was sent to pathology.

The entire chest cavity was inspected. Hemostasis was achieved. No evidence of residual thymus was visualized. A 19 French Blake drain was placed through one of the right-sided 5 mm ports and crossed transmediastinally to the left. All ports were removed except the camera port. Insufflation was removed and the lung was observed to expand fully. The final port was removed. The 12 mm port site fascia was closed with #2-0 Vicryl. All skin incisions were closed with running #4-0 Monocryl in a subcuticular fashion and Dermabond was placed on the skin. The chest tube was secured with #0 silk suture.

All instrument, sponge and needle counts were confirmed to be correct x 2 at the end of the operation. The patient was extubated and taken to the Post-Operative Recovery Unit in stable condition.

Dr. **[BLANK]** was present and scrubbed for [BLANK] elements of this procedure.

31. Transcervical Thymectomy

J. Matthew Reinersman, MD, and Stephen D. Cassivi, MD, MSc

Mayo Clinic, Rochester, MN

Essential Operative Steps

1. Patient Selection
   a. Partnering with an experienced neurologist specializing in myasthenia gravis and similar motor disorders is essential to preoperatively confirm the diagnosis of myasthenia gravis.
   b. Patients with suitable body habitus for this procedure are those patients who can adequately extend their neck and do not have limiting osteoarthritis of the cervical spine or significant osteophytes.
   c. Patients presenting with a presumed thymoma visible on imaging are not preferred for this approach and should be considered for thoracoscopic thymectomy.
   d. This approach can also be used to resect a thymus gland containing an active ectopic parathyroid gland.
2. Lines and Monitoring
   a. Standard peripheral venous access is usually sufficient along with standard non-invasive intraoperative monitoring. When possible, venous access should be obtained from the right upper extremity.
3. Patient Positioning and Preparation
   a. The patient is positioned supine with an inflatable pillow placed behind the shoulders to assist with neck extension.
   b. The operative table is shifted away from the usual anesthetic equipment so that the head of the bed accessible to the surgeon and surgical assistant.
   c. The patient is prepped and draped from the chin to just above the umbilicus to allow for possible conversion to median sternotomy.
4. General endotracheal anesthesia without use of neuromuscular blockade
5. Low collar incision
6. Create superior and inferior subplatysmal flaps
7. Divide midline strap muscles
8. Dissect upper poles of thymus gland from underneath the strap muscles on each side and divide between suture ligatures, leaving the ligatures on the thymus side long as means of retraction
9. Just behind the sternal notch, bluntly dissect the plane posterior to sternum, place Cooper retractor, let down inflatable shoulder pillow
10. Retract thymus forward and upward to display veins draining into innominate vein. Ligate and divide the draining thymic veins
11. Carry dissection along posterior aspect of thymus into mediastinum along anterior pericardium
12. Utilize 5-mm, 30-degree thoracoscope to improve visualization

I.General Thoracic Surgery

13. Dissection carried on the right side laterally and then the left side laterally.
14. Continue dissection anteriorly to divide the attachments of the anterior thymus to the retrosternal surface
15. Remove the specimen intact, weigh it, take to pathology
16. Re-examine thymectomy space for any residual thymus or fatty tissue and assess hemostasis
17. Reapproximate midline strap muscles, close platysma and skin

Potential Complications and Pitfalls

1. Patient selection is critical - nonthymomatous myasthenia. This approach should not be utilized for patients with thymoma or thymic carcinoma. Other relative contraindications include previous median sternotomy, severe osteoarthritis or previous cervical spine surgery, or previous thyroid surgery.
2. Prep and drape entire neck and anterior chest, have sternal saw immediately available and be prepared to perform sternotomy if difficult visualization, bleeding, or other problems occur.
3. Completing the posterior dissection between the thymus and the pericardium first prior to dissecting anteriorly between the thymus and sternum is highly recommended as it allows for better visualization. Maintaining the anterior attachments between the sternum and the thymus help to keep this tissue retracted anteriorly while the posterior dissection is completed down to the pericardiophrenic angles.
4. Avoid injury to phrenic nerves; Use of electrocautery in the deep lateral extent can put the phrenic nerves at risk; use low power in a patient free of muscle relaxants.
5. Entry into the pleural space can occur but is usually inconsequential and does not require a formal chest tube drainage if the lung has not been injured. Evacuation of the pleural space air can be accomplished at the end of the procedure by placing a drainage tube to underwater seal into the pleural space via the cervical incision. Sustained positive pressure breaths are obtained and the tube is pulled when the pleural air has been sufficiently cleared prior to closure of the incision.
6. If necessary, arterial monitoring line should be placed in the left upper extremity due to possible intermittent compression of the innominate artery throughout the operation may lead to false determinations of a low blood pressure. Venous lines should be placed in the right upper extremity.
7. Utilization of a 5-mm, 30-degree thoracoscope assists with visualization
8. Muscle relaxants are avoided in myasthenia gravis cases to reduce the postoperative complications due to exacerbated motor nerve disturbances, especially respiratory muscle weakness.

Template Dictation

Preoperative Diagnosis: Nonthymomatous myasthenia gravis

Postoperative Diagnosis: Same

Procedure(s) performed: Transcervical Thymectomy

Attending Surgeon: [BLANK]

Secondary Surgeon: [BLANK]

Assistants: [BLANK]

Anesthesia: [BLANK]

Indication(s) for Procedure: [AGE] year old [GENDER] with a history of [SYMPTOMS] and a diagnosis of [DIAGNOSIS] presents for transcervical thymectomy.

Description of Procedure: The patient was taken to the operating room on [DATE]. The patient's identity and planned procedure were verified, and the patient was placed on the operating room table in the supine position. Following induction of general anesthesia without the use of muscle relaxants, the patient was intubated with a single-lumen endotracheal tube. The patient's arms were tucked at the side and an inflatable pillow was placed behind the shoulders and inflated to allow extension of the neck. The entire neck and anterior chest were then prepped and draped.

A 4 cm incision was made one fingerbreadth above the sternal notch in a curvilinear transverse fashion. The platysma was incised and superior and inferior subplatysmal flaps were then created, extending to the level of the sternal notch inferiorly and to the inferior border of the thyroid superiorly. The midline between the strap muscles was then incised along the midline raphae and the upper poles of the thymus gland were detected behind these structures. The left upper pole of the thymus gland was identified, isolated, and then ligated underneath the sternohyoid and sternothyroid muscles. The pedicle was controlled between two #2-0 silk ligatures and then divided. The silk ligatures on the thymus were left long for traction purposes. Similarly the right superior pole was dissected under the right side strap muscles. The upper pole ligatures were then used to allow gentle retraction during the remainder of the procedure. Dissection was then carried down to the level of the innominate vein, posterior to the superior portions of the thymus gland. A space was cleared in the plane between the posterior sternal notch and the anterior thymus gland for placement of the Cooper retractor. With the Cooper retractor in place, the sternum was elevated anteriorly and the inflatable cushion was deflated allowing the mediastinal contents to fall away from the sternum. The thymus was then carefully dissected off of the innominate vein. Multiple small venous branches of the innominate vein were carefully ligated and divided. A 5-mm, 30-degree thoracoscope was then inserted through our incision to aid in visualization and dissection. The dissection was then continued along the anterior pericardium all of the way down to the diaphragm. The right side was then dissected free laterally, followed by the left side. We then carried our dissection anteriorly to divide the attachments of the anterior thymus to the retrosternal surface. The thymus was then able to be completely delivered through the cervical incision. It was removed intact within its capsule. It weighed [WEIGHT] grams. Pathology revealed [PATHOLOGY DIAGNOSIS]. At this point after sending the specimen off, we reinserted the thoracoscope and reinspected the mediastinum for any further thymic or fatty tissue. We assured hemostasis. Once we were satisfied, the Cooper retractor was removed, the strap muscles were reapproximated with two interrupted Vicryl sutures. The platysma was then closed with a running Vicryl suture. The incision was then irrigated and the skin was closed with #4-0 Monocryl suture. The incision was washed, dried, and dressed. The patient was recovered from anesthesia, extubated and brought to the recovery room in stable condition. At the end of the case, both sponge and instrument counts were correct, and the estimated blood loss was [**BLOOD LOSS**].

Dr. [**BLANK**] was present and scrubbed for [**BLANK**] elements of this procedure.

32. Trans-Sternal Thymectomy

Geoffrey T. Lam, MD, and Jessica S. Donington, MD

NYU School of Medicine, New York, NY

Essential Operative Steps

1. Lines and monitoring
2. General endotracheal anesthesia with double-lumen tube: preferable but not essential
3. Bronchoscopy: to confirm placement of double-lumen tube
4. Median sternotomy
5. Thymectomy
6. Preservation of phrenic nerve
7. Chest tube placement
8. Sternotomy closure

Potential Complications and Pitfalls

1. Straying off midline during sternotomy
2. Injury to innominate vein
3. Injury to phrenic nerve
4. Failure to remove the entire thymus
5. Inadequate hemostasis prior to sternotomy closure

Template Dictation

Preoperative Diagnosis: [INDICATION – e.g. mediastinal mass, thymoma, thymic carcinoma]

Postoperative Diagnosis: Same

Procedure(s) Performed: Trans-sternal thymectomy, fiberoptic bronchoscopy

Attending Surgeon: [BLANK]

Secondary Surgeon: [BLANK]

Assistants: [BLANK]

Anesthesia: [BLANK]

Fluids: [BLANK]

EBL: [BLANK]

Specimens: [BLANK]

Drains: [BLANK]

Indication(s) for Procedure: [AGE] year old [GENDER] with [THYMOMA/THYMIC CARCINOMA]. Preoperative imaging revealed [FINDINGS].

Description of Procedure: Informed consent for surgery was obtained from the patient, including a discussion of risks, benefits and alternatives, and the form was documented in the chart. The patient was taken to the operating room on [DATE] and placed on the operating room table in supine position. Anesthesia inserted appropriate intravascular access and hemodynamic monitoring lines. Preoperative IV antibiotics were administered. A time out was called to identify the correct patient, procedure and anatomic location. Following the induction of teneral endotracheal anesthesia, the patient was intubated with a double-lumen endotracheal tube. Bronchoscopy was performed. Proper placement of the endotracheal tube was confirmed. The airways were examined. Normal endobronchial anatomy was noted. There were no endobronchial abnormalities. The patient was left in the supine position, a transverse shoulder roll was placed, and the arms were tucked. A lower Bair Hugger was applied and all pressure points were padded. The neck and chest were prepped and draped in sterile fashion.

The endotracheal tube was disconnected from the ventilator. A median sternotomy was performed. Mechanical ventilation was resumed. Hemostasis of the sternum was obtained, and a sternotomy retractor was placed. The [RIGHT/LEFT] side was approached first. The ipsilateral lung was isolated, the sternal table was elevated and the pleural space was widely opened. Dissection was started inferiorly and care taken to identify and preserve the phrenic nerve. Small thymic branches were doubly clipped with medium clips and divided using Bovie electrocautery. The mass was elevated off the pericardium [THE PERICARDIUM WAS RESECTED EN BLOC IF ADHERENT] and dissection continued over the pericardial surface, superiorly up to the level of the innominate vein and laterally out to the phrenic nerve. Attention was turned to the superior horn, which was dissected free, clipped superiorly and brought inferiorly to the level of the innominate vein. Prior to beginning dissection on the contralateral side, a 28-French straight chest tube was placed into the pleural space via a separate lateral stab incision, directed anteriorly and superiorly and secured to the skin using #1 silk. Anesthesia then switched the lung isolation. The sternal table was elevated and the contralateral pleural space was opened widely. The dissection was started inferiorly and carried in a superior direction, taking care to identify and preserve the phrenic nerve. All thymic tissue and mediastinal fat between the phrenic nerves was dissected free up to the level of the innominate vein. The second superior horn was dissected free and clipped at its highest point and then dissected inferiorly down to the level of the innominate vein. The thymus was dissected off the innominate vein, and the draining vein was identified, clipped and divided. The thymus was passed off the field.

Hemostasis was achieved using Bovie electrocautery. A 28-French straight chest tube was placed into the contralateral pleural space via a separate lateral stab incision, directed anteriorly and superiorly and secured to the skin using #1 silk. The lung was reinflated and the patient left on two-lung ventilation. The sternum was reapproximated using [NUMBER] #5 stainless steel wires. The sternotomy incision was closed in layers, using #0 PDS for the fascia, #2-0 PDS for the deep dermal layer and a running #3-0 Monocryl subcuticular stitch for the skin. Sterile dry dressings were applied. The chest tubes were connected to Pleur-Evac drainage.

The patient tolerated the procedure well. The patient was extubated in the operating room and transferred in stable condition to the recovery room. At the end of the case, the sponge, needle and instrument counts were correct x2.

Dr. [BLANK] was present and scrubbed for [BLANK] elements of this procedure.

33. Open Lobectomies

Erin Gillaspie, MD and K. Robert Shen, MD

Mayo Clinic, Rochester, MN

Note: There are a variety of surgical options for managing the pulmonary vasculature and the bronchus. Different methods are described throughout the chapter.

Right Upper Lobectomy

Essential Operative Steps

1. Place an arterial line and Foley catheter.
2. General endotracheal anesthesia and thoracic epidural catheter.
3. Flexible bronchoscopy to assess airway for secretions, pus, blood, bronchial anatomical abnormalities and endobronchial lesions.
4. Exchange single lumen for dual lumen tube or place bronchial blocker.
5. Confirm tube positioning with bronchoscopy.
6. Place patient in lateral decubitus positioning with table flexed cephalad to xiphoid process.
7. Perform muscle sparing postero-lateral thoracotomy dividing the latissimus dorsi but sparing the serratus anterior muscle which is reflected anteriorly. Chest is entered in the 4th or 5th intercostal space.
8. Divide inferior pulmonary ligament up to the inferior pulmonary vein.
9. Open mediastinal pleura circumferentially around the hilum.
10. Open fissure to expose the pulmonary artery at the junction of the major and minor fissure.
11. Transect superior pulmonary vein after verifying that there is a separate inferior pulmonary vein.
12. Transect the truncus anterior artery and posterior ascending artery.
13. Transect bronchus after test clamping the right upper lobe and having the anesthesia team reinflate the right lung to verify that the bronchi to the middle and lower lobes have unobstructed flow.
14. Complete fissure posteriorly and complete parenchymal division anteriorly.
15. Perform thoracic lymphadenectomy with sampling or removal of lymph nodes from stations 4, 7, 8, 9 as well as peribronchial nodes around the bronchus of the right upper lobe.
16. Test bronchial stump for pneumostasis.
17. Check for hemostasis.
18. Tack right middle lobe to lower lobe to prevent middle lobe torsion.
19. Place chest tubes.
20. Close thoracotomy.

Potential Complications and Pitfalls
1. Traditionally, the pulmonary vein is transected first. However, if exposure is difficult, the artery or bronchus may be transected initially to provide adequate exposure to complete the lobectomy safely.
2. If the bronchus is divided first, the vein and artery are at risk for injury due to the lack the structural support of the bronchus; special care must be taken.
3. Prior to dividing any venous branches, verification of a separate inferior pulmonary vein is mandatory
4. The right upper lobe artery anatomy is variable. The posterior ascending artery typically originates from the main PA just opposite to the middle lobe artery. It may also originate from the superior segment to the right lower lobe.
5. The venous anatomy is also variable. The middle lobe vein may be a tributary of either (or both) the superior or inferior pulmonary vein. Special attention must be taken when performing a middle lobectomy to assure that the middle lobe vein isn't sacrificed.
6. Removal of the "sump node" (level 11R node), which resides between the right upper lobe bronchus and bronchus intermedius, is helpful to expose the posterior ascending artery.
7. Avoid devascularization of the whole bronchus as this impairs healing and results in higher rates of broncho-pleural fistula formation.

Template Dictation

Preoperative Diagnosis: [INDICATION]

Postoperative Diagnosis: Same

Procedure(s) Performed: Right upper lobectomy

Attending Surgeon: [BLANK]

Assistant Surgeon: [BLANK]

Assistants: [BLANK]

Anesthesia: [GENERAL ENDOTRACHEAL, THORACIC EPIDURAL]

Indication(s) for Procedure: [AGE] year old [GENDER] who presented with [DURATION] history of [COMPLAINT]. Workup included [CXR, CT, PET] which demonstrated [WORKUP FINDINGS]. Pulmonary functions tests demonstrated patient to be a candidate for lobectomy.

Description of Procedure: The patient was taken to the operating room on [DATE]. The patient's identity and planned procedure were confirmed. The patient was transferred to the operating room table and placed in supine position. General endotracheal anesthesia was induced. Flexible bronchoscopy was performed. There were no secretions, pus, blood, bronchial anatomical

I. General Thoracic Surgery

abnormalities, or endobronchial lesions. The single lumen tube was exchanged for a dual lumen endotracheal tube. Tube position was verified with bronchoscopy. A radial arterial line and additional peripheral IVs were placed.

The patient was placed in the left lateral decubitus position and prepped and draped in the usual sterile fashion. A time out was performed. All members of the surgical team were present and were in agreement.

The right lung was isolated. A serratus-sparing right posterolateral thoracotomy was performed. The chest was entered. The [FIFTH/SIXTH] rib was shingled posteriorly. The inferior pulmonary ligament was divided to the level of the inferior pulmonary vein. A station 9 lymph node was sampled. The lung and pleura were examined; the lesion was identified in the upper lobe. The lung was retracted posteriorly and the mediastinal pleura opened circumferentially around the hilum. The sump node (station 11R) was removed. The horizontal fissure was opened using electrocautery and completed with the GIA stapler to expose the underlying pulmonary artery. The superior pulmonary vein was identified and the apical, anterior and posterior branches were skeletonized, ligated proximally and distally with [TIE/SUTURE/STAPLE] and divided. The truncus anterior and posterior ascending branches of the pulmonary artery were skeletonized, ligated proximally and distally with [TIE/SUTURE/STAPLE] and divided. The upper lobe was retracted superiorly and posteriorly to identify the right upper lobe bronchus. The bronchus was exposed circumferentially with lymphatic tissue being swept up towards the specimen. The upper lobe bronchus was occluded just distal to the takeoff from the mainstem bronchus with a curved clamp. The middle and lower lobe expanded, thereby confirming unobstructed flow. The bronchus was transected and over-sewn with #3-0 PDS [SUTURE MATERIAL]. The upper was sent to Pathology. Frozen sections demonstrated negative bronchial margins

Mediastinal lymph nodes from stations 2R, 4R, 7, 8, 9, 10R, and 11R were sampled during the dissection.

The bronchial stump was submerged under water, the lung was inflated to 40 cm water pressure and the stump was found to be pneumostatic. The right middle lobe was sutured to the right lower lobe to prevent torsion. The chest was re-evaluated for bleeding and excellent hemostasis was assured.

Two 28 french chest tubes were placed in the pleural cavity and sutured into place.

The lung was allowed to re-expand under direct vision.

The ribs were re-approximated with figure of 8 peri-costal sutures. The serratus anterior layer was re-approximated with running suture. The latissimus dorsi was closed in two layers with running suture. The subcutaneous tissue and skin were closed in running fashion.

Dr. [BLANK] was present and scrubbed for [BLANK] elements of this procedure.

Right Middle Lobectomy

Essential Operative Steps
1. Place an arterial line and Foley catheter.
2. General endotracheal anesthesia and thoracic epidural catheter.
3. Flexible bronchoscopy to assess airway for secretions, pus, blood, bronchial anatomical abnormalities and endobronchial lesions.
4. Exchange single lumen for dual lumen tube or place bronchial blocker.
5. Confirm tube positioning with bronchoscopy.
6. Place patient in lateral decubitus positioning with table flexed cephalad to xiphoid process.
7. Perform a muscle sparing posterolateral thoracotomy, dividing the latissimus dorsi but sparing the serratus anterior muscle, which is reflected anteriorly. Chest is entered in the 4th or 5th intercostal space.
8. Divide inferior pulmonary ligament up to the inferior pulmonary vein.
9. Open mediastinal pleura circumferentially around the hilum.
10. Open horizontal fissure.
11. Transect venous branch to the middle lobe.
12. Transect artery (or arteries). There may be one or two middle lobe arterial branches.
13. Transect the bronchus after test clamping the right middle lobe and having the anesthesia team reinflate the right lung to verify that the bronchi to the upper and lower lobes have unobstructed flow.
14. Complete the horizontal and oblique fissures.
15. Perform thoracic lymphadenectomy with sampling or removal of lymph nodes from stations 4R, 7, 8, 9 as well as peribronchial nodes around the bronchus of the right middle lobe.
16. Test bronchial stump for pneumostasis.
17. Check for hemostasis.
18. Place chest tubes.
19. Close thoracotomy.

Potential Complications and Pitfalls
1. There may be one or two arterial branches to the middle lobe. The posterior ascending branch to the RUL should not be confused with a second branch.
2. Venous anatomy is variable. The middle lobe vein can be a tributary of the superior or inferior pulmonary vein and at times both.
3. Avoid devascularization of the whole bronchus as this impairs healing and results in higher rates of broncho-pleural fistula formation.

Template Dictation
Preoperative Diagnosis: [INDICATION]

Postoperative Diagnosis: Same

Procedure(s) Performed: Right middle lobectomy

Attending Surgeon: [BLANK]

Assistant Surgeon: [BLANK]

Assistants: [BLANK]

Anesthesia: [**GENERAL ENDOTRACHEAL, THORACIC EPIDURAL**]

Indication(s) for Procedure: [**AGE**] year old [**GENDER**] who presented with [**DURATION**] history of [**COMPLAINT**]. Workup included [**CXR, CT, PET**] which demonstrated [**WORKUP FINDINGS**]. The patient's pulmonary function tests indicate that a lobectomy could be safely performed.

Description of Procedure: The patient was taken to the operating room on [**DATE**]. The patient's identity and planned procedure were confirmed. The patient was transferred to the operating room table and placed in supine position. General endotracheal anesthesia was induced. Flexible bronchoscopy was performed. There were no secretions, pus, blood, bronchial anatomical abnormalities, or endobronchial lesions. The single lumen tube was exchanged for a dual lumen endotracheal tube. Tube position was verified with bronchoscopy. A radial arterial line and additional peripheral IVs were placed.

The patient was placed in the left lateral decubitus position and prepped and draped in the usual sterile fashion. A time out was performed. All members of the surgical team were present and were in agreement.

The right lung was isolated. A serratus-sparing right posterolateral thoracotomy was performed. The chest was entered. The [**FIFTH/SIXTH**] rib was shingled posteriorly. The inferior pulmonary ligament was divided to the level of the inferior pulmonary vein. A station 9 lymph node was sampled. The lung and pleura were examined; the lesion was identified in the upper lobe. The lung was retracted posteriorly and the mediastinal pleura was opened circumferentially around the hilum. The horizontal fissure was opened and completed with a GIA stapler to expose underlying pulmonary artery branches. The lung was rotated posteriorly and middle lobe vein identified from its takeoff from the [**SUPERIOR/INFERIOR**] pulmonary vein. The vein was skeletonized and transected with vascular load stapler. The [**ONE/TWO**] arterial branches to the right middle lobe were identified, skeletonized and divided with a vascular load stapler. The oblique fissure was completed using serial applications of GIA stapler. Finally, the middle lobe was rotated superiorly to expose the right middle lobe bronchus at the origin of the bronchus intermedius. The bronchus was exposed circumferentially. All lymphatic tissue was swept up towards the specimen. A 4.8 mm TA stapler applied to the right middle lobe bronchus. The lung allowed to re-inflate. Unobstructed airflow to the right upper and lower lobes was confirmed. The bronchus was transected, and the specimen was removed from the chest. Frozen sections demonstrated negative bronchial margins.

Station 2R, 4R, 7, 8, 9 and 10R lymph nodes were sampled.

The bronchial stump was submerged under water, the lung was inflated to 40 cm water pressure, and the stump was found to be pneumostatic. The chest was irrigated. Hemostasis was assured.

Two 28 French chest tubes were placed in the pleural cavity.

The lung was allowed to re-expand.

The ribs were re-approximated with figure of 8 peri-costal sutures. The serratus anterior layer was re-approximated with running suture. The latissimus dorsi was closed in two layers with running suture. Subcutaneous tissue and skin were closed in a running fashion.

Dr. [BLANK] was present and scrubbed for [BLANK] elements of this procedure.

Right Lower Lobectomy

Essential Operative Steps
1. Place an arterial line and Foley catheter.
2. General endotracheal anesthesia and thoracic epidural catheter.
3. Flexible bronchoscopy to assess airway for secretions, pus, blood, bronchial anatomical abnormalities and endobronchial lesions.
4. Exchange single lumen for dual lumen tube or place bronchial blocker
5. Confirm tube positioning with bronchoscopy.
6. Place patient in lateral decubitus positioning with table flexed cephalad to xiphoid process.
7. Perform muscle sparing posterolateral thoracotomy, dividing the latissimus dorsi and sparing the serratus anterior muscle, which is reflected anteriorly. The chest is entered in the 4th or 5th intercostal space.
8. Divide the inferior pulmonary ligament up to the inferior pulmonary vein.
9. Open mediastinal pleura circumferentially around the hilum.
10. Open the fissure.
11. Transect inferior pulmonary vein after verifying that there is a separate superior pulmonary vein.
12. Transect superior segmental artery and basial arterial branches.
13. Transect the bronchus after test clamping the right lower lobe and having the anesthesia team reinflate the right lung to verify that the bronchi to the right upper and middle lobes have unobstructed flow.
14. Complete the fissure posteriorly and complete parenchymal division anteriorly.
15. Perform thoracic lymphadenectomy with sampling or removal of lymph nodes from stations 4R, 7, 8, 9, and 10R as well as peribronchial nodes around the bronchus of the right lower lobe.
16. Test bronchial stump for pneumostasis.
17. Check for hemostasis.
18. Place chest tubes.

19. Close thoracotomy.

Potential Complications and Pitfalls
1. The right middle lobe bronchus is at risk when completing the fissure between the right middle lobe and lower lobe posteriorly. Care needs to be taken to ensure that the right middle lobe bronchus is not inadvertently divided or narrowed during this step.
2. Furthermore, when preparing the divide the bronchus to the right lower lobe, it is critical to ensure that the bronchus to the right middle lobe is not kinked or narrowed by the stapler since it comes off the bronchus at close to a 90 degree angle just proximal to the take-off for the right lower lobe.
3. Avoid devascularization of the whole bronchus as this impairs healing and results in higher rates of broncho-pleural fistula formation.

Template Dictation

Preoperative Diagnosis: [INDICATION]

Postoperative Diagnosis: Same

Procedure(s) Performed: Right lower lobectomy

Attending Surgeon: [BLANK]

Assistant Surgeon: [BLANK]

Assistants: [BLANK]

Anesthesia: [GENERAL ENDOTRACHEAL, THORACIC EPIDURAL]

Indication(s) for Procedure: [AGE] year old [GENDER] who presented with [DURATION] history of [COMPLAINT]. Workup included [CXR, CT, PET] which demonstrated [WORKUP FINDINGS]. The patient's pulmonary function tests indicate that a lobectomy could be safely performed.

Description of Procedure: The patient was taken to the operating room on [DATE]. The patient's identity and planned procedure were confirmed. The patient was transferred to the operating room table and placed in supine position. General endotracheal anesthesia was induced. Flexible bronchoscopy was performed. There were no secretions, pus, blood, bronchial anatomical abnormalities, or endobronchial lesions. The single lumen tube was exchanged for a dual lumen endotracheal tube. Tube position was verified with bronchoscopy. A radial arterial line and additional peripheral IVs were placed.

The patient was placed in the left lateral decubitus position and prepped and draped in the usual sterile fashion. A time out was performed. All members of the surgical team were present and were in agreement.

The right lung was isolated. A serratus-sparing right posterolateral thoracotomy was performed. The chest was entered. The sixth rib was shingled posteriorly. The inferior pulmonary ligament was divided to the level of the inferior pulmonary vein. A station 9 lymph node was sampled. The lung and pleura were examined; the lesion was identified in the upper lobe. The lung was retracted posteriorly and the mediastinal pleura was opened circumferentially around the hilum. The oblique fissure was opened using electrocautery and completed with serial GIA stapler application. The inferior pulmonary vein was encircled as it exits the pericardium and divided using a vascular load stapler. The superior and basilar segmental arterial branches to the right lower lobe were identified, encircled and ligated with a vascular load stapler. The lower lobe was rotated anteriorly; the bronchus intermedius was identified. The branch to the right middle lobe and right lower lobe were identified and the lower lobe branch exposed circumferentially with lymphatic tissue being swept up towards the specimen. A 4.8 mm TA stapler applied to the right lower lobe bronchus. The remaining was lung allowed to re-inflate to confirm unobstructed airflow. The stapler was fired, the bronchus was transected, and the specimen was removed from the chest.

Mediastinal lymph nodes from stations 4R, 7, 8, 9, and 10R and 11R were sampled.

The bronchial stump was submerged under water, the lung was inflated to 40 cm water pressure, and the stump was found to be pneumostatic. Chest was irrigated. Hemostasis was assured.

Two 28 french chest tubes were placed in the pleural cavity.

The lung was reinsufflated under direct vision.

Ribs were re-approximated with figure of 8 peri-costal sutures. The serratus anterior layer was re-approximated with running suture. The latissimus dorsi was closed in two layers with running suture. Subcutaneous tissue and skin were closed in a running fashion.

Dr. [BLANK] was present and scrubbed for [BLANK] elements of this procedure.

Left Upper Lobectomy

Essential Operative Steps
1. Place an arterial line and Foley catheter
2. General endotracheal anesthesia and thoracic epidural catheter.
3. Flexible bronchoscopy to assess airway for secretions, pus, blood, bronchial anatomical abnormalities and endobronchial lesions.
4. Exchange single lumen for dual lumen tube or place bronchial blocker. Generally, a left-sided double lumen endotracheal tube is used for most situations because it is considered technically easier to place. However, in some circumstances, such as a left pneumonectomy or a left sleeve

lobectomy, a right-sided double lumen tube may be preferable and should be discussed with the anesthesia team.
5. Confirm endotracheal tube positioning with bronchoscopy.
6. Place patient in lateral decubitus positioning with table flexed cephalad to xiphoid process.
7. Perform muscle sparing postero-lateral thoracotomy, dividing the latissimus dorsi and sparing the serratus anterior muscle, which is reflected anteriorly. The chest is entered in the 4th or 5th intercostal space.
8. Divide the inferior pulmonary ligament up to the inferior pulmonary vein.
9. Open the mediastinal pleura circumferentially around the hilum.
10. Open the fissure anteriorly and posteriorly.
11. Transect the superior pulmonary vein after verifying that there is a separate inferior pulmonary vein.
12. Transect apico-anterior, posterior and lingular arterial branches.
13. Transect bronchus after test clamping the left upper lobe and having the anesthesia team reinflate the left lung to verify that the bronchus to the lower lobe has unobstructed flow.
14. Complete the fissure.
15. Perform thoracic lymphadenectomy with sampling or removal of lymph nodes from stations 4L, 5, 6, 7, 8, 9, 10L as well as peribronchial nodes around the bronchus of the left upper lobe.
16. Test bronchial stump for pneumostasis.
17. Check for hemostasis.
18. Place chest tubes.
19. Close thoracotomy.

Potential Complications and Pitfalls

1. The left upper-lobe pulmonary artery anatomy is the most variable among the lobes. Usually, there are three branches— apico-anterior, posterior and lingular. A left upper lobectomy is the most technically challenging lobectomy in part due to this variability in the segmental arterial anatomy. In addition, the segmental arteries are quite small, and easily injured. In particular the most proximal segmental artery needs to be handled with care since an inadvertent injury can rapidly propagate into a left main pulmonary artery tear and be very difficult to control.
2. Avoid devascularization of the whole bronchus as this impairs healing and results in higher rates of broncho-pleural fistula formation.

Template Dictation

Preoperative Diagnosis: [INDICATION]

Postoperative Diagnosis: Same

Procedure(s) Performed: Left upper lobectomy

Attending Surgeon: [BLANK]

Assistant Surgeon: [BLANK]

Assistants: [BLANK]

Anesthesia: [GENERAL ENDOTRACHEAL, THORACIC EPIDURAL]

Indication(s) for Procedure: [AGE] year old [GENDER] who presented with [DURATION] history of [COMPLAINT]. Workup included [CXR, CT, PET] which demonstrated [WORKUP FINDINGS]. The patient's pulmonary function tests indicate that a lobectomy could be safely performed.

Description of Procedure: The patient was taken to the operating room on [DATE]. The patient's identity and planned procedure were confirmed. The patient was transferred to the operating room table and placed in the supine position. General endotracheal anesthesia was induced, and the patient was intubated with a single lumen endotracheal tube. Flexible bronchoscopy was performed. There were no secretions, pus, blood, bronchial anatomical abnormalities, or endobronchial lesions. The single lumen tube was exchanged for a dual lumen endotracheal tube. Tube position was verified with bronchoscopy. A radial arterial line and additional peripheral IVs were placed.

The patient was placed in the left lateral decubitus position and prepped and draped in the usual sterile fashion. A time out was performed. All members of the surgical team were present and were in agreement.

The left lung was isolated. A serratus-sparing left posterolateral thoracotomy was performed. The chest was entered. The sixth rib was shingled posteriorly. The inferior pulmonary ligament was divided to the level of the inferior pulmonary vein. The lung was retracted posteriorly and the mediastinal pleura opened circumferentially around the hilum. The fissure was opened using sharp dissection and electrocautery. The fissure was completed with serial GIA stapler applications. The superior pulmonary vein was encircled, ligated with [TIE/SUTURE], and divided. The left upper lobe pulmonary artery branches were identified, skeletonized, individually ligated proximally and distally with [TIE/SUTURE] and divided. The upper lobe was retracted anteriorly to identify the left upper lobe bronchus. The bronchus was exposed circumferentially. All lymphatic tissue was swept upwards. A curved clamp was applied to the bronchus, and the lower lobe was allowed to reinflate, thereby confirming unobstructed flow. The bronchus was transected and over-sewn with [SUTURE MATERIAL].

Mediastinal lymph node stations 4L, 5, 6, 7, 9, 10L and 11L were sampled.

The bronchial stump was submerged under water, the lung was inflated to 40 cm water pressure, and the stump was found to be pneumostatic. The chest was irrigated. Hemostasis was assured.

Two 28 French chest tubes were placed in the pleural cavity.

Lung was allowed to re-expand.

Ribs were re-approximated with figure of 8 peri-costal sutures. The serratus anterior layer was re-approximated with running suture. The latissimus dorsi was closed in two layers with running suture. Subcutaneous tissue and skin were closed in running fashion.

Dr. [BLANK] was present and scrubbed for [BLANK] elements of this procedure.

Left Lower Lobectomy

Essential Operative Steps

1. Place an arterial line and Foley catheter.
2. General endotracheal anesthesia and thoracic epidural catheter.
3. Flexible bronchoscopy to assess airway for secretions, pus, blood, bronchial anatomical abnormalities and endobronchial lesions.
4. Exchange single lumen for dual lumen tube or place bronchial blocker. Generally, a left-sided double lumen endotracheal tube is used for most situations because it is considered technically easier to place. However, in some circumstances, such as a left pneumonectomy or a left sleeve lobectomy, a right sided double lumen tube may be preferable and should be considered or discussed with the anesthesia team.
5. Confirm tube positioning with bronchoscopy.
6. Place patient in lateral decubitus positioning with table flexed cephalad to xiphoid process.
7. Perform muscle sparing postero-lateral thoracotomy dividing the latissimus dorsi but sparing the serratus anterior muscle which is reflected anteriorly. Chest is entered in the 5th intercostal space.
8. Divide inferior pulmonary ligament up to the inferior pulmonary vein.
9. Open mediastinal pleural circumferentially around the hilum.
10. Open fissure anteriorly and posteriorly.
11. Transect inferior pulmonary vein after verifying that there is a separate superior pulmonary vein.
12. Transect superior segmental (one or two branches) and basilar segmental arterial branches.
13. Transect bronchus after test clamping the left lower lobe and having the anesthesia team reinflate the left lung to verify that the bronchus to the upper lobe has unobstructed flow.
14. Complete the fissure.
15. Perform thoracic lymphadenectomy with sampling or removal of lymph nodes from stations 4, 5, 6, 7, 8, 9 as well as peribronchial nodes around the bronchus of the left lower lobe.
16. Test bronchial stump for pneumostasis.
17. Check for hemostasis.
18. Place chest tubes.
19. Close thoracotomy.

Potential Complications and Pitfalls
1. Must be careful not to compromise the pulmonary artery branch to the lingula, which originates just proximally to the lower lobe branches.
2. Avoid devascularization of the whole bronchus as this impairs healing and results in higher rates of broncho-pleural fistula formation.

Template Dictation

Preoperative Diagnosis: [INDICATION]

Postoperative Diagnosis: Same

Procedure(s) Performed: Left lower lobectomy

Attending Surgeon: [BLANK]

Assistant Surgeon: [BLANK]

Assistants: [BLANK]

Anesthesia: [GENERAL ENDOTRACHEAL, THORACIC EPIDURAL]

Indication(s) for Procedure: [AGE] year old [GENDER] who presented with [DURATION] history of [COMPLAINT]. Workup included [CXR, CT, PET] which demonstrated [WORKUP FINDINGS]. The patient's pulmonary function tests indicate that a lobectomy could be safely performed.

Description of Procedure: The patient was taken to the operating room on [DATE]. The patient's identity and planned procedure were confirmed. The patient was transferred to the operating room table and placed in the supine position. General endotracheal anesthesia was induced, and the patient was intubated with a single lumen endotracheal tube. Flexible bronchoscopy was performed. There were no secretions, pus, blood, bronchial anatomical abnormalities, or endobronchial lesions. The single lumen tube was exchanged for a dual lumen endotracheal tube. Tube position was verified with bronchoscopy. A radial arterial line and additional peripheral IVs were placed.

The patient was placed in the left lateral decubitus position and prepped and draped in the usual sterile fashion. A time out was performed. All members of the surgical team were present and were in agreement.

The left lung was isolated. A serratus-sparing left posterolateral thoracotomy was performed. The chest was entered. The sixth rib was shingled posteriorly. The inferior pulmonary ligament was divided to the level of the inferior pulmonary vein. The lung was retracted posteriorly and the mediastinal pleura opened circumferentially around the hilum. The fissure was opened using sharp dissection and electrocautery. The fissure was completed with serial GIA stapler applications. The inferior pulmonary vein was isolated and divided with a vascular load stapler. The left lower lobe pulmonary artery branches were identified, skeletonized and ligated with a vascular load stapler. The lower lobe was retracted anteriorly to identify the lower lobe bronchus. The bronchus was exposed circumferentially; all lymphatic tissue was swept up towards the specimen. A 4.8 mm TA stapler was applied to the bronchus, and the remaining lung was allowed to re-inflate. The stapler was fired, the bronchus transected sharply and the specimen removed from the chest.

Mediastinal lymph node stations 4L, 5, 6, 7, 9, 10L and 11L were sampled.

The bronchial stump was submerged under water, the lung was inflated to 40 cm water pressure, and the stump was found to be pneumostatic. The chest was irrigated. Hemostasis was assured.

Two 28 French chest tubes were placed in the pleural cavity.

The lung was re-expanded under direct vision.

Ribs were re-approximated with figure of 8 peri-costal sutures. The serratus anterior layer was re-approximated with running suture. The latissimus dorsi was closed in two layers with running suture. Subcutaneous tissue and skin were closed in running fashion.

Dr. [BLANK] was present and scrubbed for [BLANK] elements of this procedure.

34. Segmentectomy

James E. Wiseman, MD and Samuel S. Kim, MD

University of Arizona, Tucson, AZ

Essential Operative Steps

1. Pre-operative work up including PFT with DLCO. In patients with limited lung function, quantitative V/Q scan and/or cardiopulmonary exercise test is warranted.
2. Preoperative bronchoscopy for secretion clearance and visualization of anatomy
3. Double-lumen intubation
4. Positioning (lateral decubitus, with flexion of the bed at the hips)
5. Examine hemithorax for signs of other nodules/metastases prior to performing resection
6. Location and palpation of target lesion
7. Division of inferior pulmonary ligament (for mobilization in upper lobe segmentectomy, exposure of the vein in lower lobe segmentectomy)
8. Mediastinal lymph node dissection
    a. Right-sided tumors: 4R, 7, 9, 10R, 11R
    b. Left-sided tumors: 5, 6, 9, 10L, 11L
9. Correct identification of vascular and bronchial anatomy
10. Inflation test to verify isolation of target segment
11. Verification of negative surgical margins prior to closure
12. Placement of chest tubes
13. Visualization of full lung expansion at the end of the operation, including recruitment maneuvers performed by anesthesiologist

Potential Complications and Pitfalls

1. Distortion of lung anatomy by tumor or inflammation can interfere with identification of the target segment → The bronchus is the most reliable structural component; initial identification, dissection, and division of the bronchus may facilitate the operation.
2. Identification and separation of the intersegmental plane is performed by differential inflation after occluding the target bronchus and ventilating the lung. Intersegmental veins travel along this plane, and meticulous dissection along this plane to define routes of venous drainage is imperative. The presence of significant collateral ventilation can make deciphering this plane difficult. In these cases, the entire lung can be inflated initially, the target bronchus occluded, and the lung deflated. The target segment is identified as the portion of lung that remains expanded.
3. The identification and division of correct segmental vein is essential.
4. Meticulous dissection and careful handling of the tissues are essential, especially in patients with pre-existing emphysema, to avoid significant air leak which can complicate the post-operative course. Traditional

dissection of the intersegmetal plane using scissors or cautery increases the risk of postoperative airleak and bleeding. Surgical staplers, while less prone to these complications, are limited by the thickness of the lung parenchyma, and thus vulnerable to staple line disruption. This risk can be reduced by careful reinforcement of the staple line with interrupted, vertical mattress sutures.
5. Right upper anterior segmentectomy is difficult to perform due to inaccessibility of the anterior segmental bronchus from a posterior approach. Formal lobectomy is a safer approach to lesions in this anatomical division.

Template Dictation

Thoracotomy

Preoperative Diagnosis: [INDICATION for operation; typically neoplasm, but may be done for lesions with infectious or benign etiology, particularly if diagnostic uncertainty is present]

Postoperative Diagnosis: specific diagnosis (i.e. cancer histology, if not known preoperatively and if frozen section performed), other intraoperative findings

Procedure(s) Performed:

1. Thoracotomy (with laterality)
2. Segmentectomy (specify segment removed)
3. Mediastinal lymph node dissection (if done for malignancy)

Attending Surgeon: [BLANK]

Assistant Surgeon: [BLANK]

Assistants: [BLANK]

Anesthesia: [GENERAL ENDOTRACHEAL, THORACIC EPIDURAL]

Operative Findings: [Include results of frozen section specimens, anatomic variants, surgical margins]

Specimens: [Include an accurate description of all specimens sent. Typically will include mediastinal lymph nodes and levels, tissue biopsies sent to rule out metastatic disease, and the target lung segment.]

Indication(s) for Procedure: This is a [AGE] year-old [GENDER] who presented with history of [COMPLAINT/DURATION]. The patient was noted on diagnostic [CHEST RADIOGRAPHY] to have a [SIZE] nodule in the [SIDE, LOBE, AND SEGMENT]. A CT-guided biopsy was performed, which was noted to be suspicious for [TISSUE DIAGNOSIS]. (If no biopsy was performed—e.g. recent history of other malignancy with high suspicion for lung metastasis—this should be stated here.)

[MEDIASTINOSCOPY/ENDOBRONCHIAL ULTRASOUND] (if performed) did not show mediastinal lymph node involvement. Based upon the patient's presentation and preoperative workup, it was determined that (he/she) would benefit from [SIDE, LOBE, AND SEGMENT] segmentectomy [with mediastinal lymph node dissection if performed for malignancy]. The patient was informed of the risks and benefits of proceeding, including, but not limited to: pain, bleeding, scarring, poor cosmetic outcome, inadvertent injury to adjacent structures necessitating a more complex operation for repair, infection, either at the incision sites or elsewhere, persistent air leak from the lung or bronchus, recurrence of the cancer (if appropriate), as well as those risks associated with the induction of general anesthesia, up to and including death. All questions were answered to the satisfaction of the patient and family, including all alternatives to operative intervention. The patient agreed with the need for the procedure, and informed consent was obtained.

Description of procedure: The patient was taken to the operating room and placed supine on the operating table. Following induction of general anesthesia and intubation with a single-lumen endotracheal tube, a "time out" was performed, verifying correct patient, correct procedure, and correct site. Antibiotics were then given to ensure delivery within one hour of incision. Bronchoscopy was then performed; all segments were identified bilaterally, and all visible secretions were cleared. [FINDINGS]. The single-lumen endotracheal tube was then exchanged for a double-lumen tube with bronchoscopic guidance to ensure total lung isolation.

The patient was then placed in the [SIDE] lateral decubitus position. All vulnerable pressure points were appropriately padded, the bed flexed to extend the intercostal spaces, the up arm was extended cephalad to expose the axilla and secured into place, and the patient secured to the operating table using a belt and cloth tape. After positioning was completed, correct placement of the double-lumen endotracheal tube was again bronchoscopically confirmed, and the operative lung excluded. The patient was then prepped and draped in the usual sterile fashion. A standard, posterolateral thoracotomy skin incision was made overlying the fifth intercostal space, just inferior to the tip of the scapula. Using electrocautery, subcutaneous flaps were created superiorly and inferiorly, and the dissection was carried down to the level of the latissimus dorsi, which was then divided in hemostatic fashion. The serratus anterior muscle was encountered and mobilized from the chest wall by incising its soft tissue attachments along the free edge of the muscle. The sixth rib was identified by palpation, and the 5th intercostal muscle opened anteriorly and posteriorly to the paraspinous muscles using electrocautery while staying flush with the top of the sixth rib. The pleura was then sharply incised, and digital palpation used to confirm the absence of adhesions. The fifth rib was then shingled by removing a 0.5 cm segment of the rib at the level of the paraspinal muscles.

The entire lung was then mobilized using a combination of electrocautery and sharp dissection to divide attachments to the chest wall. All lung parenchyma was visualized and palpated to rule out the presence of metastatic disease. The target nodule was then palpated. Using monopolar cautery, the inferior pulmonary ligament was divided to a point just caudal to the inferior pulmonary vein. During this maneuver, the level IX lymph node basin was identified. The overlying pleura incised, and all nodes removed after ligation of the lymphatic pedicle. We then turned our attention to dissection of the mediastinal lymph node basins. Using **[ALLISON RETRACTORS/SPONGE STICKS/DUVAL GRASPERS/RING FORCEPS]**, the lung was retracted inferiorly, exposing the superior mediastinal structures.

For Right Lung Segmentectomies

The pleura immediately cephalad to the azygous vein was sharply incised, the level III and IVR lymph nodes were bluntly skeletonized and retrieved following ligation of their lymphatic pedicles. These were sent to pathology for identification and microscopic analysis.

The lung was then retracted anteriorly and the mainstem bronchus identified. The pleura overlying the hilum was sharply incised, and the soft tissue immediately caudal to the bronchus was bluntly dissected. The level VII nodes were encountered and retrieved after ligation of their lymphatic pedicles. These were sent to pathology for identification and microscopic analysis.

For Right Upper Lobe Segmentectomies

Apical Segment: The superior venous trunk was identified and dissection continued until the apical segmental branch could be identified and isolated using a blunt clamp. The dissection was then continued over the main pulmonary artery distally, exposing its segmental branches. The apical segmental branch was identified as the first division of the main pulmonary artery. This was circumferentially dissected and divided using an endoscopic stapler with a 45-millimeter vascular load. The apical segmental branch of the superior pulmonary vein was then ligated and divided in a similar fashion. The lung was then retracted medially, allowing identification of the upper lobe bronchus. Dissection was then carried distally along the bronchus until the bifurcation of the apical and the posterior segmental divisions were visualized. The apical segmental division was then isolated and divided using an endoscopic stapler.

Posterior Segment: The superior venous trunk was identified and dissection continued until the posterior segmental branch could be identified and isolated using a blunt clamp. The dissection was then continued over the main pulmonary artery distally, exposing its segmental branches. The posterior segmental branch was identified, circumferentially dissected, and divided using an endoscopic stapler with a 45-millimeter vascular load. The posterior segmental branch of the superior pulmonary vein was then ligated and divided in a similar fashion. The lung was then retracted medially, allowing identification of the upper lobe bronchus. Dissection was then carried distally along the bronchus until the bifurcation of the apical and the posterior segmental divisions were visualized. The posterior segmental division was then isolated and divided using an endoscopic stapler.

For Right Lower Lobe Segmentectomies

Superior Segment: The oblique fissure was bluntly opened, exposing the interlobar pulmonary artery. Dissection was carried out distally along the Plane of Leriche, and the overlying lung parenchymal divided with an endoscopic stapler using successive 60-millimeter parenchymal loads. The superior segmental artery(ies) were identified and divided using vascular loads following circumferential dissection. Dissection was then carried along the inferior pulmonary vein distally until the superior segmental branch was identified as the most superior branch. This was divided in a similar fashion as the segmental artery. The bronchus intermedius was then identified and dissection carried distally until the superior segmental division was encountered. This was skeletonized and divided in similar fashion using an endoscopic stapler.

Basilar Segment: The oblique fissure was bluntly opened to expose the interlobar pulmonary artery. Dissection was continued distally along the artery, exposing the basilar segmental branch. The basilar segmental pulmonary artery was then circumferentially dissected and divided using an endoscopic stapler, taking care to preserve the branch to the middle lobe. Dissection was then carried along the inferior pulmonary vein distally until the basilar segmental branch was identified. This was divided in a similar fashion, taking care to preserve the superior pulmonary vein. The basilar division of the lower lobe bronchus was then identified and divided using an endoscopic stapler.

The intersegmental boundaries were demarcated by gentle ventilation of the lung. Successive 60 millimeter stapler loads were then used to completely divide the lung parenchyma along the line of demarcation. The lung segment was then delivered through the thoracotomy incision, the surgical margin marked with a sterile marker, and the specimen sent to pathology for identification and margin analysis.

The thoracic cavity was copiously irrigated with sterile water and hemostasis achieved. Two 28-french straight chest tubes were brought through the chest wall using stab incisions immediately inferior to the thoracotomy incision anterior to the midaxillary line. The medial chest tube was positioned posteriorly, the lateral chest tube was positioned anteriorly, and both tubes were secured to the chest wall using 0-silk sutures. These were both connected to continuous suction at 20 cm H2O pressure prior to closure of the chest wall. The lung was then inflated using recruitment maneuvers to confirm full expansion. Following confirmation of negative surgical margins, the ribs were loosely reapproximated using interrupted pericardial sutures in a figure-of-eight fashion. The serratus muscle was reattached to the chest wall using a single, 0-vicryl running suture, and the latissimus dorsi was reapproximated in 2 layers using running 0-vicryl stitches.

The subdermal tissue was closed using a running, 2-0 vicryl stitch, and the skin reapproximated using 4-0 monocryl in a running, subcuticular fashion. At the end of the operation, all sponge, needle, and instrument counts were correct. The patient was placed back in supine position and bronchoscopic clearance of all secretions was performed prior to extubation.

For All Left Lung Segmentectomies

The aortopulmonary window was identified overlying the aortic arch. The pleura overlying this area was incised sharply, the level V and VI lymph nodes were bluntly skeletonized and retrieved following ligation of their lymphatic pedicles. These were sent to pathology for identification and microscopic analysis.

For Left Upper Lobe Segmentectomies

Apicoposterior Segment: The superior venous trunk was identified and dissected circumferentially using a blunt clamp. This was then divided using an endoscopic stapler with a 45-millimeter vascular load. The dissection was then continued over the main pulmonary artery distally, exposing the segmental branches. The oblique fissure was then opened, allowing identification of the lingular branch of the pulmonary artery. All branches to the apicoposterior segment were then sequentially divided using a 45-millimeter vascular load after circumferential dissection. The segmental division of the apicoposterior segmental bronchus was then identified and divided using an endoscopic stapler.

Lingula: The oblique fissure was bluntly opened and the interlobar pulmonary artery identified. The lingular branch(es) were identified and dissected circumferentially. These were then divided using a 45-millimeter vascular load on an endoscopic stapler. The lingular bronchus was then identified and divided in a similar fashion. Attention was then turned to identification of the superior pulmonary vein from a medial approach. Dissection was continued along the vein until the lingular branch could be identified, at which point it was bluntly skeletonized and ligated using an endoscopic stapler.

For Left Lower Lobe Segmentectomies

Superior Segment: The oblique fissure was bluntly opened and dissection performed on areolar plane distally until the superior segmental artery could be positively identified, taking care to also identify the lingular and basilar branches. This was circumferentially dissected and divided. The superior segmental vein was then identified as the most superior branch of the inferior vein. This was divided in a similar fashion as the segmental artery. The bronchus intermedius was then identified and dissection carried distally until the superior segmental division was encountered. This was skeletonized and divided in similar fashion using an endoscopic stapler.

Basilar Segment: The oblique fissure was bluntly opened and dissection continued until all branches of the pulmonary artery could be identified. The basilar segmental pulmonary artery was then circumferentially dissected and divided. The basilar segmental vein was then identified at its origin from the inferior pulmonary vein. This was divided in a similar fashion, taking care to preserve the superior pulmonary vein. The basilar division of the lower lobe bronchus was then identified and divided using an endoscopic stapler.

Video-Assisted Thoracoscopic Surgery

Preoperative Diagnosis: [INDICATION for operation; typically neoplasm, but may be done for lesions with infectious or benign etiology, particularly if diagnostic uncertainty is present]

Postoperative Diagnosis: specific diagnosis (i.e. cancer histology, if not known preoperatively and if frozen section performed), other intraoperative findings

Procedure(s) Performed:
1. Thoracotomy (with laterality)
2. Segmentectomy (specify segment removed)
3. Mediastinal lymph node dissection (if done for malignancy)

Attending Surgeon: [BLANK]

Assistant Surgeon: [BLANK]

Assistants: [BLANK]

Anesthesia: [GENERAL ENDOTRACHEAL, THORACIC EPIDURAL]

Operative Findings: [Include results of frozen section specimens, anatomic variants, surgical margins]

Specimens: [Include an accurate description of all specimens sent. Typically will include mediastinal lymph nodes and levels, tissue biopsies sent to rule out metastatic disease, and the target lung segment.]

Indication(s) for Procedure: This is a [AGE] year-old [GENDER] who presented with history of [COMPLAINT/DURATION]. The patient was noted on diagnostic [CHEST RADIOGRAPHY] to have a [SIZE] nodule in the [SIDE, LOBE, AND SEGMENT]. A CT-guided biopsy was performed, which was noted to be suspicious for [TISSUE DIAGNOSIS]. (If no biopsy was performed—e.g. recent history of other malignancy with high suspicion for lung metastasis—this should be stated here.) [MEDIASTINOSCOPY/ENDOBRONCHIAL ULTRASOUND] (if performed) did not show mediastinal lymph node involvement. Based upon the patient's presentation and preoperative workup, it was determined that (he/she) would benefit from [SIDE, LOBE, AND SEGMENT] segmentectomy with mediastinal lymph node dissection (if performed for malignancy). The patient was informed of the risks and benefits of proceeding, including, but not limited to: pain, bleeding, scarring, poor cosmetic outcome, inadvertent injury to adjacent structures necessitating a more complex operation for repair, infection, either at the incision sites or elsewhere, persistent air leak from the lung or bronchus, recurrence of the cancer (if appropriate), inability to complete the operation thoracoscopically requiring conversion to an open operation, as well as those risks associated with the induction of general anesthesia, up to and including death. All questions were answered to the satisfaction of the patient and family, including all alternatives to operative intervention. The patient agreed with the need for the procedure, and informed consent was obtained.

Description of procedure: The patient was taken to the operating room and placed supine on the operating table. Following induction of general anesthesia and intubation with a single-lumen endotracheal tube, a "time out" was performed, verifying correct patient, correct procedure, and correct site. Antibiotics were then given to ensure delivery within one hour of incision. Bronchoscopy was then performed; all segments were identified bilaterally, and all visible secretions were cleared. The single-lumen endotracheal tube was then exchanged for a double-lumen tube with bronchoscopic guidance to ensure total lung isolation. The patient was then placed in the [SIDE] lateral decubitus position. All vulnerable pressure points were appropriately padded, the bed flexed to extend the intercostal spaces, the up arm was extended cephalad to expose the axilla and secured into place, and the patient secured to the operating table using a belt and cloth tape. After positioning was completed, correct placement of the double-lumen endotracheal tube was again bronchoscopically confirmed, and the operative lung excluded. The patient was then prepped and draped in the usual sterile fashion. A 1-centimeter incision was made overlying the 7th rib along the mid-axillary line. The port is placed, and a 10 millimeter, 30-degree thoracoscope was then advanced through an endoport inserted into the intercostal space, and the thoracic cavity was assessed visually. Under direct visualization, the utility port (4 cm in length) is created in anterior axillary line at the level of hilum (usually 4th intercostal space for upperlobe disease and 5th for lower lobe disease). Additional traction port is created at posterior axillary line about one hand breath away from the camera port.

The dissection and pulmonary resection is essentially identical to open operation.

Dr. [BLANK] was present and scrubbed for [BLANK] elements of this procedure.

35. Carinal Pneumonectomy

Lloyd M. Felmly, Walter F. DeNino, MD, and Chadrick E. Denlinger, MD

Medical University of South Carolina, Charleston, SC

Essential Operative Steps

(Written for right pneumonectomy, but steps that differ in action or laterality during left pneumonectomy are noted)

1. Supine positioning
2. Lines and monitoring
3. General endotracheal anesthesia (can use double lumen tube or single lumen tube advanced into the left main stem bronchus prior to accessing the pleural cavity)
4. Mediastinoscopy and node sampling
5. Positioning in the left lateral decubitus position (right lateral decubitus for left pneumonectomy)
6. Right posterolateral thoracotomy (left thoracotomy if left pneumonectomy)
7. Takedown of the ipsilateral inferior pulmonary ligament and mobilization of the lung
8. Encircle and ligate ipsilateral pulmonary veins and arteries
9. **Right:** Divide the azygos vein
10. **Left:** Mobilize and retract aortic arch laterally and cephalad (division of ligamentum arteriosum)
11. Lymphadenectomy and mobilization of the airway
12. Dissection and encircling of trachea, right main bronchus, and left main bronchus
13. **Right:** If SVC has been invaded by tumor, then heparinize, clamp the vessel proximally and distally, excise the invaded portion, and replace with appropriate available graft material
14. Withdraw endotracheal tube to the distal cervical trachea (after pre-oxygenation and hyperventilation)
15. Incise trachea (guided by flexible bronchoscopy, send frozen section for tumor-free margins)
16. Incise left main bronchus (frozen section for tumor-free margins; right main bronchus if left pneumonectomy)
17. Remove right lung and carina (or appropriate lobes; left lung if left pneumonectomy)
18. Insert small catheter into left main bronchus for ventilation (right bronchus for left pneumonectomy)
19. Contralateral node dissection
20. Traction sutures to approximate distal trachea and left main bronchus (takedown of contralateral pulmonary ligament if excess tension between apposed airways; right main bronchus if left pneumonectomy)

I. General Thoracic Surgery

21. Running sutures to parachute trachea and bronchus
22. Interrupted sutures to complete end-to-end anastomosis (avoid placing sutures on the cartilage-membranous angle or through membranous trachea)
23. Terminate cross-field ventilation and re-advance endotracheal tube
24. Test anastomosis for air leaks (ventilate up to 40cm of pressure)
25. If desired, reinforce with pedicled flap
26. **Right:** End-to-side anastomosis if residual right lung lobes are left In place (at least 2cm from previous anastomotic suture line)
27. Chest tube placement
28. Assess hemostasis
29. Thoracotomy closure
30. A guardian or "Grillo" stitch can be placed between chin and sternum (decreases airway tension)
31. Extubate in the OR

Potential Complications and Pitfalls

1. Appropriate pre-operative evaluation including PFTs
2. Mediastinoscopy should be performed in the same OR session to avoid healing and subsequent pre-tracheal scarring
3. Injury to the left recurrent laryngeal nerve during dissection
4. Injury to the thoracic duct during aortic mobilization
5. Improper deairing if SVC is resected and grafted
6. Excessive lateral dissection along the airway resulting in inadequate blood supply to the anastomosis
7. No attempt should be made to crimp or wedge the edges of the anastomosis to correct the size discrepancy between the trachea and bronchus, as this can predispose the anastomosis to development of a fistula
8. Size discrepancy between the trachea and the right main stem bronchus is common and should be corrected progressively with each suture
9. Tension on the airways leading to failure of the anastomosis
10. Tearing of the anastomosis at the cartilage-membranous angle

Template Dictation

Preoperative Diagnosis: [INDICATION – e.g. Centrally located right middle lobe nonsquamous-cell lung cancer, NSCLC invading carina]

Postoperative Diagnosis: Same

Procedure(s) Performed:

1. Cervical mediastinoscopy
2. Right/Left posterolateral thoracotomy with right/left-sided carinal pneumonectomy

Attending Surgeon: [BLANK]

Secondary Surgeon: [BLANK]

Assistants: [BLANK]

Anesthesia: [BLANK]

Indication(s) for Procedure: The patient is a [AGE] [GENDER], who presented to us in the clinic with a concerning lesion on the [RIGHT/LEFT SIDE], was [LOCATION], which demonstrated on biopsy to be consistent with [FINDINGS]. Preoperative assessment of the mediastinum including [TESTS/SCANS ORDERED] [FINDINGS]. Pre-operative PFTS included FEV1 of [VALUE] and FVC of [VALUE] with a DLCO of [VALUE]. As such, the patient was consented for mediastinoscopy, a [RIGHT/LEFT]-sided thoracotomy and pneumonectomy given [RELEVANT PREOPERATIVE EVALUATION].

Description of Procedure: The patient was brought to the operating room and placed in the supine position. Monitoring lines were positioned, and a single lumen endotracheal tube was placed after the induction of general anesthesia, a time-out confirmed the correct procedure for the correct patient and site. The patient was treated with 2G Ancef and 5000 units of subcutaneous heparin.

The patient was prepared for mediastinoscopy by positioning him/her with the head at the top of the OR table. A shoulder roll was placed behind the shoulders and the neck was maximally extended. The neck and anterior chest were prepped and draped below the level of the xiphoid process to achieve a sterile field that would allow a sternotomy if necessary. The procedure was commenced with a 2-cm incision in a horizontal fashion one fingerbreadth cranial to the suprasternal notch. The platysma was divided transversely with electrocautery and the strap muscles were divided in the midline to expose the anterior surface of the trachea. Using Metzenbaum scissors, the anterior tracheal fascia was incised, and with the fingers bluntly, a plane anterior to the trachea was developed into the thoracic inlet.

The mediastinoscope was advanced into the pretracheal plane to the level of the carina. The proximal right and left main bronchi were bluntly dissected. The azygos vein was identified cranial to the right main bronchus and the right pulmonary artery was visualized crossing over the right bronchus. Lymph node biopsies were taken from the subcarinal region and were sent for frozen section analysis labeled as level 7 lymph nodes. Additional lymph nodes were removed from above the right bronchus and were sent for analysis labeled as level 4R lymph nodes. Hemostasis was achieved in both the level 4R and 7 regions using electrocautery. Additional lymph nodes were taken just above the left main bronchus and these were sent labeled as level 4L lymph nodes. The use of electrocautery was minimized while sampling the level 4L lymph nodes in order to avoid injury to the recurrent laryngeal nerve. Frozen section analysis of the resected lymph nodes did not show any evidence of metastatic disease. [FINDINGS].

The mediastinoscope was withdrawn after hemostasis was achieved and Surgicel was placed. The incision was closed in three layers. Interrupted Vicryl sutures were used to reapproximate the strap muscles. The platysma was also closed with interrupted Vicryl sutures and the skin was closed with a running subcuticular Vicryl. The skin was sealed with topical glue. The patient was then repositioned to a left lateral decubitus position and the right chest was prepped and draped in the usual manner.

After a standard right posterolateral thoracotomy incision, electrocautery was utilized to divide the subcutaneous tissues and latissimus dorsi and enter the chest cavity at the fifth intercostal space. The serratus anterior muscle was spared in this dissection. The sixth rib was divided posteriorly to help facilitate exposure. The right lung was deflated by advancing the endotracheal tube into the left bronchus using a bronchoscope for guidance. A Finochietto retractor was used to spread the ribs and a Tuffier retractor was positioned at a right angle to the Finochietto to retract the soft tissues. The chest was visually and manually explored and there were no additional lung or pleural nodules noted.

The right inferior pulmonary ligament was divided with electrocautery to the level of the inferior pulmonary vein. Lymph nodes in the inferior pulmonary ligament were sent for pathological evaluation labeled as level 9 lymph nodes. The lung was then retracted anteriorly while the pleura overlying the posterior aspect of the hilum was divided with cautery. This provided exposure to the inferior pulmonary vein, the bronchus intermedius, upper lobe bronchus and right main bronchus. The subcarinal lymph nodes were resected and sent for evaluation labeled as level 7 lymph nodes. The carina as well as the proximal left main bronchus was identified. The azygos vein was divided and the mediastinal pleura overlying the trachea was divided as well. The lung was then retracted posteriorly while the pleura overlying the anterior aspect of the hilum was divided sharply with a Metzenbaum scissors in order to avoid thermal injury to the phrenic nerve. This provided exposure to the anterior surface of the superior and inferior pulmonary veins as well as the upper aspect of the right pulmonary artery.

The inferior pulmonary vein was then dissected circumferentially using blunt dissection. An endo-GIA stapler with a vascular load was then used to divide the vein. The superior pulmonary vein was then circumferentially dissected bluntly prior to its division with the endo-GIA stapler using a second vascular load. The proximal right main pulmonary artery was then carefully dissected away from the right bronchus. The pulmonary artery was stapled twice with a linear stapler prior to its division was a #15 blade knife.

At this point a sterile ventilation circuit was passed off the field and prepared for the use of cross-field ventilation. After adequate pre-oxygenation, the ventilator was turned off and the endotracheal tube was withdrawn to the midlevel of the trachea. The left main bronchus was divided sharply with a #10 blade knife in an area that was as close to the carina as possible, but also free of gross tumor involvement. The transected bronchial lumen was then visually inspected to ensure that there was no gross evidence of disease. Two 2-0 silk sutures were then placed in the left main bronchus at the junction between the cartilaginous and membranous portions as traction sutures. An 8-0 armored endotracheal tube was then advanced into the transected bronchus to ventilate the left lung using the sterile circuit which had been passed off the field to the anesthesiologists. The trachea was then transected above the tumor. At this point the lung was completely free from the mediastinal structures and it was passed off the field and sent for pathological evaluation. The tracheal and left bronchial margins were both marked and frozen section analysis was performed. The mediastinal resection bed was examined to confirm meticulous hemostasis.

After confirming negative bronchial margins, the airway anastomosis was undertaken. The entire anastomosis was completed using interrupted 3-0 Vicryl sutures. The first sutures were placed between the left side of the trachea and the most superior margin of the left bronchus. Care was taken to compensate for the difference in luminal diameter between the trachea and bronchus. Each of these sutures were pre-placed and tied with the knots inside the lumen after they all were placed. Each of the sutures approximating the membranous portion of airway was placed. While these sutures were placed the endotracheal tube was intermittently removed from bronchus to facilitate better visualization. After each of the sutures was placed the bronchial endotracheal tube was removed and the trans-oral endotracheal tube was advanced by the anesthesiologist across the anastomosis into the left bronchus. This was manually directed from the surgical field. The sutures on the membranous airway were then tied with knots on the outside of the lumen. Finally, sutures were placed to re-approximate the remaining cartilaginous portion of the airway between the right wall of the trachea and the inferior aspect of the bronchus. After each of these sutures was placed, they were tied with the knots on the outside of the lumen.

The endotracheal tube was then withdrawn back into the trachea and the chest cavity was filled with warm saline. The airway was pressurized to 30 cm of water and the anastomosis was observed for an air leak. No bubbles were seen and the saline was aspirated. [SOFT TISSUE COVERAGE OF ANASTOMOSIS MAY BE PERFORMED AS WELL]. The chest cavity was again thoroughly inspected to assure complete hemostasis. A single 28 French chest tube was placed into the chest cavity and it was secured at the skin with a 0-silk suture.

The ribs were re-approximated with #2 Vicryl sutures. The serratus anterior was re-approximated to the tissues inferior to the muscle belly with #0 Vicryl and the latissimus dorsi fascia was closed with a running #0 Vicryl. The deep dermal and subcuticular layers were closed with running 2-0 and 3-0 sutures respectively. A sterile dressing was placed over the incision. The chest tube was then clamped and attached to a collection chamber without suction. The patient was then placed in the supine position on the operating table and a #0 prolene suture was placed between his chin and the skin overlying the sternal angle of Louis to prevent the head from being extended beyond the neutral position. The patient was then extubated in the operating room and transferred to the intensive care unit for routine monitoring.

At the end the procedure, all sponge, instrument, and needle counts were reported correct.

Dr. **[BLANK]** was present and scrubbed for **[BLANK]** elements of this procedure.

36. Extrapleural Pneumonectomy for Mesothelioma

George Makdisi, MD, Francis C. Nichols III, MD

Mayo Clinic, Rochester, MN

Essential Operative Steps

1. Lines and Monitoring
2. General endotracheal anesthesia and thoracic epidural
3. Double-lumen endotracheal tube (left-sided for right pneumonectomy and right-sided if possible for left pneumonectomy)
4. Excise the tract of previous biopsy procedure, or Pleurx tract
5. Extended posterolateral thoracotomy, divide the latissimus and serratus
6. Excise the sixth rib for improved exposure
7. Begin extrapleural dissection around the circumference of the incision, separating the tumor from the endothoracic fascia. Envision creating an envelope consisting of the parietal pleura with the lung on the inside
8. Continue the dissection up to and over the apex, avoiding injuries to the subclavian artery on the left and the innominate artery and SVC on the right. Continue along the descending aorta, along the diaphragm and along the mediastinum
9. On the left, careful sharp dissection lateral and anterior to the descending thoracic aorta performed up to about the level of the aortic arch taking care to not injure the vagus nerve, recurrent laryngeal nerve and again any intercostal arteries.
10. The tumor is unresectable if there is an invasion of vital mediastinal structures, (e.g., aorta, vena cava, esophagus, epicardium, or trachea) or chest wall. If the tumor is deemed unresectable, chest tubes are placed and the chest closed
11. The diaphragm is circumferentially excised (or, alternatively, avulsed from the chest wall). Care is taken to avoid entering the peritoneum. Sometimes entry into the peritoneal cavity is unavoidable in which case the peritoneum is closed with absorbable suture.
12. The crura are preserved protecting.
13. The pericardium is opened anteriorly and resected form inferior to superior and anterior to posterior down to the level of the hilum.
14. Intrapericardial division of the pulmonary veins
15. Division of the pulmonary artery (intrapericardially on the right and extrapericardially on the left)
16. The mainstem bronchus is divided almost flush with the carina using a TA 30 thick staple load. Just prior to firing the staple load, a breath is given by the anesthesiologist confirming no obstruction of the contralateral left mainstem bronchus.
17. The entire en bloc specimen is removed.
18. Chest is copiously irrigated with warm saline and sterile water.
19. Hemostasis is assured.

20. Ipsilateral divided bronchial stump is tested to rule out air leaks by submerging beneath saline and having anesthesia insufflate the ipsilateral side to 40 mm Hg.
21. Thoracic lymphadenectomy or lymph node sampling: stations 2R, 4R, 7, 8, 9, 10R for right sided tumors and stations 4L, 5, 6, 7, 8, 9, and 10L for left sided tumors.
22. Consider prophylactic ligation of the thoracic duct for right sided tumors, especially if there is a high suspicion for duct injury.
23. There often isn't local tissue to routinely cover the bronchus. Consider bringing up an omental pedicle through the diaphragmatic opening.
24. The diaphragm is reconstructed with a somewhat floppy 2 mm thick polytetrafluoroethylene (PTFE) patch. The patch is reimplanted into the chest wall anteriorly, laterally, and posteriorly with individually placed #1 nonabsorbable suture. Medially the patch is secured to the crura and remaining pericardium with 0 nonabsorbable suture. A laparoscopic tacking device can be helpful to secure the patch posteriorly.
25. The pericardial defect is reconstructed with a 1 mm thick fenestrated PTFE patch. The patch is secured in place with either running or interrupted #2-0 nonabsorbable suture.
26. Hemostasis is again meticulously checked for and the chest again irrigated with several liters of warm saline.
27. 500 - 750 cc of antibiotic solution similar to a Clagett closure is left within the chest cavity at the discretion of the surgeon.
28. An angled 28 Fr. straight chest tube is tunneled, placed in the chest cavity, and loosely secured in place with a #0-silk pursestring suture. The chest tube is placed to water seal (AND NEVER TO SUCTION).
29. The chest is then closed in the usual fashion with multiple layers of running # 1 absorbable suture. The skin is closed with a running #4-0 subcuticular suture. A sterile dressing is applied
30. The patient is rolled to the supine position. The authors prefer removing the chest tube at this point. With a breath given by the anesthesiologist and held at 40 mm Hg pressure, the chest tube is removed in the usual fashion, the #0-silk pursestring suture tied and a sterile dressing applied.
31. Chest x-ray obtained to assess the contralateral lung and pleural space and confirm appropriate midline positioning of the mediastinal structures.
32. Patient is taken to the recovery room and extubated when appropriate.

Potential Complications and Pitfalls

1. The authors do not routinely perform laparoscopy unless there are concerns raised on the preoperative imaging in which case laparoscopy is performed to rule out peritoneal involvement
2. The position of the operating table will change during various phases of the operation from steep Trendelenburg (apical dissection) to reverse Trendelenburg (diaphragmatic dissection), to tilted left and right for anterior and posterior mediastinal dissections

3. Excise the previous biopsy tracts
4. Place an NG tube to facilitate identification of the esophagus during the dissection
5. The tumor is unresectable if there is an invasion of vital mediastinal structures (e.g., aorta, vena cava, esophagus, epicardium, or trachea) or diffuse chest wall involvement.
6. Pericardial invasion does not preclude resection; however, if myocardial invasion is found the tumor is deemed unresectable. Open the pericardium medial to the area of concern and palpate for myocardial invasion.
7. For right sided EPPs, avoid ligating the azygous vein. If the vein is ligated, it can increase venous hypertension and possibly contribute to bleeding and to lymphatic leaks.
8. For right EPPs, take care to avoid injuring the IVC and retrohepatic veins during the extrapleural dissection and diaphragmatic reconstruction.
9. Avoid injury to the internal mammary artery and vein.
10. For patients who have had prior CABG with an ipsilateral IMA graft, special care must be taken to avoid injuring the graft.
11. Avoid ligation of intercostal arteries
12. Avoid injury to the recurrent laryngeal nerves, which can lead to aspiration or other pulmonary complications.
13. Prior to dividing the PA, check for a rise in the PA pressures. An undue rise may preclude an EPP.
14. Argon beam coagulation to the endothoracic fascia is helpful both for tumorlysis and for hemostasis.
15. Assure adequate pain control, aggressive chest physiotherapy and early mobility, physical therapy and effective pulmonary hygiene are very important factors in postoperative period.
16. Bronchoscopy is used liberally to clear secretions
17. In the absence of bleeding, hemodynamic instability in the OR may be due to an overly constrictive pericardial patch or undue constriction on the IVC (for right-sided diaphragmatic reconstructions)

Template Dictation

Preoperative Diagnosis: Biopsy proven malignant mesothelioma of the [left/ right] chest

Postoperative Diagnosis: Same

Procedure(s) Performed:

1. Partial excision sixth rib
2. [LEFT/ RIGHT] extrapleural pneumonectomy
3. left/right thoracic lymphadenectomy

Attending Surgeon: [BLANK]

I. General Thoracic Surgery

Secondary Surgeon: [BLANK]

Assistants: [BLANK]

Anesthesia: [eg: Thoracic epidural and general endotracheal anesthesia with double lumen endotracheal tube.]

Indication(s) for Procedure: [INDICATION – e.g.[MR/ MRS.] [BLANK] is a [AGE] year-old [gender] who presented biopsy proven malignant [EPITHELIOID, SARCOMATOID OR BIPHASIC TYPE] mesothelioma. Workup included: [CXR, CT, PET, Echocardiography, and PFTs-]. There was no evidence of diffuse metastatic cancer, and [Mr/Mrs.] [BLANK] was deemed an appropriate surgical candidate.[He/She] are now brought to the operating room in satisfactory condition for planned surgical resection.

Description of Procedure:

Left-Sided Extrapleural Pneumonectomy

After a team surgical briefing, the patient was brought to the operating room in satisfactory condition. Under general endotracheal anesthesia with a double-lumen endotracheal tube in place, the patient was placed in the right lateral decubitus position and prepared and draped in the usual fashion. After the surgical pause, an extended left posterolateral thoracotomy incision was made. Both the latissimus dorsi and serratus anterior were divided. The 6th rib was excised, taking care not to enter to pleural space. We began the extrapleural dissection, separating the pleura from the endothoracic fascia. We immediately encountered marked thickening of the parietal pleura. Dissection was carried posteriorly and superiorly and then anteriorly and superiorly. Attention was directed to the apex of the left chest, we were able to further dissect things free and ultimately separate the subclavian artery from the apex of the lung. The dissection was then carried inferiorly. The aortic arch was identified. The vagus nerve was identified and care taken to protect the recurrent laryngeal nerve. Using a combination of blunt and sharp dissection to separate the pleura from the aorta, we continued the dissection caudally along the descending thoracic aorta down to the costophrenic recess. The extrapleural dissection continued along the diaphragm and then along the mediastinum. Pericardium was entered anteromedially. The pericardial space was palpated. There was no evidence of tumor invasion into the epicardium. The pericardial opening was then extended from the level of the inferior pulmonary vein to the PA. The diaphragm was then incised from its lateral margin and dissected bluntly off the underlying peritoneum, circumferential resection of the diaphragm ensued. [**Description of the Disease Burden – i.e. *Overall, there was diffuse tumor involvement of the pleura. However, most of the disease burden was on the diaphragm and the pleura overlying the lower lobe.***]

The pulmonary artery isolated extrapericardially. The PA was clamped with a TA-30 vascular load stapler. There was no significant increase in the PA pressure. The stapler was fired, and the PA was divided. The superior pulmonary vein and inferior pulmonary veins were divided intrapericardially using separate firings of a TA-30 vascular load stapler. The posterior pericardial resection continued down to the left mainstem bronchus. The left mainstem bronchus was dissected free from the mediastinal tissues and divided flush with the carina using a TA-30 green load stapler under direct bronchoscopic visualization. The EPP specimen was sent to pathology as a permanent specimen. No gross residual mesothelioma was left in the pleural cavity upon completion of this radical resection. The bronchus was submerged in saline. There was no bubbling with a 40 mm Hg breath hold, indicating that the bronchial stump was completely intact.

A thoracic lymphadenectomy was completed. All lymph nodes were removed from stations 5, 6, 7, 8L, 9L, and 10L. The chest was copiously irrigated with several liters of warm saline and water. Hemostasis was secure.

We then proceeded with our reconstruction. The diaphragm was rebuilt with 2-mm thick PTFE patch secured in place with numerous #1 Polypropylene sutures. The pericardium was then rebuilt also with fenestrated piece of 1-mm thick PTFE secured in place with running #2-0 Polypropylene suture. The chest was irrigated again, and hemostasis was assured. The chest was irrigated with 1000 cc of modified DABS solution (Gentamicin/Polymyxin B irrigation solution). A third of the modified DABS solution was left in the pleural cavity. A single 28-French straight chest tube was placed. A surgical pause confirmed that all needle, sponge, and instrument counts were correct. No. 1 absorbable pericostal sutures were utilized and the muscle layers closed with multiple running #1 absorbable suture. The subcutaneous layer closed with running #2-0 absorbable suture and the skin reapproximated with #4-0 subcuticular suture. Sterile pressure dressings were applied. The patient was rolled to the supine position with positive pressure ventilation to 40 mm Hg. The chest tube was removed without difficulty. The chest tube site was closed with a# 2-0 polypropylene suture. The patient tolerated the operative procedures and left the operating room in satisfactory condition.

Dr. [BLANK] was present and scrubbed for [BLANK] elements of this procedure.

Right-Sided Extrapleural Pneumonectomy

Same as above except for the following:

- Insertion of NG tube to aid in identification and protection of the esophagus.
- The posterior dissection proceeds along the azygos vein instead of the descending thoracic aorta.
- Watch for the thoracic duct, if there is concern for a lymph leak then the thoracic duct is mass ligated with a #2-0 silk suture near the hiatus
- Thoracic lymphadenectomy on the right side includes lymph node stations 2R, 4R, 7, 8R, 9R, and 10R.

37. Lung Procurement

Mara B. Antonoff, MD and Michael K. Pasque, MD

Washington University, St. Louis, MO

Essential Operative Steps

1. Initial on-site donor evaluation
2. Bronchoscopy
3. Incision / access
4. Visualization
5. Lung recruitment
6. Thoracic organ dissection
7. Cardioplegia/pulmoplegia cannula placement
8. Heparinization
9. PGE
10. SVC ligation
11. Left atrial venting
12. IVC hemi-transection
13. Aortic crossclamp
14. Infusion of cardioplegia/pulmoplegia
15. Extubation
16. Dissection / removal of heart
17. Retrograde flush
18. Division of mediastinal tissue
19. Tracheal transection
20. Esophageal transection
21. Pericardial division
22. Division of inferior pulmonary ligaments
23. Esophageal transection
24. Aortic transection
25. Division of remaining mediastinal posterior attachments
26. Lung block removal and packaging

Note that the above steps presume that the heart is being removed for either recipient implantation or for research purposes. If the heart is not to be used at all, minor adjustments apply, which are addressed below.

Potential Complications and Pitfalls

1. Standard midline sternotomies are aesthetically displeasing and limit options for open-casket funerals. Y-shaped midline skin incisions sparing the neck and upper chest are appreciated by families, frequently requested by funeral homes, and mandated by some organ procurement organizations.
2. The practice of sequentially eviscerating the lungs from the pleural cavity to perform recruitment of the atelectatic areas of the lungs is strongly

discouraged. In situ recruitment or slight lung displacement is more than adequate to clear atelectasis and lessens the possibility of severe lung hyperinflation, injury to hilar structures, and the hemodynamic compromise that is always associated with unilateral lung evisceration. Although the routine donor may tolerate short periods of transient hemodynamic compromise, the downward spiral that can be initiated by such maneuvers in the borderline donor can place all organs—and thus their potential recipients—at immediate and unnecessary risk.

3. The practice of routine division of the azygos vein by inexperienced operators has resulted in a significant incidence of unnecessary hemorrhage, as well as damage to the adjacent upper lobe branch of the right pulmonary artery. In most cases, a single suture tie can be placed around it near its junction with the superior vena cava and the azygos can be divided later during organ extraction.

4. The pulmonary artery cannulation site should be a minimum of 1.5 cm from the pulmonary valve to guarantee a generous cuff of main pulmonary artery for the subsequent cardiac implantation procedure. Placement near or even at the bifurca- tion of the main pulmonary artery still leaves more than enough right and left pulmonary artery length for bilateral lung transplantation. When the pulmoplegia cannula is being placed in the distal main pulmonary artery, the tip of the cannula is pointed backward toward the pulmonary valve. This prevents the preferential perfusion of one lung that may otherwise occur. If the heart is not being used for implantation in a live recipient, the pulmoplegia cannula can be placed in the proximal main pulmonary artery near the pulmonary valve instead of distally near the pulmonary artery bifurcation. When placed more proximally, the tip of the pulmoplegia cannula is directed toward the bifurcation of the main pulmonary artery

5. It is not necessary to dissect the fascial attachments between the trachea and esophagus during the initial organ dissection *prior to* organ preservation. Overzealous manipulation can result in several untoward events, including dislodgment of the endotracheal tube or perforation of the esophagus or membranous trachea with mediastinal soiling.

6. Venting through the left atrium adjacent to the right superior pulmonary vein in Waterston's groove will provide excellent left heart decompression as long as a sucker is immediately placed through it into the left atrium. The primary advantage of this vent site location is the elimination of the need for suture closure of the left atrial appendage vent site. It also assures an adequate right pulmonary vein cuff.

7. It is important to carry out the organ preservation procedure in the correct order. Left ventricular distention invariably occurs if the aortic crossclamp is applied (thus preventing left ventricular emptying) as the first step in the organ preservation procedure, before reduction in left atrial and ventricular return.

8. The adequacy of cardioplegic solution delivery must be assured by a rapid cessation of cardiac contractile and electrical activity. The adequacy

of aortic root pressure and absence of ventricular distention must be continually monitored during infusion of cardioplegic solution. Left ventricular distention during infusion of cardioplegic solution mandates immediate attention. Simply passing the left atrial sucker across the mitral valve (like a standard left ventricular vent) is the most efficient method to eliminate this problem. Repeated distention of the heart suggests that either aortic insufficiency is present or that the vena caval and left atrial venting maneuvers are not adequate and in need of immediate further attention.

9. The flow of gradually clearing pulmoplegia solution from the left atrial vent site must be monitored during its infusion. Equal distribution of perfusate to both lungs must be assured, and both lungs should "blanch" equally. The midline positioning of the tip of the pulmonary artery perfusion cannula must be intermittently confirmed to assure that differential flow to one lung over the other is not occurring secondary to inadvertent cannula displacement.

10. During the retrograde pulmoplegia flush, the return of clear solution into the ipsilateral pulmonary artery assures that the infusion is proceeding correctly. One should be sure to watch for the occasional pulmonary embolus as it is flushed from the pulmonary artery, which should be noted, but is, of yet, of unclear clinical significance.

11. If the heart is not being used for a live recipient, there is no need to preserve a left atrial cuff for cardiac implantation. The left atrial incision can therefore be initiated immediately adjacent to the interatrial groove posteriorly. This maneuver optimizes the size of the left atrial cuff that remains attached to the pulmonary veins. The incision is continued in the atrioventricular groove circumferentially around the heart, leaving the entire left atrium with the lung block.

Template Dictation

Preoperative Diagnosis: [INDICATION—e.g. brain death secondary to trauma, etc.]

Postoperative Diagnosis: Same

Procedure(s) Performed: Bilateral donor pneumonectomy (+/- CARDIECTOMY)

Attending Surgeon: [BLANK]

Secondary Surgeon: [BLANK]

Assistants: [BLANK]

Anesthesia: General Endotracheal

Indication(s) for Procedure: [AGE] year old [GENDER] with [DURATION] history of [INDICATION]. A suitable recipient was identified and the family provided proper informed consent for organ donation.

Description of Procedure: Donor/Recipient blood typing and compatibility were confirmed with a review of all pertinent donor history. The patient was brought to the operating room with a single-lumen endotracheal tube already in place. Standard monitoring lines were already in place, including [**LINE TYPES**] in the [**LATERALITY**] [**VESSEL**].

Donor hemodynamics, inotrope/pressor infusions, telemetry monitoring, echocardiogram, and chest CT, and latest arterial blood gas were reviewed. The patient was positioned supine. Both arms were tucked. Bronchoscopy was performed and the airways were examined to ensure suitability for donation. Bronchoscopic examination revealed [**BRONCHOCSCOPIC FINDINGS**—e.g. normal, healthy airways; thick/thin secretions which cleared easily/recurred after clearance, minor suctioning trauma, etc]. After prepping and draping, access was obtained through a Y-shaped midline skin incision sparing the neck and upper chest. Using electrocautery, tissues were dissected down to the sternum, and a median sternotomy was performed in standard fashion.

Bilateral pleural spaces were entered, and the lungs were palpated and visually inspected. Findings including [**FINDINGS**—e.g. apical scarring, granulomas, adhesions, normal healthy lungs, etc] were reported to the recipient team along with the anticipated cross-clamp time.

Recruitment was attempted of all atelectatic lung segments via gentle massage and sustained inflation to 20-30 cm H2O pressure. A pericardial well was created, and the heart and great vessels were examined for anatomic abnormalities and injuries [**NOTE ANY SUCH FINDINGS**].

Thoracic organ dissection was initiated by carefully separating the main and right pulmonary arteries from the ascending aorta, followed by taking down of the attachments of the right pulmonary artery to the superior vena cava. The superior vena cava was further dissected free of all circumferential mediastinal attachments up to and including the innominate vein (if cardiac transplantation is anticipated). The azygos vein was ligated near its juncture with the superior vena cava. A heavy silk suture was passed around the superior vena cava above the level of the azygos vein.

Attention was turned toward careful sharp dissection of Waterston's inter-atrial groove in order to allow easier subsequent differentiation of the cardiac and pulmonary left atrial cuffs, as well as to facilitate left atrial venting.

A horizontal mattress #4-0 Prolene stitch was placed in the anterior midportion of the ascending aorta to later secure the cardioplegia cannula. An identical stitch was placed in the [**DISTAL** if taking the heart vs PROXIMAL if not using the heart] pulmonary artery. The posterior pericardium overlying the trachea (between the superior vena cava and ascending aorta) was incised cephalad to the right pulmonary artery, allowing gentle dissection of the trachea above the carina.

With careful finger dissection, the anterior, lateral, and medial surfaces of the trachea were cleared to facilitate more rapid tracheal access during actual organ excision.

Careful communication occurred between our team and [**THE ABDOMINAL TRANSPLANT TEAM AND ALL**] receiving team[S] in order to assure appropriate timing of heparinization and cross-clamp. 30,000 units of heparin [**OR OTHER DOSE IF APPROPRIATE**] were administered via central venous access. After 3 minutes, the cardioplegia and pulmoplegia cannulae were placed and connected to their respective infusion tubing. A high-flow 6.5 mm metal-tip cannula was used for the pulmoplegia, and a standard cardioplegia cannula for the heart preservation. The lung was reexamined for significant atelectasis, and [**NONE WAS FOUND** vs **ADDITIONAL RECRUITMENT MANEUVERS WERE UNDERTAKEN.**] A syringe of prostaglandin E1 was injected into the main pulmonary artery immediately adjacent to the pulmoplegia cannula. The superior vena cava was occluded with the previously placed supra-azygos silk suture by [**TYING THE SUTURE** vs **COMING DOWN ON THE RIMMEL TOURNIQUETTE**]. The left atrium was vented by [**ATRIAL VENTING TECHNIQUE**—e.g. transecting the tip of the left atrial appendage, making the initial portion of the left atrial incision between the atrioventricular groove and the left inferior pulmonary vein, or **ideally** (see pitfalls above) making the initial portal of the left atrial incision adjacent to the right superior pulmonary vein in the previously dissected Waterston inter-atrial groove]. The inferior vena cava was then vented with hemitransection (one centimeter above the diaphragmatic reflection if the heart is being used for transplantation).

The aortic cross-clamp was applied and the cardioplegic infusion was begun at a pressure of approximately 80 mm Hg, while the pulmoplegia was initiated through the high-flow cannula at gravity pressure. Tidal volume was reduced by half to allow a large volume of saline slush to be placed into both pleural spaces and the pericardial well. 5.6 liters of pulmoplegia were infused in an antegrade fashion, with cardioplegia infused until the pulmoplegia was done [**WITH A TOTAL OF BLANK ML GIVEN**—should be at least a liter in an adult, but variable maximum depending on how long the lung perfusion takes). During this period, the adequacy of pulmoplegia [+/- **CARDIOPLEGIA**] was ensured by monitoring the direction of the pulmoplegia catheter and equal blanching of both lungs [+/- **ADEQUATE AORTIC ROOT PRESSURE**].

After the completion of preservation infusion, the apex of the heart was elevated and the inferior vena caval transection was completed. The left atrial incision was extended from the vent site in Waterston's groove. Extension of this initial left atrial incision was carried out under the inferior edge of the inferior vena cava. The incision was further extended on the undersurface of the left atrium parallel to the AV groove, halfway between the inferior pulmonary veins and the AV groove. It was extended to the base of the left atrial appendage. The left atrial incision was then completed from inside the left atrium, allowing visualization of the orifices of all 4 pulmonary veins. The right and left innominate veins were transected along with the azygos vein. The arch vessels were each transected and the descending aorta divided just beyond the left subclavian with care taken not to injure the pulmonary artery near the ligamentum arteriosum. The main pulmonary artery was then transected at the level of the pulmoplegia cannulation site. The heart was removed from the field [**AND SUBMERGED IN A STERILE PLASTIC TRANSPORTATION CANISTER FILLED WITH PRESERVATION FLUID AND SEALED IN A STERILE PLASTIC TRANSPORT BAG FILLED WITH ICE**].

After removal of the heart, the lung perfusion was completed by instilling another 250 mL of retrograde flush to each of the 4 pulmonary veins, with care taken to examine for pulmonary emboli coming up through retrograde flushing. [**PE'S NOTED**—no PE's were seen, one large PE was extracted from a specific side, etc].

After completing the retrograde flush, all mediastinal tissue was divided at the level of the aortic arch vessels down to the level of the mid-trachea. The donor was extubated and all tubes including temperature probes and gastric tubes were removed from the esophagus. The trachea was digitally separated from the esophagus and divided between 2 TA-30 staple loads. The esophagus was mobilized and divided with a 45 mm GIA stapler. All remaining mediastinal tissue was then divided straight back to the thoracic spine, and the remaining organ block was gently lifted up as it was sharply dissected off of the spine down to the level of the mid-thorax.

Attention was then turned to the lower thorax, where the pericardium was divided near its diaphragmatic attachments. Both inferior pulmonary ligaments were mobilized and divided sharply. The lower esophagus was divided with a second firing of the GIA 45 mm stapler. The descending aorta was sharply transected. All remaining lower mediastinal tissue was then divided straight back to the spine, being careful to protect lung parenchyma. The remaining posterior mediastinal attachments were taken sharply against the spine, moving cephalad, until the double-lung block was free.

[**DESCRIBE BACK TABLE DISSECTION, IF PERFORMED, I.E. IF THE TWO LUNGS ARE DESTINED FOR 2 SEPARATE INSTITUTIONS**: The donor aorta and esophagus were resected posteriorly. The left atrial cuff was divided in the midline, pericardium divided in the midline, the pulmonary artery was divided at its bifurcation, and the left main bronchus was amputated. Both hila were then fully prepared, mobilizing the pulmonary artery to the first upper lobe branch, and dividing the bronchus one ring proximal to the upper lobe takeoff.

Excessive pericardium on both sides was then resected.]

The double-lung block [vs **EACH SINGLE LUNG SEPARATELY**] was placed in a sterile plastic transport bag filled with cold perfusate solution, while the lungs were examined for any unexpected pathology or surgical damage. The sterile plastic transport bag was sealed and placed into a second bag, with added ice slush. This bag was then placed into a third sealed bag. The bag was labeled, placed in a secure ice chest, and covered with ice. All relevant documentation from the donor was secured into the ice chest. Final updates were communicated to the receiving team.

Our team then left the donor operating room with the lungs [vs **HEART AND LUNGS**] **[WHILE THE ABDOMINAL TEAM CONTINUED TO WORK]**. The cooler was expeditiously taken from the facility accompanied by Dr. **[NAME]**.

Complications: There were no complications noted. **[OR NOTE IF THERE WERE AND WHAT THEY WERE]**

Dr. **[BLANK]** was present and scrubbed for **[BLANK]** elements of this procedure.

38. Lung Transplantation

Mara B. Antonoff, MD and G. Alexander Patterson, MD

Washington University, St. Louis, MO

Essential Operative Steps
1. Lines and monitoring, including femoral arterial line placed by surgical team
2. General endotracheal anesthesia
3. +/- Preoperative bronchoscopy
4. Intraoperative transesophageal echocardiogram
5. Incision: Bilateral anterior thoracotomy vs. clamshell thoracotomy vs. median sternotomy vs. posterolateral thoracotomy
6. Dissect out recipient lung(s). Isolate the main pulmonary arteries, pulmonary veins, and mainstem bronchi.
7. Back-table donor lung preparation
8. CPB decision, +/- cannulation and initiation of bypass
9. Explant lungs
10. Anastomoses in the following order: 1). Bronchus, 2). Pulmonary artery, 3). Vein (left atrial cuff)
11. Reperfusion
12. +/- CPB weaning and decannulation
13. Closure
14. Bronchoscopy

Potential Complications and Pitfalls
1. Decision of single vs. bilateral lung transplant: it is generally accepted that patients with septic lung disease, particularly cystic fibrosis and bronchiectasis, require a bilateral lung transplants in order to remove the entire focus of sepsis and prevent soiling of the allograft lung. However, patients with diseases such as emphysema tend to have favorable outcomes with either single or bilateral lung transplants. Considerations for single vs. bilateral transplant may be based on age, size, and co-morbidities. Bilateral lung transplants emphasized among those who are younger, fitter, and taller.
2. For patients with emphysema, it is important to avoid hyperinflation of the native lungs. If hypotension occurs prior to chest opening, positive pressure ventilation should be disconnected allowing intrathoracic pressure to return to normal.
3. For any patients whose indication is septic lung disease, preoperative bronchoscopy using an adult bronchoscope through a single-lumen tube is a critical step. All attempts should be made to thoroughly clear the airways of purulent secretions, which helps reduce the need for cardiopulmonary bypass. If preoperative bronchoscopy is not warranted, the patient may be intubated with a standard left-sided double lumen tube

upon induction.
4. During incision and entry into thoracic cavity, avoid internal mammary artery injury. Care should also be taken to avoid injury to recipient lungs.
5. For bilateral lung transplants, the decision as to which lung should be done first is based on the quantitative V/Q scan. The lung that contributes a small percentage of the total ventilation and perfusion should be removed first. This allows greater success with single-lung ventilation, using the healthier native lung during the transplant of the more diseased side, and ventilation through the new donor lung during the dissection and implantation of the second lung. This strategy aids in avoidance of cardiopulmonary bypass. Further, if there were to be an event that would mandate aborting the procedure prior to completing the implantation of both lungs, it would be advantageous to transplant the more diseased lung first.
6. Attempts should be made to detach all pleural adhesions and fully mobilize both hila prior to explantation of the first lung. Careful attention must be directed toward managing travel times for organ procurement, in order to minimize the ischemic time of the transplanted lungs and to also minimize the amount of time that the first implanted lung is exposed to the entire cardiac output (thereby decreasing risk of reperfusion edema in that lung).
7. The decision regarding the use of cardiopulmonary bypass is made based on data obtained from the pulmonary artery catheter, arterial blood gases, and trans-esophageal echocardiography. Hemodynamic instability, inability to adequately oxygenate or ventilate with one lung, dramatic increases in pulmonary arterial pressures with unilateral pulmonary artery clamping, and deterioration of right ventricular function are all potential reasons for cardiopulmonary bypass. In order to minimize perioperative hemorrhage, all attempts should be made to do as much of the dissection as possible and achieve optimal hemostasis on the chest well prior to systemic heparinization and entry onto bypass.
8. Size-mismatched lungs: if oversized, and recognized on the back table, a lobectomy can be performed; if appreciated after implantation, appropriate wedge resections can be performed, targeting the lingula and right middle lobe using stapling devices.
9. Perioperative hemorrhage: may be related to large raw surface area created after explantation of septic lungs or those that were previously pleurodesed, and is exacerbated by cardiopulmonary bypass. This may be avoided with meticulous attention to stopping all surgically correctable bleeding and aggressive correction of coagulopathies. Leaving the chest open (and covered with a temporary dressing) followed by delayed chest closure 24 to 48 hours later is useful in some circumstances.
10. Technically unsatisfactory bronchial anastomosis: easily identified in the OR at postimplantation bronchoscopy. Immediate revision should be performed for inaccurate alignment and inadequate caliber.
11. PA or PV anastomotic problems: may be identified via persistent

pulmonary hypertension, unexplained hypoxemia, pulmonary edema or findings on intraoperative TEE. Nuclear perfusion scans can be performed immediately post-op in the ICU or even in the OR to identify any issues with flow to either lung. Gradients can be identified with comparison of pressures on either side of the anastomosis measured intraoperatively or with contrast angiography postoperatively. Surgical correction must be performed if clinically relevant gradient exists.

12. Primary graft dysfunction: compromised PaO2 to FiO2 ratio in the first 48 hours and the findings of panlobar infiltrates on postoperative CXRs. (ISHLT grading system) Managed with aggressive cardiopulmonary support in ICU, using PEEP, diuresis, iNO, aerosolized prostacyclin, and, if otherwise unresponsive, ECMO and/or retransplantation. Avoid by ensuring absence of donor infection/aspiration/contusion, careful attention to appropriate cold storage, limiting hyperinflation during/after procurement, using optimal lung preservation strategies, and minimization of ischemic times.

Template Dictation

Preoperative Diagnosis: [INDICATION—e.g. pulmonary fibrosis, cystic fibrosis, chronic obstructive pulmonary disease, etc.]

Postoperative Diagnosis: Same

Procedure(s) Performed: [**BILATERAL** vs **LEFT SINGLE** vs **RIGHT SINGLE**] lung transplant (+/- cardiopulmonary bypass)

Attending Surgeon: [BLANK]

Secondary Surgeon: [BLANK]

Assistants: [BLANK]

Anesthesia: General Endotracheal

Indication(s) for Procedure: [AGE] year old [GENDER] with [DURATION] history of [INDICATION]. A suitable donor was identified. The harvest was conducted by our team and the organs were separated into separate lung grafts upon arrival at [HOSPITAL].

Description of Procedure: The patient was brought to the operating room and general anesthesia was induced. [**A SINGLE LUMEN ENDOTRACHEAL TUBE WAS INITIALLY PLACED IN ORDER TO ALLOW THOROUGH SECRETION CLEARANCE VIA BRONCHOSCOPY. THE TUBE WAS SUBSEQUENTLY CHANGED OVER TO A STANDARD LEFT-SIDED DOUBLE LUMEN TUBE**] or [**THE PATIENT WAS INTUBATED WITH A LEFT-SIDED DOUBLE LUMEN ENDOTRACHEAL TUBE**] to allow lung-isolation. Standard monitoring lines were inserted, including [**LINE TYPES**] in the [**LATERALITY**] [**VESSEL**]. The patient received [**DOSE**] of

[ANTIBIOTICS] at the time of anesthetic induction. Subcutaneous heparin was given for deep venous thrombosis prophylaxis, and sequential compression devices were placed on bilateral lower extremities.

The patient was positioned supine with the arms tucked into the sides. All bony prominences were appropriately padded. After suitable prepping and draping, [BILATERAL ANTEROLATERAL THORACOTOMIES] or [MEDIAN STERNOTOMY] or [LATERALITY, POSTEROLATERAL THORACOTOMY] was/were made [IN THE FOURTH VS FIFTH INTERSPACE]. The sternum was divided transversely. The mammary vessels were divided between silk ligatures. Both pleural spaces were entered and found [FREE OF ADHESIONS VS SCARRED WITH ADHESIONS]. We noted [INTRAOPERATIVE ANATOMIC AND HEMODYNAMIC FINDINGS AND ASSESSMENT TO INCLUDE OR EXCLUDE CARDIOPULMONARY BYPASS... Consider pulmonary pressures, oxygenation, echo findings, etc.].

[Entry onto cardiopulmonary bypass, if used: The pericardium was opened in a hockey stick-shaped incision, extending down the ascending aorta and angling over toward the right atrial appendage. The patient was fully heparinized. Two non-pledgeted 2-0 Prolene pursestring sutures were placed in the ascending aorta, and it was cannulated without difficulty. The cannula was secured at the sternum with silk suture to prevent dislodgement of the cannula during the transplant procedure. In a similar fashion, a 2-0 Prolene non-pledgeted pursestring suture was placed in the right atrial appendage and it was was secured to the sternum to prevent dislodgement during the transplant procedure. The patient was then placed on cardiopulmonary bypass without difficulty.]

[Backtable dissection, if performed: A donor/recipient time-out was performed. The lungs were brought from the cooler and kept cold using topical application of crushed ice. The donor aorta and esophagus were resected posteriorly. The left atrial cuff was divided in the midline, pericardium divided in the midline, the pulmonary artery was divided at its bifurcation, the left main bronchus was amputated. Both hila were then fully prepared, mobilizing the pulmonary artery to the first upper lobe branch, and dividing the bronchus one ring proximal to the upper lobe takeoff.

Excessive pericardium on both sides was then resected. The lungs were kept cold until the appropriate time for implantation.]

Based on the quantitative V/Q scan, the [**RIGHT** vs **LEFT**] lung was resected first [+/-**AFTER THE PATIENT WAS SAFELY PLACED ON CARDIOPULMONARY BYPASS**]. Pulmonary vein branches were divided between silk ligatures. The upper lobar pulmonary artery was divided between silk ligatures. The distal pulmonary artery was transected beyond a vascular staple line. Bronchial tissue was divided with cautery. The bronchus was divided well up in the mediastinum at a site suitable for anastomosis. The pericardium was opened circumferentially. Hemostasis was achieved. Attention was then directed to the

[LEFT vs RIGHT] side where an identical extraction of the other lung was performed. [IF NOT ON CARDIOPULMONARY BYPASS, THE FIRST LUNG IS ISOLATED, EXPLANTED, AND DONOR LUNG IMPLANTED; NOTE APPROPRIATE MODIFICATIONS IF NO CARDIOPULMONARY BYPASS.]

The donor [LEFT VS RIGHT] lung was brought up into the field. It was kept cold using topical application of crushed ice. The donor and recipient bronchi were approximated with a running suture of 4-0 PDS. A central Satinsky clamp was placed. The pulmonary arteries were trimmed to size and an end-to-end anastomosis constructed using 5-0 Prolene. Both vein stumps were grasped and retracted laterally. A central Satinsky clamp was placed, the veins stumps were amputated, and the bridging atrial tissue between the vein stumps was divided to create an atriotomy suitable for the venous anastomosis. A left atrial anastomosis was then performed using a running suture of 4-0 Prolene with sutures placed in such a manner as to evert all muscle from the lumen. The suture line was left open on its anterior aspect while the pulmonary artery clamp was released and the lung de-aired antegrade.

The suture line was then secured. Partial perfusion was restored to the [LEFT VS RIGHT] lung and low volume ventilation established (*if done on bypass*). [*(If done without bypass):* **FULL VENTILATION AND PERFUSION WERE RESTORED TO THE IMPLANTED LUNG.**]

Attention was then directed to the [RIGHT VS LEFT] side where an identical implantation was performed. After restoration of ventilation and perfusion of both lungs, gas exchange was [**EXCELLENT, MODERATE, POOR?**], hemodynamics were [**UNSATISFACTORY VS SATISFACTORY**—additional steps taken if unsatisfactory].

[IF BYPASS USED: Both lungs were then fully ventilated, and the patient was weaned from cardiopulmonary bypass. [**DESCRIBE USE OF INOTROPES, PRESSORS, AND CORRESPONDING HEMODYNAMIC/ECHO FINDINGS.**] With this, [HE/SHE] was weaned from cardiopulmonary bypass and maintained stable hemodynamics with a s ystemicpressure of [NUMBER], and a pulmonary artery systolic pressure in the [NUMBER]. The saturations initially were in the [NUMBERS]. The lungs appeared to be in [BLANK] condition with [no] erythema or edema. We observed [HIM/HER] for quite some time and [HE/SHE] remained hemodynamically stable and was decannulated in the standard fashion. Protamine sulfate was administered. Both the cannulation sites were both carefully examined and found to be completely hemostatic. The pericardium was then loosely approximated in the midline with multiple interrupted 2-0 Vicryl sutures.]

Hemostasis was achieved in both pleural spaces. Two #24 Blake drains were brought through separate stab wounds into each pleural space. The chest was then closed using heavy polypropylene pericostal sutures and two heavy figure-of-eight sternal wires. Fascial sutures of Dexon and subcuticular closure and a Dermabond dressing completed the wound closure.

The patient was then extubated and re-intubated using a single-lumen tube. Flexible bronchoscopy was performed. The airways were examined. Both bronchial anastomoses were widely patent. The donor airways were viable. Blood and secretions were aspirated. The patient was then transferred directly to the Cardiothoracic Intensive Care Unit in stable condition.

Estimated Blood Loss: [Blank]

Approximately [NUMBER] mL.

Sponge/instrument/needle counts: Correct.

Condition upon discharge from the operating room: The patient remained stable throughout.

Complications: There were no complications noted. **[OR NOTE IF THERE WERE]**

Dr. **[BLANK]** was present and scrubbed for **[BLANK]** elements of this procedure.

39. Bronchial and Arterial Sleeve Resection

George Makdisi, MD, Dennis Wigle, MD, PhD

Mayo Clinic, Rochester, MN

Essential Operative Steps

1. Lines and Monitoring
2. General endotracheal anesthesia / Single lumen tube for bronchoscopy
3. Flexible bronchoscopy is mandatory to examine the extent of the tumor
4. Double-lumen endotracheal tube (left sided for sleeve resection on the right and right sided for sleeve resections on the left).
5. Serratus-sparing posterolateral thoracotomy/ or lateral thoracotomy. Enter through the 5th intercostal space. Harvest the intercostal muscle flap for coverage of the anastomosis.
6. Assess for pleural metastases
7. Open posterior and anterior mediastinal pleura to expose the main stem bronchus
8. Assess for local invasion and resectability
9. Dissect and divide the pulmonary veins, arteries and the fissure as usual.
10. Sharply divide the distal main bronchus and proximal bronchus for anastomosis perpendicular to the long axis
11. Get frozen section to assure negative margins, if positive resect further
12. If an arterial sleeve needs to be done, give 5000 IU of heparin before clamping the artery
13. Decide your best type of arterial reconstruction,
14. Get proximal and distal control of the pulmonary artery
15. Clamp superior and inferior pulmonary veins
16. Do Infrahilar pericardial release to decrease tension
17. End to end anastomosis, with interrupted polypropylene sutures with knots outside
18. Complete lymph node dissection
19. Check for vascular kinking when the rest of the lung is expanded
20. Cover anastomosis with intercostal muscle flap
21. Chest tube drains
22. Redo bronchoscopy to check anastomosis
23. Repeat bronchoscopy before discharge

Potential Complications and Pitfalls

1. The orientation of the proximal and distal airways should be maintained by traction suture at the junction of membranous and cartilaginous airways
2. The main pulmonary artery is usually clamped after administration of 5000 U heparin. Heparin is not reversed at the end of the operation. No further heparin; just is standard DVT prophylaxis postop
3. Bronchial fistula can be avoided by:

a. Anastomosis tension free: do hilar release
b. Lumen disparity: Bronchial size matching can be a problem; use intussusception techniques as required
c. Protect the anastomosis by wrapping with a vascularized pedicle of autologous tissue (pericardial fat, intercostal muscle, or pleura). An intercostal flap should not cover 360 degrees of the circumference.
4. Segmental bronchial patency. It is important to check that all segmental bronchi are patent and that all the sutures are placed in a way that does not jeopardize the patency of the segmental bronchi
5. Postoperative hemoptysis. Rule out bronchial-arterial fistula immediately. This can be avoided by isolating the arterial reconstruction from the bronchial anastomosis
6. Vascular and bronchial kinking. It is critical to examine the anastomoses after lung reexpansion to ensure there is no rotation or kinking
7. The main pitfalls of the use of a conduit are its sizing and length
8. Postoperative bronchial stenosis treated by dilatation or stenting if needed

Template Dictation

Preoperative Diagnosis: Endobronchial tumor involving the orifice of the [BLANK] lobe.

Postoperative Diagnosis: Same

Procedure(s) Performed: Bronchial and arterial Sleeve resection of [BLANK]

Attending Surgeon: [BLANK]

Secondary Surgeon: [BLANK]

Assistants: [BLANK]

Anesthesia: Thoracic epidural and general endotracheal anesthesia.

Indication(s) for Procedure: [Mr/ Mrs.] [BLANK] is a [age] year-old [gender] who presented [right/ left] lung mass. Workup included [CXR, CT, PET], biopsy had been performed, and the findings are consistent with a **[pathology e.g. endobronchial tumor involving the orifice or the [BLANK] lobe].** [Mr/ Mrs.] [BLANK] is brought now for surgical resection

Description of Procedure: Bronchial sleeve resection of the right upper lobe

The patient was brought to the operating room and had a thoracic epidural catheter placed by the anesthesia team. The patient was then placed in the supine position on the operating table. Following an uneventful induction of general endotracheal anesthesia, the patient was intubated with a single-lumen endotracheal tube. We performed flexible videobronchoscopy. The left-sided airways had normal anatomy. There were no endobronchial lesions, significant secretions, blood, pus or other abnormalities. In the right-sided airways, there was an obvious tumor mass that had completely occluded the entire orifice of the right upper lobe of the lung. There was tumor coming out of the orifice into the mid bronchus intermedius bronchus.

The single-lumen endotracheal tube was exchanged for a double-lumen endotracheal tube by the Anesthesia Team. He was turned into left lateral decubitus position with the right side up. The left chest was sterilely prepped and draped in the usual manner for a standard right posterolateral thoracotomy. We made a serratus-sparing right posterolateral thoracotomy incision and entered the chest through fifth intercostal space. The 5th intercostal muscle pedicle was harvested for future coverage of the anastomosis. There was no evidence of pleural disease in the chest. The tumor could be palpated centrally at the takeoff to the right upper lobe bronchus. We took the inferior pulmonary ligament down with Bovie electrocautery up to the inferior pulmonary vein and harvested station 9 lymph nodes. Then we started our dissection in the fissure by identifying the pulmonary arterial branches heading down to the right lower lobe, and the middle lobe. We next proceeded with our right upper lobectomy. The superior pulmonary vein was dissected free and ligated using an endovascular stapler. A number of pulmonary arterial branches were identified heading to the right upper lobe. We were able to identify a large pulmonary arterial truncal branch heading up to the right upper lobe coming off the main PA relatively proximal. This was ligated using an endovascular stapler. As a consequence, we proceeded with dissecting out the bronchus. Given our prior bronchoscopy, it was clear that a sleeve lobectomy would be required in order to obtain an adequate margin. Proximally, we then transected the distal right main bronchus just proximal to the take-off of the right upper with a No. 10 blade. This allowed us to look inside the airway, and we could see that we were grossly clear of the tumor originating from the orifice of the right upper lobe of the lung. Then we transected the bronchus intermedius just above the takeoff of the superior segmental bronchus of the lower lobe. The right upper lobe bronchus was now separated with the corresponding portion of the right mainstem attached. The right main bronchial margin and the bronchus intermedius margin on the sleeve part of the airway were marked with stitches for Pathology for orientation. The final margins were clear of tumor. We completed the fissure posteriorly with a single firing of a blue load Endo GIA stapler. We then swept lymph nodes up toward the specimen. With the bronchus now ligated, all of the attachments at the hilum for the right upper lobe were now free; we then performed an end-to-end anastomosis using #2-0 absorbable stay sutures placed around one cartilaginous ring at 3 and 9 o'clock on both the right main bronchus side as well as on the intermedius bronchus side. We then used interrupted #4-0 absorbable suture. We began on the cartilaginous wall at the 12 o'clock position on both sides and then continued laterally with interrupted suture technique. Once all the cartilaginous sutures had been placed, we then also reapproximated the membranous walls with interrupted #4-0 absorbable suture sutures and then tied the sutures in the reverse order (the back wall tied first then the anterior wall) after tying the stay sutures down. The bronchial anastomosis was tested under saline and was found to be pneumostatic to 35 mm of water pressure. We then harvested a vascularized pericardial fat pad and then passed it circumferentially around our bronchial anastomosis and tacked it to the airway in several places with mattress #3-0 silk sutures. We then completed a thoracic lymphadenectomy with harvesting lymph nodes from station 9, 7, 2, 4, 10, and 11. The lung was reinflated. There was minimal air leak. The intercostal muscle flap was passed around the anastomosis posteriorly taking care not to completely encircle the anastomosis. We placed two 28-French chest tubes and closed the chest in layers with figure-of-eight #1 pericostal absorbable suture. The lung was re-expanded under direct vision. We closed the serratus with a running #1 absorbable suture, and we closed the latissimus in two layers with running #1 absorbable suture. The subdermal tissues were closed using #2-0 absorbable suture. The skin was closed with a #4-0 absorbable subcuticular suture. The patient tolerated the procedure well. There were no intraoperative complications. All needle, sponge, and instrument counts were correct on two occasions.

[Mr/Mrs.] [BLANK] appeared to tolerate the procedure well and was transferred to the recovery room in stable condition.

Left upper lobe with arterial sleeve resections:

Same as above except using right-sided double lumen endotracheal tube

We were able to completely mobilize the left lung, and the tumor did appear mobile within the left upper lobe and potentially resectable.

We first began with an intrapericardial dissection in order to identify the relevant anatomy. The inferior and superior pulmonary veins and the left main pulmonary artery were dissected free and umbilical tapes placed round them for vascular control. We were able to readily identify the superior pulmonary vein, and it was ligated between two fires of a TA-30 vascular stapler. Working out along the pulmonary artery, we were able to identify a number of branches heading to the left upper lobe. These were ligated in succession using silk ties. We did encounter some pulmonary artery branches where the tumor was flush up against the pulmonary artery.

Working in the fissure, it was clear that there was extension of tumor and associated fibrotic tissue over on to the superior segment. As a consequence, we dissected out the left main stem bronchus posteriorly. We were able to identify the separation point where the bronchus bifurcated into the left upper and left lower lobes. At this point we dissected free the left upper lobe bronchus and ligated this using a TA-30 bronchial stapler and we were only still attached to two relatively large pulmonary arterial branches that were flush against the pulmonary artery. In order to resect this safely, 5000 U of heparin was given, and we clamped the remaining left inferior pulmonary vein and the left main pulmonary artery in order to have vascular control. The tumor was cut free off of the pulmonary artery with an appropriate margin on the artery. We had adequate hemostasis while this took place. The tumor was now successfully removed with all of its attachments and sent to pathology. We reconstructed the pulmonary artery with a primary anastomosis with running sutures of [#5-0 or 6-0] nonabsorbable monofilament. After removal of the clamps, it appeared as though we had adequate hemostasis.

We then completed a thoracic lymphadenectomy. Lymph nodes were harvested from stations 2L, 4L, 5, 6, 7, 9, 10L and 11L. In order to separate the area of our pulmonary sleeve from the bronchial stump we harvested a pleural flap in order to interpose this between the artery and the bronchus. The pleural flap was tacked down on to the bronchus and surrounding tissue using a number of #3-0 silk sutures. Once this was complete we carefully irrigated with many liters of warm saline. Our bronchial stump was intact under saline immersion. We had adequate hemostasis. The lung was reinflated. There was minimal air leak. We placed two 28-French chest tubes and closed the chest in layers with figure-of-eight #1 pericostal absorbable suture. The lung was re-expanded under direct vision. We closed the serratus with a running #1 absorbable suture, and we closed the latissimus in two layers with running #1 absorbable suture. The subdermal tissues were closed using #2-0 absorbable suture. The skin was closed with a #4-0 absorbable subcuticular suture. The patient tolerated the procedure well. There were no intraoperative complications. A surgical pause confirmed that all needle, sponge, and instrument counts were correct. [Mr/ Mrs.] [BLANK] appeared to tolerate the procedure well and was transferred to the recovery room in stable condition.

Techniques of Pulmonary Artery Reconstruction

1. <u>Patch reconstruction after partial resection</u>. The wall of the vessel on the opposite side should be free of tumor. It can be associated with a standard lobectomy or a lobectomy with a sleeve resection of the bronchus. The patch (autologous or Bovine pericardium) is held in place by two stay sutures of polypropylene #5-0. We tie the lower stay suture then continue running sutures while keeping some degree of looseness on the patch which is desirable at this stage, the looseness will disappear after declamping. The upper stay suture is not tied but simply keeps the patch in the correct place. The pericardium is usually harvested anteriorly to the phrenic nerve; the defect is small and can be left open with no fear of cardiac herniation.
2. <u>Sleeve resection with end-to-end-anastomosis</u> (as described in our case). Sleeve resection of the artery is usually required when the circumference of the vessel is extensively invaded. It is required also when vascular and bronchial reconstructions are performed simultaneously, with a marked shortening of the bronchial axis. After the resection the ensuing defect can be reconstructed by end-to-end anastomosis after bronchial reconstruction, caliber discrepancy is compensated by the elasticity of the wall of the vessel. Sectioning the vessel can improve exposure of the bronchial side. In this situation, the vascular anastomosis should be completed after performing the bronchial reconstruction. It is accomplished with a #5-0 or 6-0 nonabsorbable monofilament. Caliber

discrepancy between the two sides of the anastomosis is typically not a problem and matching is greatly helped by the elasticity of the vessel
3. <u>Sleeve resection followed by reconstruction with a prosthetic conduit</u> as polytetrafluoroethylene (PTFE) can be used when a long bronchial segment separates the two pulmonary artery stumps such that an end-to-end anastomosis is not feasible. The proximal anastomosis between the pulmonary artery and the conduit is performed first. The distal anastomosis is performed last
4. <u>Reconstruction of the main PA at its origin under cardiopulmonary bypass.</u> This is an option of last resort

II. Adult Cardiac Surgery

1. Aortic Root Replacement for Ascending Aortic Aneurysm

Fawwaz R. Shaw, MD and Edward D. Verrier, MD

University of Washington, Seattle, WA.

Essential Operative Steps

1. Placement of appropriate monitoring lines and induction of general endotracheal anesthesia.
2. Review of the preoperative CT scan or MRI identifying annulus size, location of sinotubular junction, extension of disease into aortic arch and coronary anatomy.
3. Operating room briefing with Anesthesia, Perfusion, and Nursing teams regarding intraoperative plans, cannulation strategies, myocardial protection plans, possible inotropic needs, antibiotic coverage, post-operative coagulation, local hemostatic agents planned, type of conduit and valve planned, annular and button stitches planned and need for left ventricular vent.
4. Evaluation of the heart and valve function with intraoperative transesophageal echocardiography.
5. Venous and appropriate arterial cannulation (distal ascending aorta versus femoral or right axillary arteries).
6. Cardiopulmonary bypass. (Depth of cooling, possible deep hypothermic circulatory arrest (DHCA) and re-warming timing.)
7. Myocardial protection strategy (solution, timing and mode of delivery).
8. Examination of the aorta and identification of the proximal and distal extents of the aneurysm.
9. Division of the proximal aorta above the sinotubular junction.
10. Examination of the aortic root and determination of the need for valve replacement versus repair/resuspension, or an aortic interposition graft versus a Bentall procedure.
11. Excision of the aortic valve, meticulously removing debris and debriding the annulus if heavily calcified.
12. Careful dissection and release of the coronary buttons from the aortic wall marking the proper orientation with a stitch.
13. Completion of the proximal division of the aorta.
14. Selection of an appropriately sized composite aortic-valved conduit.
15. Placement of the annular valve stitches. (Pledgeted versus un-pledgeted, left ventricle to aorta versus aorta to left ventricle.)
16. Securing the valved conduit via the sewing ring. (Ensure all pledgets are accounted for.)
17. Re-implantation of the coronary arteries.
18. Completion of the distal aortic anastomosis. (Determine need for Teflon felt reinforcement.)
19. De-airing the heart and conduit.
20. Remove cross clamp after hot shot.

21. Placement of temporary pacing wires.
22. Wean from cardiopulmonary bypass.
23. Examination of the heart for function and the valve for leaflet excursion, function and paravalvular leaks.
24. Ensure hemostasis, place chest/mediastinal tubes and close the chest.

Potential Complications and Pitfalls

1. If contraindication to mechanical aortic valve. (A bioprosthetic-valved conduit can be created by first selecting an appropriately sized bioprosthetic valve. An aortic conduit approximately 3-5 mm larger than the valve is selected. The sewing ring of the valve is then secured to the graft with a running 4-0 polypropylene suture creating a watertight anastomosis between the sewing ring and the aortic conduit. The valve leaflets are then examined for appropriate excursion and to ensure no leaflet impingement prior to tying the suture.)
2. Inability to place a retrograde cardioplegia cannula in the coronary sinus.
3. Inappropriately placed arterial cannula in the ascending aorta with insufficient room for cross clamp placement.
4. Injury to the conduction system as a result of deep valve stitches in the region of the right and non coronary sinuses.
5. Coronary occlusion due to suboptimal lay of the coronary arteries after reimplantation.
6. Length of conduit too long (causing kinking) or too short (causing tension).
7. Incomplete or excessive mobilization of the coronary arteries leading to tension, twisting or kinking of the coronary anastomosis.
8. Failure to completely debride a calcified aortic annulus leading to abnormal seating of the valved conduit and poor hemostasis.
9. Inadequate de-airing maneuvers or air embolus down the right coronary leading to right ventricular dysfunction.
10. Breaking a stitch during tying of conduit to annulus (leading to possible loss of pledget and need for a repair stitch).

Template Dictation

Preoperative Diagnosis: Ascending aortic aneurysm, Annuloaortic ectasia

Postoperative Diagnosis: Same

Procedure(s) Performed: Aortic Root and Valve replacement [Type of conduit/valve, e.g. #25 ATM Medical Mechanical Valved Conduit].

Attending Surgeon: [BLANK]

Secondary Surgeon: [BLANK]

Assistants: [BLANK]

II. Adult Cardiac Surgery

Anesthesia: [BLANK]

Indication(s) for Procedure: [AGE] old [GENDER] who developed [SYMPTOMS e.g. progressively worsening shortness of breath and dyspnea] and was found to have [FINDINGS e.g. 6.5 cm ascending aortic aneurysm with a bicuspid aortic valve].

Description of the Procedure: The patient was brought to the operating room where an intra-operative briefing or huddle was performed with the surgical, anesthesia, nursing and perfusion teams, confirming the correct patient, diagnosis and operative plan. The patient was placed in the supine position and general endotracheal anesthesia was instituted. Appropriate monitoring lines were then placed. Preoperative transesophageal echocardiogram was performed to evaluate cardiac and valve function. The chest, abdomen and lower extremities were prepped and draped in sterile fashion.

A midline incision was made from the sternal notch to just distal to the xiphoid process and the sternum was transected in the midline. The anterior mediastinum was entered, the pericardium was opened and a pericardial cradle was created. Mediastinal anatomy was then carefully reviewed. The aorta was dissected and inspected. Systemic heparinization was performed with 3 mg/kg of intravenous heparin via a centrally placed intravenous catheter. We instituted cardiopulmonary bypass via central cannulation with a two stage right atrial cannula and a distal ascending aortic cannula. The patient was allowed to systematically drift in temperature. We placed a cannula in the coronary sinus for retrograde cardioplegia confirmed by TEE, and one in the ascending aorta for antegrade cardioplegia. A left ventricular vent was placed via the right superior pulmonary vein and placement was also confirmed by TEE.

Both antegrade and retrograde cardioplegia were administered. Warm glutamate/aspartate blood cardioplegia was utilized for induction antegrade followed by cold blood cardioplegia for maintenance. Cold blood cardioplegia was given every 20 minutes for the duration of the operation either via the coronary sinus or directly into the orifices of the coronary arteries by hand-held cannulae. Prior to removal of the cross clamp a hot shot of substrate enriched warm blood cardioplegia was given. Carbon dioxide was infused into the operative field to minimize air accumulation in the heart.

We opened the aorta obliquely above the sinotubular junction and found [FINDINGS e.g. a congenitally bicuspid aortic valve with marked dilation of the sinuses]. We elected to proceed with the following aortic root operation [AVR with ascending aorta replacement, a Bentall procedure, a David procedure, hemi-arch replacement]. The diseased valve was carefully excised at the level of the annulus with care to remove all calcium debris. We then excised the ascending aorta, carefully creating the left and right coronary artery buttons for subsequent re-implantation. The coronary buttons were marked with temporary 4-0 Prolene sutures to maintain proper orientation.

Interrupted 2-0 pledgeted TiCron sutures were sequentially placed in the annulus of the aortic valve from below, with the pledgets on the ventricular side. We then selected an appropriate sized composite valved prosthesis **[SELECTED CONDUIT]** and placed our TiCron sutures through the sewing ring. The valved prosthesis was gently lowered into place at the level of the annulus and the sutures were carefully tied to tightly secure the prosthesis to the annulus. Full excursion of all valve leaflets was confirmed. We created holes using an ophthalmic cautery in the conduit at the appropriate height, adjacent to the left and right coronary buttons. We used a 6-0 Prolene suture in a running fashion to anastomose the coronary buttons to the conduit. The conduit was then sized for appropriate length and the distal end of the graft was anastomosed in an end to end fashion using running 4-0 Prolene suture reinforced with a Teflon felt strip.

We then placed the patient's head down, filled the heart with blood, temporarily turned off the left ventricular vent and gently ventilated the patient to remove pulmonary vein air. We also vented the ascending aorta to complete our de-airing maneuvers. The cross clamp was removed after warm substrate enhanced cardioplegic solution was administered. Temporary pacing wires were placed.

Spontaneous rhythm was ensured **[or the patient was temporarily paced]** and the patient was weaned gradually from cardiopulmonary bypass on low dose inotropic support. Transesophageal echocardiography demonstrated preserved ventricular function, no aortic insufficiency and appropriate excursion of the valve leaflets. We then decannulated the patient once all de-airing maneuvers were completed and reinforced our cannulation sites with appropriately placed sutures. Heparin was fully reversed with **[DOSE]** Protamine. We ensured adequate hemostasis and placed a **[SIZE e.g. 32 Fr]** chest tube in the mediastinum **[and pleural spaces if necessary]**. The sternum was closed with interrupted **[SIZE e.g. 22 gauge]** stainless steel wires. The fascia was closed with 0 Vicryl suture in running fashion. We closed the deep dermal layer with 2-0 Vicryl suture in running fashion and re-approximated the skin edges with 4-0 Monocryl in a subcuticular fashion. A sterile dressing was then placed over the incision and at the chest tube site.

Needle, sponge and instrument counts were reported as correct x 2. The patient was transferred to the Intensive Care Unit with stable vital signs. The post-operative huddle / debriefing was completed.

Dr. **[BLANK]** was present and scrubbed for **[BLANK]** elements of this procedure.

2. Aortic Root Replacement (Endocarditis)

Michael O. Kayatta, MD and Michael E. Halkos, MD, MSc

Emory University, Atlanta, GA

Essential Operative Steps

1. Median sternotomy
2. Open pericardium and create pericardial well
3. Arterial cannulation
4. Venous cannulation
5. Initiate CPB and place aortic cross-clamp to administer cardioplegia
6. Transect aorta and remove all infected tissue including aortic valve
7. Create coronary buttons
8. Proximal anastomosis (homograft to aortic annulus)
9. Coronary to homograft anastomoses
10. Distal homograft to aorta anastomosis
11. Remove aortic cross clamp
12. Check for hemostasis
13. Wean from CPB
14. Venous and aortic decannulation
15. Sternotomy closure

Potential Complications and Pitfalls

1. Insufficient myocardial protection
2. Inadequate LV drainage with LV vent
3. Bunching of the homograft during anastomosis leading to aortic valve incompetence
4. Injury to coronary artery ostia
5. Inadequate control of hemostasis prior to sternal closure
6. Bleeding complications

Template Dictation

Preoperative Diagnosis: [INDICATION – e.g. aortic valve endocarditis with aortic root abscess]

Postoperative Diagnosis: Same

Procedure(s) Performed: Aortic root replacement with [SIZE] homograft aortic root conduit [DETAILS – e.g. extent of tissue removed]

Attending Surgeon: [BLANK]

Secondary Surgeon: [BLANK]

Assistants: [BLANK]

Anesthesia: [BLANK]

Indication(s) for Procedure: [AGE] year old [GENDER] with [DURATION] history of [COMPLAINT – e.g. sepsis with persistent bacteremia and aortic root abscess]. Preoperative echocardiogram reveals [FINDINGS – e.g. aortic valve vegetation with aortic root dilation].

Description of Procedure: The patient was taken to the operating room on [DATE]. The patient's identity and planned procedure verified, and the patient was placed on the operating room table in the supine position. General anesthesia was obtained. A right internal jugular central venous line and pulmonary artery catheter and radial arterial line were inserted. Preoperative transesophageal echocardiogram was then performed to evaluate cardiac function, aortic valve and root pathology. We then proceeded to prep and drape the chest, abdomen, groins, and lower extremities in sterile fashion. A time out was performed. [ANTIBOTIC] was given within 60 minutes of incision. Median sternotomy was then performed. The pericardium was opened and a pericardial well was created. Epiaortic ultrasound was then performed which revealed a grade [GRADE] aorta. The aortic cannulation sutures were then placed in the ascending aorta below the level of the innominate artery. The right atrial cannulation sutures were then placed within the right atrium.

A total of [UNITS (400U per kg)] of systemic heparin was administered. The aortic cannula was then inserted, secured and de-aired. A venous cannula was then placed and secured in the right atrium. A retrograde cannula was placed through the right atrium into the coronary sinus. A DLP vent was then inserted into the ascending aorta for administration of antegrade cardioplegia. The aortic cross-clamp was placed. Antegrade cardioplegia was administered and rapid arrest of the heart followed. After 1 liter of high potassium antegrade cardioplegia, 500cc of retrograde cardioplegia was given. Ice was applied to the heart. The patient was cooled to [32-34] degrees Celsius. Additional myocardial protection was achieved with continuous retrograde cardioplegia. Additional doses of cardioplegia were administered via antegrade every thirty minutes **[or continuously]**. A left ventricular vent was placed via the right superior pulmonary vein.

After arrest of the heart with cardioplegia, the ascending aorta was opened transversely with a #15 blade just above the level of the sinotubular junction. The aortic root was then dissected free of surrounding structures. All aortic leaflets were then excised. The aortic sinus tissue was then excised to the level of the aortic annulus. The left and right coronary buttons were then created leaving adequate aortic tissue to be able to perform the anastomoses. Radical debridement of all infected tissues was then carried out **[include specifics]**. All contaminated instruments were then removed from the field. #4-0 pledgeted sutures were placed at each commissure for retraction.

Following this, a series of #2-0 Tevdek pledgeted horizontal mattress aortic-based sutures were placed circumferentially around the aortic annulus. These were then brought through the base of a [SIZE] homograft conduit. **[Alternatively a running suture technique can be utilized.]** The conduit was then seated down into the LVOT. The sutures were then tied and cut. The coronary ostia on the homograft were then enlarged, and the coronary buttons were then sewn into the homograft ostia using running [#5- or #6-0] Prolene suture. Finally, the distal homograft was anastomosed circumferentially to the ascending aorta using a running #4-0 Prolene suture.

The aortic cross-clamp was then removed. All suture lines were evaluated for hemostasis. A total of [NUMBER] chest tubes were placed in the [LEFT/RIGHT] pleural space, and [NUMBER] chest tubes were placed in the mediastinum. [ATRIAL/VENTRICULAR] pacing wires were then inserted and tested for appropriate capture. The heart was then de-aired, and the LV vent was removed. The patient was weaned from cardiopulmonary bypass and the DLP vent was removed. Transesophageal echocardiogram revealed a competent aortic valve. The venous cannula was removed, and the cannulation sutures were tied down. The aortic cannula was then removed, and the cannulation sutures tied down. Protamine was then slowly administered. Adequate hemostasis was then confirmed within the mediastinum. The sternum was then closed with stainless steel sternal wires. The fascia was then closed with a #1 PDS suture. The deep dermal layer was then closed with #3-0 PDS suture in running fashion. The skin and subcuticular layer was closed with #4-0 Monocryl in running fashion.

All instrument, sponge and needle counts were confirmed to be correct, twice, at the end of the operation. The patient was subsequently transferred to the postoperative cardiac surgical intensive care unit in critical condition.

Dr. [BLANK] was present and scrubbed for [BLANK] elements of this procedure.

3. Total Arch/Hemiarch Replacement with DHCA – Dissection

Tom P. Theruvath, MD, PhD and John S. Ikonomidis, MD, PhD

Medical University of South Carolina, Charleston, SC

Essential Operative Steps

1. ECG, pulse oximetry, bilateral upper extremity arterial monitoring, PA Catheter
2. Induce general anesthesia
3. Mark midline chest incision and bilateral groins for possible arterial access if needed
4. TEE, Foley, end-tidal CO_2, temperature probes (*nasopharyngeal, bladder, rectal*), bi-hemispheric cerebral oxygen saturation monitoring
5. Prep and drape to include both legs circumferentially
6. Pass CPB lines and prime circuit
7. Median sternotomy with 1-2 cm extension cranially to supraclavicular notch
8. Dissection superior to innominate vein to visualize innominate artery and evaluate arch to determine whether total or just proximal transverse (*hemirach*) arch needs to be replaced.
9. Systemic heparinization (400 IU/Kg)
10. Dissection of Innominate artery and construction of end/side anastomosis to a 10 mm Hemashield graft (*chimney graft*) with 5-0 Prolene for arterial cannulation
11. Confirm ACT > 460 sec and connect Hemashield graft to arterial cannula (*soft flow tip*), secure with heavy silk ties twice, de-air and connect to arterial side of pump oxygenator
12. Confirm absence of pericardial effusion/hemopericardium and prepare to control hypertension once opening pericardium. Prepare pericardial well and assess root/proximal ascending aorta to decide whether root needs to be reconstructed
13. Placement of dual stage venous cannula and connect to venous side of pump oxygenator
14. Retrograde autologous priming with placement of antegrade dual stage cardioplegia and root vent and retrograde cardioplegia tacks
15. Commence CPB and start systemic cooling to 25°C. Dose steroid for cerebral protection
16. Aorta is crossclamped proximal to innominate artery takeoff and heart arrested with a combination of antegrade and retrograde cold blood cardioplegia with topical ice saline cooling
17. Aorta is transected midway, resected back to sinotubular junction and trimmed cranially up to the crossclamp.
18. If the false lumen has caused dissection proximally into the sinuses of Valsalvae, the false lumen can be obliterated by utilizing a sandwich technique with placement of a Teflon strip in between the dissected walls

and reinforced with surgical adhesives. (*if dissection involves base of aortic root or coronary ostia, aortic root reconstruction by re-suspension, remodeling or replacement of aortic valve with coronary artery bypasses needs to be considered; this involves complex reconstruction not discussed in this chapter*)
19. Tubular Dacron graft is sized (*approximately 26 mm – 30 mm*)
20. Once 25°C is reached, Trendelenburg position is assumed, propofol is given, head is packed in ice, and a DeBakey peripheral vascular clamp is applied to the base of the innominate artery. The crossclamp is removed.
21. Selective antegrade cerebral perfusion is commenced with decreased flows to maintain a mean right brachial artery pressure of 60-70 mmHg.
22. Aorta is resected into the arch with undercutting of the proximal hemiarch such that the takeoffs of all 3 great vessels are easily visualized **OR** the aorta is resected back to the proximal descending aorta leaving an island of arch surrounding the great vessels just distal to left subclavian artery (*leave all three brachiocephalic vessels attached to a single arterial button*).
23. The tubular Dacron graft is trimmed and beveled and a proximal anastomosis is made between it and the hemiarch with running 3-0 Prolene suture to carefully include all layers with each needle bite **OR** the tubular Dacron graft is trimmed and an anastomosis between the distal aorta in a running fashion with 3-0 Prolene and the arch button using the same suture technique is constructed.
24. Anastomoses are reinforced with a small amount of surgical adhesives circumferentially (*we do not utilize Teflon felt strips*).
25. The aortic arch is carefully de-aired after removing the peripheral vascular clamp at the base of the innominate artery and a crossclamp reapplied after adequate flush to the ascending/transverse arch.
26. Anastomoses are inspected carefully and repair sutures placed were necessary
27. Rewarming is begun and full flow perfusion is re-established via innominate artery
28. The Dacron graft is trimmed to length for proximal anastomosis
29. Antegrade cardioplegia tack/root vent is placed into ascending graft and retrograde cardioplegia tack removed
30. Proximal anastomosis is performed with 3-0 Prolene
31. Following warm cardioplegia dose ventricular pacing wires are placed and crossclamp removed
32. Once rewarmed to 36°C, the patient is weaned from CPB. De-airing (*assessed by TEE*) and hemostasis is assured.
33. Antegrade cardioplegia tack/root vent and venous cannula are removed, Protamine given and the arterial cannula removed (*the Hemashield graft is tied twice with heavy silk*), and all cannulae sites reinforced with 4-0 Prolene sutures

34. Chest is closed in usual fashion after placement of mediastinal chest tube and oblique sinus/right lateral 19 Fr Blake® drain

Potential Complications and Pitfalls
1. Usual complications with sternotomy, dissection, and cannulation
2. Inability to place antegrade cardioplegia/root vent cannula due to anterior wall dissection involvement
3. Organ (*especially cerebral*) mal-perfusion and need for alternative arterial cannulation site (*e.g. right subclavicular cutdown for right axillary cannulation or groin cutdown for femoral arterial cannulation*)
4. Distal reentry tear leading to mal-perfusion after placement of crossclamp with need to pursue repair during fibrillatory arrest
5. Severe Aortic insufficiency with aortic root dilation and involvement of aortic valve with need for either aortic valve resuspension or replacement (*due to their complexity we do not describe these scenarios*)
6. Dissection involves coronary arteries and coronary button/bypass has to be constructed to proximal Dacron graft.
7. Improper de-airing
8. Too long of conduit with need to re-cross clamp, shorten and re-anastomose end/end ascending aorta graft
9. Bleeding from anastomoses (*common challenge, especially needle holes and need for adjuncts in hemostatsis including local adjuncts, e.g. surgical adhesives, and systemic adjuncts, e.g. Factor VII*)

Template Dictation

Preoperative Diagnosis: Acute Type A Aortic Dissection

Post-operative Diagnosis: Same

Procedure(s) Performed: Repair of ascending and hemiarch **[OR TOTAL ARCH]** aorta for acute type A aortic dissection utilizing profound hypothermic circulatory arrest and selective antegrade cerebral perfusion via innominate artery.

Attending Surgeon: [BLANK]

Secondary Surgeon: [BLANK]

Assistants: [BLANK]

Anesthesia: [BLANK]

Operative Findings: A [XX]-cm ascending aorta with friable tissues and a dissection flap visualized in the ascending aorta. **[SIGNIFICANT TOTAL TRANSVERSE AORTIC ARCH HEMATOMA/INTIMAL FRAGMENTATION/OR SIGNIFICANT ANEURYSMAL ENLARGEMENT WAS DEMONSTRATED NECESSITATING TOTAL ARCH REPLACEMENT].** The aortic valve was competent and without pathologic changes.

Description of Procedure: With the patient in supine position under general anesthesia with monitoring lines in place, the chest, abdomen, and lower extremities circumferentially were prepped and draped in sterile fashion. Cardiopulmonary bypass lines were passed and primed. A median sternotomy was made and extended slightly cranially in the midline towards the neck through which the innominate vein was identified and retracted with vessel loops. The innominate artery was carefully dissected and proximal and distal control was obtained. The bypass lines were cut and the patient was systematically heparinized. A side-biting clamp was placed on the innominate artery. A longitudinal arteriotomy was made in the artery and an end-to-side anastomosis was made between a 10-mm Dacron graft which was attached to a 7 mm Soft-Flow® arterial cannula. Following completion of the anastomosis, the clamp was removed and no leaks were observed. The graft and cannula were de-aired and attached to the arterial side of the pump oxygenator.

The pericardium was opened in inverted-T fashion and extended upwards to include the entire ascending aorta. A pericardial well was created. The ascending aorta was friable with a bluish hue indicating ascending aortic dissection [without or with aneurysmal dilation at **XX** cm]. **[THE ASCENDING AORTA DEMONSTRATED SIGNS OF DISSECTION WITH HEMOTAMA INVOLVEMENT OF THE TRANSVERSE ARCH WITHOUT OR WITH ANEURYSMAL DILATION AT XX CM]**. TEE confirmed [absence/presence] of a pericardial effusion and [absence/presence] of aortic insufficiency. A dual-stage venous cannula was positioned and secured through the right atrial appendage and attached to the venous side of the pump oxygenator. Retrograde autologous priming was started and antegrade and retrograde cardioplegia tacks were inserted. Following confirmation of an ACT greater than 460 seconds and completion of retrograde autologous priming, cardiopulmonary bypass was commenced and systemic cooling to 25°C was initiated in preparation for hypothermic circulatory arrest and replacement of the aorta into the proximal hemiarch **[ASCENDING AORTA AND TOTAL ARCH]**. The heart was arrested by placement of a crossclamp at the distal ascending aorta and with a combination of antegrade and retrograde cold blood cardioplegia with topical ice saline cooling. Every 20 minutes throughout the procedure 250 cc of retrograde cold blood cardioplegia was given to maintain myocardial protection.

The ascending aorta was transected in its midportion. It was dissected backwards to the crossclamp and removed leaving about 1 cm proximal to the clamp. This specimen was sent to pathology for sectioning and assessment of cystic medial degeneration. The proximal portion of the aneurysm was then dissected free and removed to the level of the sinotubular junction. At this point, it was possible to inspect the aortic valve and it was found to be a competent tricuspid aortic valve without pathologies. Both left and right coronary ostia were unobstructed and without involvement of the dissection flap. To exclude a proximal false lumen, a Teflon strip was placed in between the layers of the proximal aortic wall, and reinforced carefully with BioGlue®.

At this time, the patient's systematic temperature had reached 25°C. The head of the patient was packed in ice and propofol and steroids were applied for cerebral protection adjuncts. A small right angle clamp was placed at the innominate artery proximal to the graft and flows were reduced to approximately 1 to 1.5 L/min to maintain a right brachial artery pressure of approximately 60 to 70mmHg mean. The main crossclamp was removed and cardiotomy suction was used to clear the operative field. The ascending aorta was then resected more distally with undercutting of the proximal hemiarch such that all 3 great vessels were easily visualized. [THE AORTA WAS THEN RESECTED FURTHER TO JUST DISTAL TO THE LEFT SUBCLAVIAN ARTERY TAKEOFF LEAVING AN ISLAND OF ARCH SURROUNDING THE GREAT VESSELS, LEAVING ALL THREE BRACHIOCEPHALIC VESSELS ATTACHED TO A SINGLE ARTERIAL BUTTON. CAREFULL DISSECTION WAS PERFOMED TO SPARE THE LEFT RECURRENT LARYNGEAL NERVE] A [XX]-mm tubular Dacron graft was brought into the operative field and trimmed accordingly. The distal anastomosis was made between it and the hemiarch with a running 3-0 Prolene suture. This anastomosis proceeded smoothly and was reinforced with a small amount of BioGlue® circumferentially. [THE DISTAL ANASTOMOSIS WAS FIRST CREATED BETWEEN THE ARTERIAL ISLAND AND THE GRAFT WITH A CIRCULAR RUNNING 3-0 PROLENE AFTER WHICH THE DACRON GRAFT WAS TRIMMED TO CREATE THE DESCENDING AORTIC ORIFICE TO DACRON GRAFT ANASTAMOSIS WITH A RUNNING 3-0 PROLENE IN THE SAME FASHION. ANASTOMOSES WERE REINFORCED WITH A SMALL AMOUNT OF BIOGLUE® CIRCUMFERENTIALLY]. The newly constructed distal anastomosis was de-aired by removal of the innominate artery clamp, ending the selective antegrade cerebral perfusion and a crossclamp was reapplied to the more proximal Dacron graft, reestablishing full bypass flow. The anastomosis was inspected for leaks and repair sutures with 4-0 Prolene were placed as necessary. Systemic rewarming was begun.

Attention was turned to the proximal portion of the ascending aorta. The Dacron graft was trimmed to length for a tight fit to the sinotubular junction of the aorta. The retrograde cardioplegia catheter was removed and the site tied down. An antegrade cardioplegia tack/root vent was placed into the anterior midportion of the Dacron graft to which the cardioplegia line was attached. The proximal anastomosis was then created with a 3-0 Prolene suture in the usual circumferential running fashion. Prior to tying the suture the heart was allowed to refill for de-airing and a 500 cc dose of warm cardioplegia was delivered. Ventricular pacing wires were placed.

The crossclamp was removed and the patient was defibrillated into normal sinus rhythm/resumed spontaneous normal sinus rhythm. After an appropriate period of rewarming and de-airing, ventilation was begun and the patient was weaned off cardiopulmonary bypass. Once the systemic temperature had reached 36°C, the cannulae were removed with uneventful protamine administration. Hemostasis

II. Adult Cardiac Surgery

was obtained and confirmed at all cannulation, anastomoses, and dissection sites. A 36 Fr mediastinal chest tube was left in the mediastinum followed by a 19 Fr Blake® drain in the posterior pericardium. The sternum was closed with a total of X stainless steel wires followed by wound irrigation and closure of fascia, soft tissue, and skin anatomically with running Vicryl sutures in layers. The skin was cleaned and sterile dressings applied. The sterile drapes were removed and the patient was transferred to the Cardiothoracic Intensive Care Unit in critical but stable condition having tolerated the procedure well.

At the end of the procedure all sponge, instrument and needle counts were counted twice and reported to be correct. Dr. [XX] was scrubbed for [XX] parts of the procedure

PERFUSION DATA: Cardiopulmonary bypass time [XX] minutes with a crossclamp time of [XX] minutes and a hypothermic circulatory arrest time with selective antegrade cerebral perfusion of [XX] minutes.

All instrument, sponge and needle counts were confirmed to be correct, twice, at the end of the operation. The patient was subsequently transferred to the postoperative cardiac surgical intensive care unit in critical condition.

Dr. [BLANK] was present and scrubbed for [BLANK] elements of this procedure.

4. Elephant Trunk Part 1

Parth Amin MD and Jeffrey Schwartz MD

Loyola University Medical Center, Maywood, IL

Essential Operative Steps

1. Invasive monitoring and general anesthesia
2. Right femoral arterial line
3. TEE to evaluate for aortic regurgitation
4. Right axillary exposure
5. Heparinization for axillary conduit/graft
6. Sternotomy
7. Atrial pursestring
8. Initiate cardiopulmonary bypass
9. Begin cooling
10. SVC pursestring for retrograde cerebral perfusion
11. Right superior pulmonary venous vent
12. Cross clamp (if associated procedures)
13. Administration of antegrade [possible retrograde] cardioplegia
14. Trendelenberg position
15. Snare cerebral vessels
16. Excise aneurysm
17. Create island [possible separate grafts]
18. Wean patient from cardiopulmonary bypass when cooled
19. Invaginate graft 5-10 cm
20. Sew distal anastomosis
21. Cannulate graft after de-airing
22. Resume lower body flow/bypass
23. Sew island to graft
24. De-air and resume full cardiopulmonary bypass flow
25. Re-warm
26. Sew proximal anastomosis
27. De-air
28. Wean off cardiopulmonary bypass
29. Pacer wires
30. Chest and mediastinal tubes
31. Hemostasis
32. Close sternotomy and axillary cannulation site

Potential Complications and Pitfalls

1. Sternotomy/wound problems
2. Cooling/rewarming too rapidly
3. Inadequate de-airing
4. Prolonged circulatory arrest time
5. Incomplete occlusion of the SVC with tourniquet

II. Adult Cardiac Surgery

6. Inadequate length of elephant trunk
7. Bleeding

Template Dictation

Preoperative Diagnosis: Arch and descending aortic aneurysm

Post-operative Diagnosis: Same

Procedure(s) Performed:

Attending Surgeon: [BLANK]

Secondary Surgeon: [BLANK]

Assistants: [BLANK]

Anesthesia: [BLANK]

Circulatory Arrest Time: [Minutes]

Products: [FFP/Platelets/PRBCs]

Indication(s) for Procedure: [AGE] year old [GENDER] with a past history of [dissection, aneurysm], who presents with an arch and descending thoracic aneurysm with maximal diameter [cm]. Given the risk of rupture, and the risk and benefit profile, repair was discussed. Concomitant **[coronary artery disease and/or valvular pathology was/was not]** noted on cardiac catheterization and preoperative echocardiography.

Description of Procedure: The patient was brought to the operating room, positioned in a supine manner, and underwent induction of general anesthesia. Pulmonary artery catheter, radial and femoral arterial lines, adequate intravenous access, and foley catheter were placed. The patient was then prepped and draped in a sterile fashion. A right infraclavicular incision was made, deepened through pectoralis fascia, and the axillary vein exposed. The vein was then dissected circumferentially and retracted such that the axillary artery was exposed and circumferentially controlled. 100 units/kg heparin was then systemically administered. The axillary artery was clamped, an arteriotomy made, and a standard 5-0 Prolene continuous anastomosis was fashioned in an end-to-side manner to an 8 mm Dacron graft. The graft was then clamped after flushing and de-airing. The anesthesiologist then confirmed **[no aortic insufficiency]** with transesophageal echocardiography.

A median sternotomy was performed extending from below the sternal notch to the tip of the xiphoid process. A pursestring was then placed at the right atrial appendage. The innominate, left common carotid artery, and left subclavian arteries were then circumferentially dissected and controlled. The remainder of the total dose heparin was then administered directly into the right atrium. The ACT was then maintained at greater than 450 seconds. The right axillary conduit was then cannulated and de-aired. A dual-staged venous cannula was inserted into the right atrium and directed to the inferior vena cava. Cardiopulmonary bypass was initiated with concomitant cooling to 18 degrees centigrade. A right superior pulmonary vent was then placed through a 4-0 prolene pursestring suture. A 4-0 Prolene pursestring was then placed in the superior vena cava for retrograde cerebral perfusion. The SVC was encircled with an umbilical tape. An antegrade cardioplegia suture was also placed in the ascending aorta.

If additional procedures or ventricular distension. Upon fibrillation of the heart, the ascending aorta was cross-clamped just proximal to the innominate artery. Ice was placed upon the heart and 1200 cc of cold blood cardioplegia was administered. [If aortic valve or significant coronary disease pathology present, describe procedure during cooling].

After approximately 45 minutes of cooling, the patient was placed in steep Trendelenburg position. Cardiopulmonary bypass was weaned and the patient separated from cardiopulmonary bypass. The ascending aorta and aortic arch were then excised, leaving an island for the cerebral and upper extremity vessels. The aorta was then transected just beyond the left subclavian artery. [In the case of a previous dissection, describe dissection flap fenestration into the descending thoracic aorta.] The innominate and left common carotid artery were then snared, and antegrade cerebral perfusion initiated at a rate of 10 cc/kg/min.

A [size mm] Dacron graft was then invaginated and delivered into the descending thoracic aorta in order to create an elephant trunk. The distal portion of the elephant trunk was approximately 5-10 cm in length and marked with multiple metal clips. The distal anastomosis was then fashioned with a running 3-0 Prolene suture with felt reinforcement. The left vagus nerve and esophagus were protected during dissection. The graft was then withdrawn from inside the outer and cut to length. The graft was then filled with saline irrigation and after adequate de-airing, the graft was cannulated and flow resumed to the lower body. Antegrade cardioplegia was then delivered directly into the coronary ostia. A circumferential patch was cut from the Dacron graft which corresponded to the cerebral and upper extremity vessel island. A 3-0 Prolene continuous anastomosis was then performed. The tourniquets were released from the innominate, left common carotid, and the left subclavian artery as the axillary. The graft was de-aired, clamped proximal to the takeoff of the innominate artery, and warming instituted. Total circulatory arrest time was [minutes].

The proximal anastomosis was performed using 3-0 prolene suture with Teflon strips. Warm antegrade cardioplegia was then given and the cross-clamp released. After 50 minutes of re-warming, ventricular pacing wires were placed, and mediastinal and pleural tubes were placed and secured to the skin. Cardiopulmonary bypass was weaned and the venous pursestring secured. The axillary conduit was tied off with a large silk suture. Hemostasis was obtained. The right axillary incision was closed with multiple layers of absorbable suture. The pericardium was re-approximated and the sternotomy was closed with alternating single and double sternal wires. The fascial closure was performed with absorbable suture, as was the dermal, and subcuticular layer. Sterile dressings were placed on the wounds. The patient was then taken to ICU in stable condition having tolerating the procedure well.

Dr. **[BLANK]** was present and scrubbed for **[BLANK]** elements of this procedure.

5. Elephant Trunk Part 2

Parth Amin MD and Jeffrey Schwartz MD

Loyola University Medical Center, Maywood, IL

Essential Operative Steps

1. Appropriate invasive monitoring
2. Spinal drain
3. Right lateral decubitus positioning with hips supine
4. Left femoral arterial and venous access
5. Confirm lines by transesophageal echocardiography
6. Thoracoabdominal exposure
7. Divide diaphragm radially
8. Initiate cardiopulmonary bypass
9. Clamp proximal descending aorta
10. Open aorta
11. Identify elephant trunk
12. Clamp elephant trunk
13. Perform anastomosis with new graft
14. Determine extent of aneurysm
15. Maintain femoral flows greater than 60 mmHg
16. Maintain systemic perfusion greater than 70-80 mmHg
17. Open aorta and identify visceral vessels
18. Maintain cold blood cardioplegia at 10 cc/kg/min to each visceral segment
19. Create beveled anastomosis for visceral segment
20. Sew distal anastomosis onto visceral segment
21. Perform left renal anastomosis
22. Wean off cardiopulmonary bypass
23. Reverse anticoagulation
24. Obtain hemostasis.
25. Close femoral exposure
26. Re-approximate diaphragm
27. Place chest tubes and peri-aortic drain
28. Close thoracoabdominal incision

Potential Complications and Pitfalls

1. Renal failure
2. Mesenteric ischemia
3. Spinal ischemia/paraplegia
4. Disruption of proximal Elephant trunk anastomosis
5. Bleeding
6. Lower extremity ischemia

II. Adult Cardiac Surgery

Template Dictation

Preoperative Diagnosis: Arch and descending aortic aneurysm

Post-operative Diagnosis: Same

Procedure(s) Performed:

Attending Surgeon: [BLANK]

Secondary Surgeon: [BLANK]

Assistants: [BLANK]

Anesthesia: [BLANK]

Circulatory Arrest Time: [Minutes]

Products: [FFP/Platelets/PRBCs]

Indication(s) for Procedure: [AGE] year old [GENDER] with aortic arch aneurysm extending to the distal descending thoracic aorta. The first operation was performed to repair the ascending and aortic arch. The patient now presents to complete the repair of the aneurysm.

Description of Procedure: The patient was brought to the operating room and positioned in a supine manner. After induction of general anesthesia, a right femoral arterial line, and right radial arterial line were placed. Spinal drain was then placed. Right internal jugular approach was then used for placement of pulmonary artery catheter. After exchange to a double lumen tube, bronchoscopy was performed to assure appropriate positioning. A transesophageal echo probe was then inserted. The patient was then positioned in a right lateral decubitus position with access to the left groin. The patient was then prepped and draped in a sterile manner.

An oblique left groin incision was made for femoral arterial and venous exposure. The femoral vein and artery were circumferentially dissected and controlled. Concentric 5-0 Prolene pursestring sutures were placed in both vessels. A thoracoabdominal incision was made extending through the left chest in the 7th intercostals space, across the costal margin, and ending midway between the anterosuperior iliac spine and umbilicus. The diaphragm was divided radially, with a 2-3 centimeters left off the chest wall. The retroperitoneum was dissected free and the left common iliac was encircled. The left renal artery was identified and encircled.

A counter incision was made in the 4th intercostal space and the aorta dissected free of the surrounding tissue. The proximal descending thoracic aorta was encircled. The patient was then given 300 units/kg of heparin with repeat assessment throughout the procedure to maintain ACT greater than 450 seconds. The femoral artery and vein were then cannulated using Seldinger technique and echocardiographic confirmation of venous line in the right atrium. Cardiopulmonary bypass was then initiated with cooling to 32 degrees Centigrade.

A clamp was placed on the proximal descending aorta and another clamp placed just above the visceral segment. The proximal descending aorta was opened and the previously placed elephant trunk/Dacron graft identified. The graft was clamped. Intercostals were identified and oversewn with 3-0 Prolene suture. A [size mm] Dacron graft with 10 mm sidearm was then sewn to the previously placed graft an end-to-end, 4-0 Prolene, standard continuous anastomosis. The proximal clamp was then moved down to the distal graft to assess the hemostasis of the anastomosis. Once hemostasis was assured, the femoral flow was decreased and the aorta was then opened its entire length. Below the visceral segment, the aorta was normal. Pruitt catheters were placed in the right renal, celiac, SMA, and left renal. The distal aorta was clamped and flow was then resumed to maintain femoral arterial pressures in excess of 60 mm Hg, with systemic pressure greater than 80 mmHg. Cold blood at 20 degrees Centigrade was administered to each visceral at a rate of 200 cc/branch vessel/minute.

An side-to-side anastomosis was then performed to the visceral segment with a 3-0 Prolene standard continuous fashion. The graft was de-aired through the side-arm. After completing the suture line, clamp was released and the viscera were reperfused. The side arm of the Dacron graft was then anastomosed to the left renal with running 6-0 Prolene suture. At this point, the distal graft was cut to length and anastomosed to the aortic bifurcation.

Cardiopulmonary bypass was then weaned off. Arterial and venous cannula were removed and the femoral pursestrings secured. Protamine reversal was given. Hemostasis was excellent. The aneurysm sac was then reapproximated over the graft. A right angle and straight chest tube were positioned and secured to the skin. A Blake drain was left around the aneurysm itself. The diaphragm was reapproximated using large PDS sure. The ribs were then reapproximated using large Vicryl sutures. The fascia, dermis, and subcuticiular skin layer were then closed with absorbable suture. Sterile dressing was placed on the wound. The patient tolerated the procedure well and was transferred to ICU in stable condition.

Dr. [BLANK] was present and scrubbed for [BLANK] elements of this procedure.

6. Endovascular Management of Acute Type B Dissection

Parth Amin, MD[1], and Joss Fernandez, MD[2]

[1]Loyola University Medical Center, Maywood, IL

[2]Missouri Heart Center, Columbia, MO

Essential Operative Steps

1. Invasive arterial pressure monitoring
2. Spinal drain placement
3. Femoral arterial exposure
4. Contralateral percutaneous femoral access
5. Intravascular Ultrasound (IVUS)
6. True lumen sheath placement
7. Wire access into true lumen
8. Confirmation of true lumen wire access with IVUS
9. Ultrasound evaluation of mesenteric arteries
10. Ultrasound evaluation of renal arteries
11. Delivery device for thoracic graft into true lumen
12. Fluoroscopic confirmation of perfusion to all vessels

Potential Complications and Pitfalls

1. Access site complications
2. Stenting of false lumen
3. Persistent Malperfusion of Viscera
4. Lower extremity ischemia
5. Renal failure
6. Mesenteric ischemia
7. Paralysis
8. Cerebrovascular Accident

Template Dictation

Preoperative Diagnosis: Acute Type B Dissection with Malperfusion

Post-operative Diagnosis: Same

Attending Surgeon: [BLANK]

Secondary Surgeon: [BLANK]

Assistants: [BLANK]

Anesthesia: [BLANK]

Contrast: [mL Type of contrast]

Indication(s) for Procedure: Patient is a [age /gender] with an acute Type B dissection. Despite medical management, the patient was found to have arterial malperfusion to the kidneys, intestine, and/or lower extremity. As a result of the malperfusion, urgent intervention was indicated. The goal of endovascular vascular management of acute type B dissections was to decompression the false lumen, re-pressurize the true lumen and assure perfusion of visceral vessels whether through individual vessel stenting from true lumen to branch or fenestration of the obstructing intimal flap. Discussion included open and endovascular fenestration, thoracic stent graft placement, and bypass. The risk/benefit profile favored endovascular stent placement.

Description of procedure: The patient was brought to the operating room, positioned in a supine manner, and had left radial arterial line and large bore venous access placed. The patient's right arm, abdomen and groins were then prepped and draped in a sterile manner. The preoperative CT scan revealed that the [**right/left**] femoral artery was perfused by the true lumen. A right femoral cut down was performed using a transverse incision 1 cm below the inguinal ligament. The femoral artery was circumferentially dissected and controlled. Systemic heparin 100 units/kg was then administered. A Micropuncture system was used for femoral access, and exchanged for a 9 French sheath. Contralateral percutaneous femoral access was then obtained with a micropuncture system. An 0.035 inch guidewire and pigtail catheter were taken to the aortic arch from this approach.

If femoral access vessels too small for delivery device: A transverse incision was made in between the anterior superior iliac spine and the umbilicus. The anterior fascia was incised, the muscle split, and the retroperitoneal plane entered. The iliac bifurcation was identified, circumferentially dissected, and controlled. After adequate heparinization, the iliac artery was clamped, an arteriotomy made, and a standard 6-0 prolene running anastomosis performed to an 10 mm Dacron graft.

An 0.035 inch Glidewire was then advanced to the arch of the aorta under fluoroscopic guidance. An intravascular ultrasound was then used to confirm location of the wire in the true lumen. The left renal vein was used as a landmark to identify the celiac artery, the superior mesenteric artery, and the right and left renal arteries. The following vessels were fed by the true lumen [**mesenterics, renals, lower extremity**]. Malperfusion to the [**mesenterics, renals, lower extremity**] was noted on IVUS. Pressure measurements were also taken in the true lumen using a standard 5F catheter.

If difficulty in assessing true lumen: Right brachial access was performed using a micropuncture system and exchange performed to a 5 French sheath. A 300 cm angled 035 inch Glidewire was advanced from the right arm into the aortic arch. A snare was then brought from the femoral approach and used to bring the right arm wire to the [right/left] femoral artery. An IVUS was then used to confirm the wire location in the true lumen].

Measurements of the diameter and length of the thoracic stent graft were taken from the preoperative CT scan. The diameter was oversized by < 10% of the approximate normal native aortic diameter. Based on IVUS localization the intimal defects or fenestrations were marked. The proximal and distal landing zones were then marked at minimum 2 cm proximal and distally. After the access wire was exchanged for a stiffer wire, the delivery device was taken to the descending thoracic aorta.

The blood pressure was brought down to a systolic pressure in the 100-110 mmHg range. After a breath hold, the thoracic stent graft was deployed. The pigtail catheter was taken to the aortic arch and then another angiogram was taken. The graft was deployed in the appropriate position. Significant reduction in perfusion of the false lumen was noted. Additional angiographic views of the mesenteric, renals, and iliac vessels were undertaken. Contrast was noted to fill in an antegrade fashion, with no delay, in all the vessels noted.

If individual branch vessel malperfusion is still present: Wire access was then obtained into the [**mesenteric, renal**] artery with malperfusion. A Guidecath system was then used to access the orifice of the vessel. Once in the vessel, the system was exchanged to an 0.014 platform. An angiogram was performed and sizing determined. A balloon expandable stent was then deployed from the true lumen into the branch vessel. Repeat angiogram showed perfusion of the stented artery.

If the true lumen of the visceral aorta is still compressed compromising multiple branch vessels: Endovascular fenestration is performed. IVUS is introduced into the right femoral access where the wire has been confirmed to be in the true lumen. After a wire was placed across a more proximal fenestration, a snare was brought to capture the wire from below. The snared wire was then pulled down, causing a tear in the intimal flap. Once the fenestration was created, IVUS was repeated to confirm fenestration and branch vessel patency.

The wires and catheters were removed. The arterial exposure was closed with a running 5-0 prolene suture. The wound was then closed in multiple layers. The distal pulses were evaluated and were [**palpable/dopplerable**]. The patient was taken to ICU in stable condition, having tolerated the procedure well.

Dr. [**BLANK**] was present and scrubbed for [**BLANK**] elements of this procedure.

7. Aortic Valve Replacement for Aortic Insufficiency or Aortic Stenosis

Amy Fiedler, MD, and Frederick Y. Chen, MD, Ph.D

Brigham and Women's Hospital, Boston MA

Essential Operative Steps

1. Lines and monitoring
2. General endotracheal anesthesia
3. Intraoperative transesophageal echocardiogram
4. Median sternotomy
5. Open pericardium, pericardial well, survey ascending aorta cannulation and clamp sites for plaque burden with epi aortic ultrasound
6. Systemic heparanization (400 u/kg)
7. Check ACT
8. Arterial cannulation
9. Venous cannulation
10. Myocardial protection cannula placement (antegrade and/or retrograde cardioplegia)
11. Initiate CPB
12. Aortic cross clamp
13. Arrest heart with antegrade cardioplegia (1200 mL) and topical cooling for cardiac arrest (+/- retrograde cardioplegia)
14. Place LV vent
15. Aortotomy
16. Excise valve and debride calcium from annulus
17. Irrigate and inspect LVOT, anterior leaflets of mitral valve for debris.
18. Size valve
19. Seat and tie valve in place Close ascending aorta in layers
20. Initial De-airing
21. Remove aortic cross clamp
22. Check for hemostasis
23. Arterial and ventricular pacer wire placement and pace heart
24. Complete de-airing
25. Wean from CPB
26. Protamine administration for heparin reversal (test dose first)
27. Aortic and Venous decannulation
28. Assess hemostasis
29. Sternotomy closure

Potential Complications and Pitfalls

1. Stay midline during sternotomy
2. Avoid injury to innominate vein while making pericardial well
3. Gentle tissue handling important to avoid

4. cannulation complications such as aortic dissection/bleeding, right atrial tear
5. Avoid areas of calcification for cannulation and clamp site leading to stroke
6. Insufficient myocardial protection and cardiac arrest (cross clamp not across, aortic insufficiency, insufficient venous drainage)
7. Coronary sinus injury with retrograde cardioplegia cannulation
8. Inadequate decalcification leading to paravalvular leak
9. Undersizing of the valve leading to patient/prosthetic mismatch.
10. Oversizing of the valve leading to coronary artery compromise
11. Poor strut placement obstructing the coronary artery ostia.
12. Improper deairing prior to removal of aortic root vent
13. Inadequate control of hemostasis prior to sternal closure/bleeding from cannulation sites

Template Dictation

Preoperative Diagnosis: Severe, symptomatic aortic stenosis, aortic insufficiency, acute on chronic systolic heart failure
Postoperative Diagnosis: Same

Procedure(s) Performed: Aortic valve replacement (specify valve type, specify technique i.e: supra-annular technique)

Attending Surgeon: [BLANK]

Secondary Surgeon: [BLANK]

Assistants: [BLANK]

Anesthesia: [BLANK]

Indication(s) for Procedure: [AGE] year old [GENDER] with [DURATION] history of [COMPLAINT- i.e: increasing shortness of breath, dyspnea on exertion, chest pain]. Pre-operative echocardiography reveals [FINDINGS].

Description of Procedure: The patient was taken to the Operating Theatre on [DATE]. The patient's identity and planned procedure verified, and the patient was placed on the operating room table in supine position. General anesthesia was obtained and invasive hemodynamic monitoring lines were placed. A transesophageal echocardiogram was then performed to evaluate cardiac and valve function. We then prepped and draped the chest, abdomen, groins, and lower extremities in the standard sterile fashion. A time out was performed, with patient and procedure again verified. Median sternotomy was performed and a pericardial cradle was hung. We then adequately heparinized the patient and cannulated the ascending aorta in an area free of calcification and cannulated the right atrium as well. Antegrade cardioplegia cannula was placed. We then went on cardiopulmonary bypass with an ACT greater than 450 and delivered cold antegrade cardioplegia directly into the root after crossclamping the aorta. The heart went into a quick diastolic arrest. An LV vent was placed. Aortotomy was performed and the valve visualized. The calcified aortic valve was removed and passed off the table as specimen. Calcification at the level of the annulus was carefully debrided. The annulus, LVOT, and anterior leaflets of the mitral valve were then copiously irrigated to remove any extra particulate debris. The valve annulus was measured. It would comfortably accommodate a **[INSERT VALVE TYPE AND SIZE HERE]** appropriately and using horizontal mattress pledgeted sutures, secured it in place via the supra-annular technique. We then performed aggressive de-airing maneuvers and closed the ascending aorta in two layers with 4-0 Prolene suture. We placed the patient in Trendelenburg position and removed the aortic cross clamp with the aortic vent on high. We placed atrial and ventricular pacing wires and began pacing appropriately and subsequently separated from CPB without difficulty after final de airing. We removed the venous cannula and inspected the valve grossly and found it to be free of paravalvular leak with appropriate gradients. We then gave protamine. After half the dose of protamine was administered, the aortic cannula were removed. All cannulation sites were further reinforced with additional suture. We closed the thymic tissues over the ascending aorta. **[NUMBER OF]** mediastinal drains were then placed. The sternum was then closed with **[INSERT NUMBER]** sternal wires. The fascia was closed with #1 PDS in a running fashion. The deep dermal layer was then closed with #2-0 Vicryl suture in running fashion. The skin and subcuticular layer was closed with #3-0 Monocryl in a running fashion. The skin was then cleansed with sterile saline and dressed with an antibiotic ointment and a Primapore dressing.

All instrument, sponge, and needle counts were confirmed to be correct x 2 at the end of the surgical procedure. The patient was subsequently transferred to the postoperative cardiac surgical intensive care unit in critical condition.

Dr. **[BLANK]** was present and scrubbed for **[BLANK]** elements of this procedure.

8. Aortic Valve Replacement with Aortic Root Enlargement

Sandeep Sainathan, MD, and David D. Yuh MD

Yale University, New Haven, CT.

Essential Operative Steps

1. Informed consent
2. Large bore IV insertion and general endotracheal anesthesia. Watch for ventricular fibrillation on induction
3. Intraoperative monitoring line insertion (arterial line and pulmonary artery catheter) and Foley catheter insertion
4. Intraoperative transesophageal echocardiogram. Confirm valvular morphology, gradients, valve area, annular dimensions, assess left ventricular dimension, and function.
5. Median sternotomy
6. Open pericardium, pericardial stay sutures
7. Survey ascending aorta for plaque burden either with palpation or epiaortic ultrasound. Mobilize the ascending aorta from the main pulmonary artery.
8. Systemic heparinization (400 u/kg)
9. Arterial cannulation
10. Venous cannulation with a two stage venous cannula inserted via the right atrial appendage
11. Antegrade aortic cannula insertion and +/- retrograde coronary sinus cannula
12. Check ACT (>400 sec)
13. Initiate CPB, cool to 32 degrees centigrade
14. LV vent via the RSPV
15. Aortic cross clamp (reduce CPB flow rate, apply cross clamp, and increase CPB flow to 2.0-2.5L/min/m2)
16. Antegrade cardioplegia and topical cooling with cold saline for cardiac arrest (+/-Retrograde cardioplegia)
17. Asses for adequacy of antegrade cardioplegia by adequate distension of the aortic root with rapid myocardial arrest and lack of left ventricular distention. If there is significant AI, can use either direct administration of the cardioplegia after aortotomy via ostial cannula or use retrograde cardiologic arrest. However, the adequacy of right ventricular protection needs to be confirmed after performing an aortotomy and observing good retrograde flow from the right coronary ostia. If poor, supplement with antegrade ostial injection
18. Saturate the field with CO_2 gas
19. Aortotomy in oblique manner starting 10-20 mm above the right coronary artery. Excise aortic valve leaflets. Debride and size the annulus. Calculate the EOA (Effective Orifice Area) for the prosthetic valve indexed to the body surface area with chart provided by the manufacture.

A value less than 0.85 cm2/m2 can lead to a patient-prosthesis mismatch and a value below 0.65 cm2/m2 represents severe patient-prosthesis mismatch. A value between 0.85 to 0.65 cm2/m2 may be acceptable in a sedentary high-risk patient with significant annular calcification, as compared to the risk from a more extensive aortic root enlargement procedure

20. Option to deal with a small aortic annulus include: Use a valve one size up than measured size by placing the valve with canted up in the non-coronary sinus, use of a Medtronic Freestyle valve, aortic annular enlargement, aortic root replacement, and left ventricle apical to descending aortic conduit. In adults, annular enlargements are made posteriorly (Nicks and Manougian's techniques), in the fibrous part of the aortic annulus in the region of the aortic –mitral valve continuity. In children, annular enlargements are generally made anteriorly (Konno), in the muscular part of the aortic annulus as generally there is an associated subannular obstructive component.
21. Once a decision is made to perform an aortic annular enlargement, carry the oblique aortotomy towards the middle of the non-coronary sinus (Nick's method). This provides an annular enlargement to accommodate a valve one size larger than originally sized. When the aortotomy is carried down the commissure between the non-coronary and left coronary cusp into the anterior mitral leaflet (Manougian's method), a much larger annular enlargement to accommodate a prosthesis two sizes larger than originally sized can be obtained. The Konno, which is a method used predominantly in children provides the maximum enlargement but with more technical complexity. Each of the resultant defects is repaired with native pericardium, bovine pericardium or Dacron graft. Care needs to be taken to repair the roof of the left atrium in Manougian's method.
22. Valve replacement and closure of the aortotomy after deairing the aorta.
23. Antegrade warm blood cardioplegia "hot shot" administration for rewarming
24. Remove aortic cross clamp with continued deairing of the left heart.
25. Check for hemostasis
26. Arterial and ventricular pacer wire placement
27. Chest tube placement
28. Wean from CPB
29. Venous decannulation
30. Protamine administration for heparin reversal (test dose first)
31. Aortic decannulation
32. Assess hemostasis
33. Sternotomy closure

Potential Complications and Pitfalls

1. Ventricular fibrillation on induction of general anesthesia in AS

2. Inability to arrest a hypertrophied left ventricle with significant AI with antegrade cardioplegia. Use ostial antegrade injection or a retrograde coronary sinus injection.
3. Avoid fracturing a plaque during aortic cross clamping. If not able to avoid the plaque, avoid application of the cross clamp perpendicular to the plaque to prevent a fracture.
4. Injury to the pulmonary artery during aortotomy due to inadequate mobilization of the ascending aorta from it.
5. Injuring the right and left coronary ostia during aortotomy, due to either a low incision or abnormally located high ostial position.
6. Aggressive annular debridement resulting in annular disruption, injury to AV nodal conduction tissue, and injury to the anterior leaflet of the mitral valve.
7. Injury to the left atrial dome during annular enlargement.
8. Injury to anterior mitral subvalvar apparatus and extensive enlargement of the anterior mitral intertrigonal area causing mitral insufficiency.
9. Poorly controllable hemorrhage from the posterior annular area or left atrial dome after removal of the cross clamp with poor access.
10. Insufficient aortic wall to securely close an aortomy due to extension of the aortomy less than 10 mm from the annulus.
11. Narrow sino-tubular junction preventing adequate closure of the aortotomy around the stent posts of the bioprosthetic aortic valve.
12. Improper deairing prior to removal of aortic root vent
13. Inadequate control of hemostasis prior to sternal closure/ bleeding from cannulation sites and aortic suture line.

Template Dictation

Preoperative Diagnosis: [INDICATION – e.g. severe aortic stenosis, aortic regurgitation]

Postoperative Diagnosis: Same

Procedure(s) Performed: Aortic valve replacement (bioprosthetic/mechanical) with root enlargement

Attending Surgeon: [BLANK]

Secondary Surgeon: [BLANK]

Assistants: [BLANK]

Anesthesia: [BLANK]

Indication(s) for Procedure: [AGE] year old [GENDER] with [DURATION] history of [COMPLAINT] –E.g. shortness of breath, syncope, chest pain]. Preoperative echocardiography revealed

Operative Findings: [- e.g. AS – Trileaflet/bileaflet aortic valve with an area of 0.8 cm2 with a mean gradient of 40 mm Hg with an annulus size of 19 mm and preserved LV function. Preoperative coronary angiography revealed no significant obstructive disease. AR- Trileaflet/bileaflet aortic valve with a central regurgitation jet, vena contracta of > 6mm with a regurgitant volume > 50%, annulus size of 19 mm, and preserved LV function.]

Description of Procedure: The patient was taken to the operating room on [**DATE**]. The patient's identity and planned procedure verified, and the patient was placed on the operating room table in the supine position. General anesthesia was administered via an endotracheal tube. A right internal jugular central venous line, pulmonary artery catheter, radial arterial lines were inserted, and a urinary catheter was placed.

Preoperative transesophageal echocardiogram was then performed to evaluate cardiac and valvular function. It confirmed the preoperative transthoracic findings. We then proceeded to prep and drape the chest, abdomen, groins, and lower extremities in sterile fashion. A time out was performed.

Median sternotomy was then performed. After identification of the innominate vein, the pericardium was opened. There were no pericardial adhesions and pericardial stay sutures were placed. The ascending aorta was mobilized from the main pulmonary artery. The ascending aorta was measured at the root and the sinotubular junction and was [**cms**]. In addition, there was no palpable calcification in the ascending aorta. The aortic cannulation sutures were then placed in the ascending aorta below the level of the innominate artery. The right atrial cannulation sutures were then placed within the right atrial appendage. A total of [**UNITS**] of systemic heparin was administered. The aortic cannula was then inserted, secured and de-aired. A two-stage venous cannula was then placed and secured in the right atrial appendage. A DLP (dual lumen aortic root cannula with vent) cannula was then inserted into the ascending aorta for administration of antegrade cardioplegia. A retrograde cannula was placed in the coronary sinus through a pursestring suture placed in the low right atrium.

Cardiopulmonary bypass was initiated and the patient was cooled to 32 degrees centigrade. A left ventricular vent was placed via the right superior pulmonary vein. The aortic cross-clamp was placed. Antegrade cardioplegia was administered and there was rapid arrest of the heart followed by administration of retrograde cardioplegia. Cooled saline was applied to the heart. (In case of AI/ AS with associated AI, after application of the aortic cross clamp, an ascending aortotomy was performed and antegrade cardioplegia was directly administered via the coronary ostia via ostial cannulas).The operative field was saturated with CO_2 gas.

After administering [**BLANK**] mL of cardioplegia, an aortotomy was made 10-20 mm above the right coronary artery and extended in an oblique fashion towards the non-coronary cusp. The aortic valve was inspected. It was tricuspid/bicuspid with severe calcification of the leaflets with/without commissural fusion. The

203

leaflets were excised keeping as close as possible to the annulus. Following this, the left ventricular outflow tract was packed with a gauze and the annulus gently debrided of calcifications. The debris was carefully collected via an open ended sucker. Following this, the left ventricular outflow tract pack was removed and thorough cold saline irrigation was delivered into the aortic root and left ventricular cavity to wash out any missed debris. The annulus was sized. The annulus was sized to 19 mm with an effective orifice area indexed to the patient's body surface area at less than 0.85 cm2/m2. Hence, a decision was made to enlarge the aortic annulus.

1. Nicks method: The oblique aortotomy was carried through the middle of the non-coronary sinus up to the base of the anterior mitral leaflet. With this incision, we were able to size the annulus up to 21 mm with the effective orifice area indexed to the body surface area of the patient now greater than 0.85 cm2/m2. The resultant defect in the sinus was repaired using a 5mm wide Dacron graft with running 4/0 polpropylene sutures. Following this, non-everting 2/0, polyester pledgeted annular sutures were placed in an interrupted fashion around the aortic annulus. In the area of the repair, in the non-coronary sinus, the plegeted sutures were placed from outside the aortic wall incorporating the Dacron graft. Following this, the annular sutures were passed through the sewing ring of the aortic prosthesis. The aortic prosthetic was gently lowered to sit upon the aortic annulus and the sutures were tied and cut. The right and left coronary ostia were inspected for adequate clearance from the prosthesis. The sinotubular junction was of an adequate size to accommodate the stent posts of the prosthesis and hence the Dacron graft was trimmed accordingly. (In case the sino-tubular junction is constrictive around the stent posts, the patch can be incorporated in the aortomy closure at this level in order to enlarge it). The aortotomy was closed with 4/0 polypropylene sutures in 2 layers, with the first deeper layer comprised of a continuous suture in a horizontal mattress fashion and the second superficial layer in a simple running fashion. Before tying the suture, the aorta and left heart were deaired through the aortotomy.

2. Manougian method: The oblique aortotomy was carried through the commissure between the left and non-coronary cusp onto the anterior leaflet of the mitral valve after opening the adjoining roof of the left atrium. The resultant defect was repaired using a 5mm wide Dacron patch starting at the apex of the anterior mitral leaflet incision with 5/0 polypropylene suture. Care was taken to incorporate the roof of the left atrium into the patch repair. Following this, non-everting 2/0 polyester plegeted annular sutures were placed in an interrupted fashion. In the area of the repair, the pledgeted sutures were placed from outside the aortic wall incorporating the Dacron graft. Following this, the annular sutures were passed through the sewing ring of the aortic prosthesis. The aortic prosthetic was gently lowered to sit upon the aortic annulus and the sutures were tied and cut. The right and left coronary ostia were inspected

for adequate clearance from the prosthesis. The sinotubular junction was of an adequate size to accommodate the stent post of the prosthesis and hence the Dacron graft was trimmed accordingly. The aortotomy was closed with 4/0 polypropylene sutures in 2 layers, with the first deeper layer comprised of a continuous suture in a horizontal mattress fashion and the second superficial layer in a simple running fashion. Before tying the suture, the aorta and left heart were deaired through the aortotomy.

A hot shot of cardioplegia was administered and the patient was rewarmed. The aortic cross-clamp was then removed. The retrograde cardioplegia cannula was removed. Two chest tubes were placed in the mediastinum. Temporary atrial and ventricular pacing wires were then inserted and tested for appropriate capture. The heart was de-aired, and the DLP vent and LV vent were removed. The patient was weaned from cardiopulmonary bypass. TEE showed a well-seated valve with no paravalvular leaks, mean gradient [**NUMBER**], and normal movement of the anterior leaflet of the mitral valve.

The venous cannula was removed, and the cannulation sutures were tied down. A test dose of protamine was administered and the patient was monitored for adverse reaction before the protamine was resumed. The aortic cannula was then removed, and the cannulation sutures tied down.

Adequate hemostasis was then confirmed within the mediastinum. All instrument, sponge and needle counts were confirmed to be correct x 2. The sternum was then closed with a total of [**NUMBER**] stainless steel sternal wires. There was no change in the hemodynamics after sternal closure. The wound was irrigated with antibiotic solution. The presternal fascia was then closed with 0-0 Polyglactin suture in a running fashion. The deep dermal layer was then closed with 2-0 Polyglactin suture in a running fashion. The skin and subcuticular layer was closed with 4-0 Polyglactin suture in a running fashion. Sterile occlusive dressing was applied to the skin incision. The mediastinal drains were connected to an underwater seal on suction. The patient was subsequently transferred to the postoperative cardiac surgical intensive care unit.

Dr. [**BLANK**] was present and scrubbed for [**BLANK**] elements of this operation.

9. Biatrial Cox-Maze Ablation for Atrial Fibrillation

Mark J. Kearns, MD and Jamil Bashir, MD

Division of Cardiovascular Surgery, St. Paul's Hospital

University of British Columbia Vancouver, BC, Canada

Essential Operative Steps

1. Right pulmonary veins bluntly dissected
2. Bipolar radiofrequency clamp device inserted around right pulmonary veins and ablation performed
3. Left pulmonary veins bluntly dissected
4. Clamp device used to ablate left pulmonary veins
5. Small incision at base of right atrial appendage
6. Clamp device used for ablation from atrial incision to superior cavoatrial junction along the atrial free wall
7. Vertical right atriotomy
8. Clamp device for ablation lines from posterior aspect of vertical atriotomy extending along superior and inferior vena cavae, respectively
9. Cryoablation probe inserted through first (small) atrial incision, to create ablation line connecting the incision to the tricuspid annulus (above the septal leaflet)
10. Cryoablation probe again used to connect anterior aspect of vertical atriotomy to tricuspid annulus (above the antero-posterior commissure)
11. Left atrial appendage amputation
12. Clamp device to ablate between amputation site and left superior pulmonary vein
13. Standard left atrial incision
14. Clamp device to create adjoining ablation lines between superior and inferior pulmonary veins, respectively
15. Clamp device oriented from inferior aspect of left atriotomy towards mitral annulus around P2; ablation performed at this site
16. Cryoablation probe used to extend above ablation line to the mitral annulus, both endocardially, and epicardially (crossing the coronary sinus)
17. Closure of left atrial appendage amputation site

Potential Complications and Pitfalls

1. Friable atrial tissue, prone to injury
2. Injury to pulmonary arteries and veins
3. Inadequate hemostasis
4. Hemorrhage
5. Blood product transfusion and related adverse effects
6. Injury to conduction tissue and need for permanent pacemaker
7. Prolonged CPB and cross-clamp times

8. Failure to achieve lesion transmurality
9. Procedural failure

Template Dictation

Preoperative Diagnosis: [INDICATION—e.g. symptomatic AF, undergoing other cardiac operations; asymptomatic AF, undergoing other cardiac operations and where the ablation can be performed with minimal additional risk.]

Postoperative Diagnosis: Same

Procedure(s) Performed: [X] and surgical AF ablation (DETAILS—e.g. cardiac incisions, energy source(s) used, extent of lesion sets employed, whether testing for exit block was performed, and additional CPB and cross-clamp times required for the ablation).

Attending Surgeon: [BLANK]

Secondary Surgeon: [BLANK]

Assistants: [BLANK]

Anesthesia: [BLANK]

Indication(s) for Procedure: [AGE] year old [GENDER] with a [DURATION] history of [**COMPLAINTS—symptoms accounted for by condition X, in addition to symptom burden associated with AF**]. In addition to preoperative investigations for condition X, include details regarding the type of AF (paroxysmal or persistent), and any past interventions used to treat it (pharmacologic, cardioversion, electrophysiology ablation attempts).

Description of Procedure: [**DETAILS of preparation for procedure X (the primary cardiac surgical indication)**]. With the arterial and bicaval cannulation sutures in place, heparin [**UNITS**] was administered intravenously. The patient remained in [**RHYTHM**] and the absence of left atrial thrombus was confirmed by trans-esophageal echocardiography [*for the patient in AF at the time of surgery, document whether they were converted to normal sinus rhythm for the purpose of testing for exit block*]. The aorta and both cavae were cannulated in standard fashion. The superior and inferior vena cavae were freed circumferentially, and ensnared with umbilical tapes just distal to both caval cannulation sites. Cardiopulmonary bypass was then instituted at normothermia.

The right superior and inferior pulmonary veins were dissected circumferentially to allow the passage of a bipolar radiofrequency clamp device [**MANUFACTURER**]. The jaws of the clamp were closed around both right-sided veins, and ablation carried out as indicated by [**MANUFACTURER**]. The clamp was removed and cleaned with saline-soaked gauze. Next the left superior and inferior pulmonary veins were identified and dissected circumferentially. The ablation clamp was carefully positioned around both veins, closed and ablation was performed as previously described. [***Document whether exit block at the*** *pulmonary veins was tested for, to ensure completeness of the ablation*]. The patient was then cooled to 34 degrees Celsius, and both caval tapes were snared securely using rubber tourniquets.

A small incision was made at the base of the right atrial appendage and the clamp device was inserted. The clamp was oriented towards the junction of the right atrium and superior vena cava, along the right atrial free wall. The clamp was closed, and ablation carried out at this site. A vertical right atriotomy was performed approximately 2cm from the first free wall ablation. The clamp was then used to perform two ablation lines, orthogonal to the right atriotomy incision, starting from its base and oriented superiorly and inferiorly along both cavae, respectively. Next, a cryoablation device was inserted through the small incision at the base of the right atrial appendage. The probe was oriented to create an endocardial line of ablation from its entry point to the tricuspid annulus (above the septal leaflet). Following copious saline irrigation to remove the cryoablation probe safely, it was repositioned to join the anterior aspect of the vertical right atriotomy with the tricuspid annulus above its antero-posterior commissure. An endocardial line of ablation was created at this site, and the probe was removed as described previously.

Cannulation sutures were placed in the aorta proximal to the arterial cannulation site, and an antegrade cardioplegia/venting catheter was introduced and secured in place. Cardiopulmonary bypass flows were reduced, and the ascending aorta was clamped prior to the resumption of full flow. Cold blood cardioplegia [**VOLUME**] was administered down the antegrade cannula to achieve complete electro-mechanical cardiac arrest. Once arrest was achieved, the left atrial appendage was identified and amputated. The bipolar radiofrequency clamp device was introduced through the appendectomy and oriented towards left superior pulmonary vein. The clamp was closed and a line of ablation was created joining the left atrial appendage base with the left superior pulmonary vein.

A standard left atrial incision was performed next, and the bipolar clamp device was used to create two adjoining ablation lines across the superior and inferior pulmonary veins, respectively. From the inferior aspect of the left atriotomy, the clamp device was used to create a line of ablation oriented towards the mitral annulus, in the region of the P2. A cryoablation probe was used to fully extend this lesion down to the mitral annulus both endocardially, and epicardially, crossing the coronary sinus. The site of left atrial appendage amputation was then closed in two layers using 5-0 prolene suture.

[DETAILS of the remainder of the cardiac operation (procedure X), including: closure of cardiac incisions, re-warming, de-airing, weaning from cardiopulmonary bypass, heparin reversal and hemostasis, drains left in situ, atrial and ventricular pacing wires, sternal and soft tissue closure, and details regarding patient stability and level of pharmacologic support at the end of the case].

Instrument, sponge, and needle counts were correct. The patient was transferred to the cardiac surgical intensive care unit in stable condition.

Dr. [BLANK] was present and scrubbed for [BLANK] elements of the case.

II. Adult Cardiac Surgery

10. Coronary Artery Bypass Grafting With Cardiopulmonary Bypass

Damien J. LaPar, MD, MSc and Gorav Ailawadi MD

University of Virginia, Charlottesville, VA

Essential Operative Steps

1. Lines and Monitoring
2. General endotracheal anesthesia
3. Intraoperative transesophageal echocardiogram
4. Median sternotomy
5. Conduit choice and LIMA harvest
6. Open pericardium, pericardial well, survey ascending aorta for plaque burden (consider epiaortic ultrasound), cannulation and proximal anastomosis sites.
7. Systemic heparinization (400 u/kg)
8. Arterial cannulation
9. Venous cannulation
10. Myocardial protection cannula placement (DLP in aortic root, +/- retrograde cannula in coronary sinus)
11. Check ACT (>400 sec)
12. Initiate CPB
13. Aortic cross clamp (reduce CPB flow rate, apply cross clamp, increase CPB flow to 2.0-2.5L/min/m2)
14. Antegrade cardioplegia (1200 ml) and topical cooling with ice for cardiac arrest (+/- retrgrograde cardioplegia)
15. Distal anastomoses (start with right side for instillation of cardioplegia down completed vein graft for better right heart myocardial protection).
16. Proximal anastomoses
17. Antegrade warm blood cardioplegia "hot shot" administration for rewarming
18. Remove aortic cross clamp
19. Check for hemostasis
20. Arterial and ventricular pacer wire placement
21. Chest tube placement
22. Wean from CPB
23. Venous decannulation
24. Protamine administration for heparin reversal (test dose first)
25. Aortic decannulation
26. Assess hemostasis
27. Sternotomy closure

Potential Complications and Pitfalls

1. Stay midline during sternotomy

2. Avoid injury to innominate vein while making pericardial well
3. Avoid IMA injury
4. Cannulation catastrophe (Aortic dissection/ bleeding, Right atrial tear)
5. Poor choice of location of aortic cannula/ crossclamp (leading to stroke)
6. Insufficient myocardial protection and cardiac arrest (cross clamp not across, aortic insufficiency, insufficient venous drainage)
7. Coronary sinus injury with retrograde cardioplegia cannulation
8. Difficulty finding coronary arteries, including intramyocardial vessels
9. Injury to coronary artery/ posterior wall while opening coronaries
10. Opening coronary proximal to lesion
11. Kinking of bypass grafts and/or insufficient graft length resulting in tension of graft
12. Improper deairing prior to removal of aortic root vent
13. Bleeding from distal anastomoses
14. Inadequate control of hemostasis prior to sternal closure/ bleeding from cannulation sites.

Template Dictation

Preoperative Diagnosis: [INDICATION – e.g. Unstable angina, 90% stenosis LAD, 80% proximal PDA]

Postoperative Diagnosis: Same

Procedure(s) Performed: Coronary artery bypass grafting **(DETAILS – e.g. LIMA to LAD, SVG to PDA)**

Attending Surgeon: [BLANK]

Secondary Surgeon: [BLANK]

Assistants: [BLANK]

Anesthesia: [BLANK]

EBL: [ml]

Products: [FFP/Platelets/PRBCs]

CPB Time: [Minutes]

Aortic Cross Clamp Time: [Minutes]

Indication(s) for Procedure: [AGE] year old [GENDER] with [DURATION] history of [COMPLAINT – e.g. increasingly worse chest pain and shortness of breath]. Preoperative coronary catheterization reveals [FINDINGS - e.g. 90% stenosis of LAD and 80% stenosis of proximal PDA with estimated ejection fraction of 50-55%].

Description of Procedure: The patient was taken to the operating room on [DATE]. The patient's identity and planned procedure verified, and the patient was placed on the operating room table in the supine position. General anesthesia was obtained. A right internal jugular central venous line and pulmonary artery catheter and radial arterial line were inserted. Preoperative transesophageal echocardiogram was then performed to evaluate cardiac function and valve function. We then proceeded to prep and drape the chest, abdomen, groins, and lower extremities in sterile fashion. A time out was performed. Median sternotomy was then performed. Simultaneous to this, a right lower extremity endoscopic saphenous vein harvest was performed, performed by physician's assistant. After performing the sternotomy, we then proceeded to harvest the left internal mammary artery in a pedicled fashion. Once dissected, 5000 units of heparin were administered prior to distal division. Hemostasis of the LIMA bed was confirmed. Following harvest of the LIMA, the IMA retractor was removed and a sternotomy retractor placed. After identification of the innominate vein, the pericardium was opened and a pericardial well was created. The aortic cannulation sutures were then placed in the ascending aorta below the level of the innominate artery. The right atrial cannulation sutures were then placed within the right atrium. A total of [UNITS] of systemic heparin was administered. The aortic cannula was then inserted, secured and de-aired. Venous cannula was then placed and secured in the right atrium. A retrograde cannula was placed through the right atrium. A DLP vent was then inserted into the ascending aorta for administration of antegrade cardioplegia. The aortic cross-clamp was placed. Antegrade cardioplegia was administered and there was rapid arrest of the heart followed by retrograde cardioplegia. Ice was applied to the heart.

After administering [BLANK] mL of cardioplegia, a suitable site on the [TARGET – e.g. posterior descending coronary artery] was located. Using a #15C blade, the artery was opened. A saphenous vein graft was trimmed, splatulated and a running #7-0 Prolene suture was used to create an end-to-side anastomosis. Antegrade cardioplegia was then administered through the SVG and hemostasis and flow through the graft was confirmed. A suitable site on the [TARGET – e.g. left anterior descending coronary artery] was identified along the mid portion. Using a #15C scalpel blade, the artery artery was opened. The LIMA was then trimmed to an appropriate length and spatulated. A bulldog was placed on the LIMA. We then performed the distal LIMA anastomosis using running #7-0 Prolene in an end-to-side fashion. We then tested the anastomosis by removing the bulldog clamp to confirm patency of the graft and hemostasis. An adequate length of the [LEFT/RIGHT] sided saphenous vein graft to the PDA was then assessed by briefly filling the heart and measuring its length to the aortic root. The vein was trimmed proximally and spatulated. The heart was then drained, and the site for proximal anastomosis was selected. A #11 blade was used to create an aortotomy and an aortic punch was then used to enlarge the aortotomy, and the proximal anastomosis was completed using running #6-0 Prolene.

Once the proximal anastomosis was complete, hot shot cardioplegia was administered and the patient was rewarmed. The bulldog was removed from the

LIMA. The aortic cross-clamp was then removed. A total of [NUMBER] chest tubes were placed in the [LEFT/RIGHT] pleural space, and [NUMBER] chest tubes were placed in the mediastinum. [ATRIAL/VENTRICULAR] pacing wires were then inserted and tested for appropriate capture. The heart was de-aired, and the DLP vent was removed and cannulation sutures tied down. The patient was weaned from cardiopulmonary bypass. The venous cannula was removed, and the cannulation sutures were tied down. A test dose of protamine was administered and the patient was monitored for adverse reaction before the protamine was resumed. The aortic cannula was then removed, and the cannulation sutures tied down. Adequate hemostasis was then confirmed within the mediastinum and left chest wall LIMA harvest site. The sternum was then closed with a total of [NUMBER] stainless steel sternal wires. The wound was irrigated with Betadine saline and antibiotic saline. The fascia was then closed with #1 Vicryl suture in running fashion. The deep dermal layer was then closed with #2-0 Vicryl suture in running fashion. The skin and subcuticular layer was closed with #3-0 Monocryl in running fashion. The skin of the wound was cleansed with sterile saline and dressed with antibiotic ointment and a Primapore dressing.

All instrument, sponge and needle counts were confirmed to be correct x 2 at the end of the operation. The patient was subsequently transferred to the postoperative cardiac surgical intensive care unit in critical condition.

Dr. [BLANK] was present and scrubbed for [BLANK] elements of this procedure.

11. Coronary Artery Bypass Grafting With Mammary and Vein Grafts - Off Pump

Uthman Aluthman, M.D, and Teresa M. Kieser, MD

Libin Cardiovascular Institute of Alberta, Division of Cardiac Surgery, University of Calgary, Calgary, Alberta, Canada

Essential Operative Steps

1. Lines and Monitoring
2. General endotracheal anesthesia
3. Intraoperative transesophageal echocardiogram
4. Median sternotomy
5. Conduit choice and LIMA harvest
6. Open pericardium, pericardial well, survey ascending aorta for plaque burden (consider epiaortic ultrasound).
7. Systemic heparinization
8. OctoBase retractor, Trendelenberg position of OR table +/-lateral rotation of OR table to expose distal target without hypotension; placement of posterior pericardial sutures and/or pericardial sling to position/elevate heart for optimal exposure for distal anastomosis; Octopus tissue stabilizer to stabilize the anastomotic site, possible use of Starfish heart positioner to aid in exposure of target site and improve hemodynamics during anastomosis completion, possible placement of temporary atrial +/- ventricular pacing wires to stabilize rhythm and/or to counteract bradycardia especially if performing RCA distal anastomosis, placement of proximal snare (retracto-tape) on native coronary artery to control bleeding during performance of distal anastomosis; use of intra-coronary shunt for signs of ischemia or for better visibility; use of blower-mister for accurate visualization during performance of distal anastomosis.
9. Distal anastomosis (es)
10. Proximal anastomosis
11. Check for hemostasis
12. Arterial and ventricular pacer wire placement
13. Chest tube placement
14. Protamine administration for heparin reversal (test dose first)
15. Assess hemostasis
16. Sternotomy closure

Potential Complications and Pitfalls

1. Stay midline during sternotomy
2. Avoid injury to innominate vein while making pericardial well
3. Avoid IMA injury
4. Difficulty finding coronary arteries, including intramyocardial vessels

5. Specific to off-pump: during performance of distal anastomosis- signs of ischemia, hypotension, hemodynamic compromise, and ventricular arrhythmia/fibrillation during performance of distal anastomosis, necessitating urgent conversion to on-pump CABG; suboptimal bypass requiring revision/redo of bypass
6. Injury to coronary artery/ posterior wall while opening coronaries
7. Opening coronary proximal to lesion
8. Kinking of bypass grafts and/or insufficient graft length resulting in tension of graft
9. Bleeding from distal anastomoses
10. Inadequate control of hemostasis prior to sternal closure/ bleeding from cannulation sites.

Template Dictation

Preoperative Diagnosis: [BLANK]

Post-operative Diagnosis: Same

Procedure(s) Performed: Elective double coronary artery bypass grafting (CABG) off pump, left internal mammary artery (LIMA) to left anterior descending artery (LAD), Great Saphenous Vein Graft (GSVG) to marginal artery.

Attending Surgeon: [BLANK]

Secondary Surgeon: [BLANK]

Assistants: [BLANK]

Anesthesia: [BLANK]

Indication(s) for Procedure: [**NAME**] is a [**AGE**]-year-old [**GENDER**] with [**DURATION**] history of [**COMPLAINT**]. Preoperative coronary catheterization reveals [**BLANK finding**]. ECHO intraoperatively [**BLANK finding**]

Operative Findings: The patient had reasonable LAD and marginal artery to bypass and excellent conduits of left internal mammary artery and saphenous vein from the left lower leg. Heart function was normal without any regional wall motion abnormalities seen on the trans-esophageal echo. She/He did have 1 unit of PRBC's.

Description of Procedure: Under general anesthesia and endotracheal intubation, a right internal jugular central venous line, pulmonary artery catheter and radial arterial line were inserted. Chest, groins and lower extremities was prepped and draped in the usual sterile fashion. The chest was opened via midline sternotomy. The left internal mammary artery was taken down via the skeletonized technique with the use of the Harmonic scalpel and the Bugge retractor. Simultaneous to this, a left lower extremity greater saphenous vein was harvested by open technique,

II. Adult Cardiac Surgery

performed by a physician's assistant. Once all conduits were harvested and hemostasis maintained, 300 IU/Kg of heparin were administered achieving ACT around 400.

The Bugge retractor used to harvest the LIMA was exchanged for the Octobase retractor. The patient was placed in deep Trendelenburg position, and with a heart sling attached to the posterior pericardium 1 cm away from the border of the left atrium and 2/3 from the inferior vena cava and 1/3 the distance from the left inferior pulmonary vein, the heart was elevated. The LIMA was brought through the hole in the pericardium. The Octopus tissue stabilizer was used to stabilize the site of the LIMA to LAD anastomosis. A retracto-tape was placed on the LAD proximal to the location of the anastomosis. LIMA was trimmed to an appropriate length and spatulated. Using a # 15 scalpel blade, LAD was opened and a 1.5 mm shunt was inserted into the LAD. A running #7-0 Prolene suture was used to create an end-to-side anastomosis. The systolic blood pressure was kept above 100 with 0.4 mg norepinephrine and the end-tidal CO_2 was carefully monitored to avoid drops of more than 2-3 mmHg. This anastomosis was hemostatic and transit-time flow was used to check the flow, resistance (Pulsatility Index) and diastolic filling and found to be adequate. Using the previously placed proximal snare to occlude the LAD, we tested for competitive flow, which there was none because the LAD had a 90% stenosis. The heart was placed in the neutral position and transit-time flows were re-measured and were found to be good.

The patient was placed deeper in the Trendelenberg position and the OR table was rotated toward the surgeon's side; the heart sling was repositioned so as to expose the later wall of the left ventricle. The reversed saphenous vein was gently distended to check for leaks. The marginal artery was identified and the Octopus tissue stabilizer was used to stabilize the intended location of the distal anastomosis. A proximal snare and intracoronary shunt was used as for the LIMA-LAD anastomosis, and the saphenous vein to marginal artery anastomosis was performed using continuous 7.0 Prolene. The heart and patient were then both placed in neutral position.

The proximal saphenous vein to ascending aorta anastomosis was then completed using the Heartstring device so as to avoid any clamping of the ascending aorta. The anastomosis was performed using 6-0 Prolene and was hemostatic. Transit-time flow was then used to measure graft flow, resistance and diastolic filling and found to be adequate.

Protamine was given to reverse the heparin. Both graft flows were checked again with transit-time flow. Blake drains were placed in the left pleural cavity and in the anterior and posterior mediastinum. Pacing wires were placed in the surface of the right atrium and right ventricle and tested for appropriate capture.

The sternum was closed with #5 stainless steel sternal wires x 8. The fascia was closed with #0 Ethibond, the subcutaneous layers with #2-0 Vicryl and the skin with #3-0 Monocryl in running fashion.

All instruments, sponge and needle counts were confirmed to be correct x2 at the end of operation. The patient tolerated the procedure well and was taken to the cardiovascular intensive care unit in stable condition on low dose Dopamine and IV nitroglycerin.

The total OR time: [BLANK]

ECHO findings: [BLANK]

Transit time flows were as follows: LIMA to LAD: [BLANK] mL per minute/PI [BLANK]/DF [BLANK%]; with proximal snare was [BLANK] mL per minute/PI [BLANK]/DF [BLANK%]. Post Protamine: [BLANK] (ml/min)/ PI [BLANK] /DF [BLANK].

The SVG to Marginal artery: [BLANK] mL per minute/PI [BLANK]/DF [BLANK%]; with proximal snare was [BLANK] mL per minute/PI [BLANK]/DF [BLANK%]. Post Protamine: [BLANK] (ml/min)/ PI [BLANK] /DF [BLANK]

Dr. [BLANK] was present and scrubbed for [BLANK] elements of this procedure.

12. Coronary Artery Bypass Grafting + Mitral Valve Repair Vs Replacement

Kenan W Yount MD MBA and Leora T Yarboro MD

University of Virginia, Charlottesville, VA

Essential Operative Steps

1. Lines & monitoring (*e.g.*, large bore central +/- pulmonary artery catheter; arterial)
2. Intraoperative transesophageal echocardiogram (*i.e.*, assess for mechanism)
3. Median sternotomy
4. Conduit harvests (*e.g.*, endoscopic saphenous vein harvest, LIMA harvest)
5. Open pericardium, pericardial well, survey ascending aorta for plaque burden (consider epiaortic ultrasound), cannulation, proximal anastomosis sites
6. Systemic heparinization
7. Arterial cannulation
8. Bicaval cannulation
9. Myocardial protection and vent placement (DLP in aortic root, retrograde cannulation in coronary sinus)
10. Check ACT
11. Initiate CPB
12. Initial interatrial groove dissection
13. Aortic cross-clamp (reduce CPB flow rate, apply cross-clamp, increase CPB flow)
14. Anterograde +/- retrograde cardioplegia +/- topical cooling for cardiac arrest
15. Distal anastomoses (consider starting with right side for instillation of cardioplegia down completed vein graft for better right myocardial protection).
16. Interatrial groove dissection and retractor (*e.g.*, Cosgrove) insertion
17. Inspect valve for pathology and mechanism; decide on repair *vs.* replacement
18. Leaflet excision with chordal sparing (or valve leaflet repair/resection); careful debridement
19. Sutures through annulus and through replacement valve (or annuloplasty ring)
20. Close atriotomy +/- leave left ventricular vent
21. Proximal anastomoses
22. Antegrade warm blood cardioplegia "hot shot" administration for rewarming
23. Remove aortic cross-clamp
24. Check for hemostasis

25. Temporary pacing wire placement
26. Chest tube placement
27. Wean from CPB
28. Venous decannulation
29. Protamine administration for heparin reversal (test dose, first)
30. Aortic decannulation
31. Assess hemostasis
32. Sternotomy closure

Potential Complications and Pitfalls

1. Entry
    i. Midline during sternotomy
    ii. Innominate vein injury while making pericardial well
2. Harvest
    i. LIMA injury during harvest
    ii. Heparinization during LIMA and saphenous harvest
3. Cannulation
    i. Aortic dissection with arterial cannula insertion
    ii. Aortic cannulation and cross-clamp site selection (to avoid stroke)
    iii. Right atrial or caval tear with bicaval venous cannula insertion
    iv. Coronary sinus injury with retrograde cannula insertion
4. Protection
    i. Inadequate myocardial protection and cardiac arrest (*e.g.*, cross-clamp not across, aortic insufficiency, insufficient venous drainage)
    ii. Ordering of bypass grafts
5. Bypass Grafting
    i. Difficulty finding coronary arteries (*e.g.*, intramyocardial segments)
    ii. Posterior injury during opening of coronary arteries
6. Mitral
    i. Consider approach (*e.g.*, generally interatrial, but may require transeptal if atria are not enlarged)
    ii. Decision to repair or replace mitral valve
    iii. Careful leaflet excision and annular debridement if calcified (*e.g.*, to avoid stroke from embolization, to avoid risk of AV dissociation)
    iv. Careful placement and tying of sutures (*e.g.*, to avoid perivavular leak, to avoid injury to surrounding structures)
    v. Adequate venting +/- Valsalva to de-air during atriotomy closure
7. Closure & Decannulation
    i. Kinking of bypass grafts and/or insufficient graft length resulting in graft tension after completion of proximal anastomosis
    ii. Avoid excessive manipulation of the heart (*e.g.*, to prevent AV dissociation—generally why distal bypasses are completed before mitral in addition to augmenting myocardial protection)
    iii. Inspecting postoperative TEE for residual regurgitation
    iv. Improper de-airing prior to vent removal

II. Adult Cardiac Surgery

v. Bleeding from atriotomy site, anastomotic sites, cannulation sites
vi. RIMA injury during sternal wire placement

Template Dictation

Preoperative Diagnoses: [INDICATION – e.g. severe mitral regurgitation, coronary artery disease, congestive heart failure]

Postoperative Diagnoses: Same

Procedure(s) Performed:

1. Coronary artery bypass grafting x [**NUMBER**], [**DETAILS** – e.g., LIMA to LAD, SVG to PDA
2. Mitral valve [**REPAIR/REPLACEMENT**] with a [**NUMBER**] mm [**TYPE OF VALVE OR ANNULOPLASTY RING**]
3. [**SIDE**] endovascular vein harvest

Attending Surgeon: [BLANK]

Secondary Surgeon: [BLANK]

Assistants: [BLANK]

Anesthesia: [BLANK]

Indication(s) for Procedure: [AGE] year old [GENDER] with a [DURATION] history of [COMPLAINT – *e.g.*, increasing worse chest pain and shortness of breath]. [HE/SHE] was found to have severe mitral insufficiency on a recent echocardiogram and a preoperative coronary catheterization revealed multi-vessel coronary artery disease with [FINDINGS – *e.g.*, 90% stenosis of LAD and 80% stenosis of the proximal PDA with an estimated ejection fraction of 35%]. After a discussion of the risks and benefits, the patient was consented for coronary artery bypass grafting with a mitral valve repair versus replacement; should replacement be necessary, the patient had a stated preference of receiving a [TISSUE/MECHANICAL] valve.

Description of the Procedure: The patient was correctly identified in the holding area and brought to the operative suite where [HE/SHE] was placed supine on the operative table. The patient's identity and planned procedure were verified. After adequate induction of general anesthesia, the patient was intubated with a single-lumen endotracheal tube. A right internal jugular central venous line with a pulmonary artery catheter was placed as well as a radial arterial line, Foley catheter, and transesophageal echocardiogram probe. A preoperative transesophageal echocardiogram was performed to evaluate cardiac function and valve function. The patient's chest, abdomen, groins, and lower extremities were then prepped and draped in the usual sterile fashion. A time-out was completed.

The physician assistant performed an endoscopic saphenous vein harvest in the right lower extremity. Concomitantly, a median sternotomy was performed using a sternal saw. The left internal mammary artery was harvested in a pedicled fashion. Once dissected, 5000 units of heparin were administered prior to distal division. There was excellent flow after distal division. The LIMA was wrapped in a lidocaine soaked sponge for use at a later time. Hemostasis of the vascular bed was confirmed. The mammary retractor was then removed and replaced with a sternal retractor.

After identification of the innominate vein, the pericardium was opened and a pericardial well was fashioned. Aortic cannulation sutures were placed in the ascending aorta below the level of the innominate artery in preparation for arterial cannulation. Right atrial cannulation sutures were then placed in the right atrial appendage and the right atrial-IVC junction in preparation for bicaval venous cannulation. The patient was systemically heparinized with [UNITS] of heparin. The aortic cannula was then inserted into the ascending aorta, de-aired, and secured. The venous cannulas were then placed through the right atrial appendage into the SVC and through the right atrial-caval junction into the IVC. A retrograde cannula was then placed into the coronary sinus without difficulty. A DLP vent was inserted into the ascending aorta. The patient was then placed on cardiopulmonary bypass. Initial dissection of the interatrial groove was performed. The cross-clamp was applied; antegrade and retrograde cardioplegia were given with immediate arrest of the heart. Cold topical solution was applied and cardioplegia was given every 20 minutes for the remainder of the case.

The bypass began with the SVG to PDA anastomosis. The PDA was opened using a #15C scalpel. The anastomosis was completed distally in an end-to-side fashion using a running #7-0 Prolene. Antegrade cardioplegia was then administered through the graft, which was found to be patent and hemostatic. The proximal graft was then left free to cardioplegia. A suitable site on the LAD was identified along its mid-portion. The LIMA graft was then trimmed to the appropriate length and clamped with a bulldog. The anastomosis was completed in an end-to-side fashion using a running #7-0 Prolene. The bulldog clamp was removed, and the graft was found to be patent and hemostatic.

To address the mitral valve, the interatrial groove was opened and the left atrium was entered sharply with a #15 blades scalpel. This incision was then extended with Metzenbaum scissors. Cosgrove retractors were placed to better visualize the mitral valve. There appeared to be normal valve leaflets but abnormal leaflet tethering in the subvalvular apparatus with nonviable left ventricular muscle inferiorly. Consequently, the decision was made to replace rather than repair the valve, and the anterior leaflet was excised while leaving the chordal attachments in place. The valve was then sized and a [SIZE] mm [TYPE] [TISSUE/MECHANICAL] valve was selected. Sutures were placed through the annulus and brought to the sewing ring of the valve, which was then tied down. The replacement valve appeared to be well-seated. It was tested and found to be hemostatic. We therefore closed the atriotomy around the left ventricular vent with a single layer of running #3-0 Prolene, and the vent was placed to suction to aid in de-airing.

II. Adult Cardiac Surgery

The patient was allowed to rewarm. A site for the proximal bypass graft anastomosis was selected on the aorta. An aortotomy for the proximal anastomosis of the saphenous vein graft was made with a #11-0 blade scalpel followed by an aortic punch to enlarge the aortotomy, and the proximal anastomosis was completed using a running #5-0 Prolene.

A hot shot was given, and the cross-clamp was removed. Ventricular pacing wires were then placed and the patient was paced at 80 beats per minute. Four chest tubes were placed: 2 in the mediastinum and 1 in each pleural space. The follow-up transesophageal echocardiogram confirmed that there was no residual air in the heart and that the mitral valve had no perivalvular leak. All vents were then removed, and the patient was subsequently weaned from bypass. The IVC and SVC cannulas were removed. Protamine was given. The aortic cannula was removed. The cannulation sites were then tied down and confirmed to be hemostatic. The patient's sternum was then reapproximated with #6-0 stainless steel wires. We irrigated the sternum with a solution of Betadine and Ancef. The fascia was closed with a running #1-0 Vicryl followed by a deep dermal layer of running #2-0 Vicryl. The skin was closed in a running subcuticular fashion using #3-0 Monocryl. Bacitracin was applied to the incision sites, which were then covered with sterile Primapore dressing.

All instrument, sponge, and needle counts were confirmed to be correct x 2 at the end of the operation. The patient was transferred to the post-operative unit in critical condition.

Dr. [BLANK] was present and scrubbed for [BLANK] elements of this procedure.

13. Coronary Artery Bypass Grafting With Aortic Valve Replacement

Michelle C. Ellis, MD and Jonathon W. Haft, MD

University of Michigan, Ann Arbor, MI

Essential Operative Steps

1. Lines and monitoring
2. General endotracheal anesthesia
3. Intraoperative transesophageal echocardiogram
4. Median sternotomy
5. Conduit choice and LIMA harvest
6. Open pericardium, pericardial well, assess ascending aorta for plaque burden (consider epiaortic ultrasound or alternative cannulation strategy)
7. Systemic heparinization (300u/kg)
8. Arterial cannulation
9. Venous cannulation
10. Cardioplegia cannula placement (antegrade via aortic root, retrograde via coronary sinus)
11. Check ACT (>350sec)
12. Initiate cardiopulmonary bypass
13. Aortic cross clamp
14. Antegrade cardioplegia +/- topical cooling, followed by retrograde cardioplegia
15. Assess and plan distal targets
16. Aortotomy, excision of aortic valve leaflets and debridement of the annulus
17. Choose prosthetic valve and size
18. Irrigate left ventricle and aortic root copiously while giving retrograde cardioplegia
19. Distal coronary anastomoses
20. Place annular sutures and implant valve
21. Close aortotomy
22. Proximal anastomoses
23. Retrograde hot shot/warm blood cardioplegia
24. Remove aortic cross clamp
25. Check for hemostasis
26. Temporary epicardial pacer wire placement
27. Wean from cardiopulmonary bypass
28. Protamine administration and decannulation
29. Assess hemostasis, place pleural/mediastinal tubes
30. Sternotomy closure

II. Adult Cardiac Surgery

Potential Complications and Pitfalls

1. Stay midline during sternotomy
2. IMA injury
3. Cannulation complication (aortic dissection/disruption, inadequate anticoagulation)
4. Poor choice of aortic cannula/cross clamp location (too low/inadequate space for aortotomy and proximals, stroke risk)
5. Insufficient myocardial protection (retrograde cannula malpositioned)
6. Coronary sinus injury
7. Quality/caliber of targets
8. Twisting, kinking, or inadequate length of graft
9. Valve-patient mismatch
10. Inadequate debridement of annulus
11. Poor seating of valve, occlusion of coronary ostia
12. Damage to prosthetic valve (commissure posts, leaflets) during suture tying
13. Inadequate de-airing prior to aortic root vent removal
14. Perivalvular leak
15. Inadequate control of hemostasis prior to sternal closure

Template Dictation

Preoperative Diagnosis: [**INDICATION** exertional or unstable angina, dyspnea]

Postoperative Diagnosis: Same

Procedure(s) Performed:

1. Endoscopic vein harvesting
2. Coronary artery bypass grafting [**DETAILS** conduit used and targets]
3. Aortic valve replacement [**PROSTHETIC IMPLANT** info]

Attending Surgeon: [BLANK]

Secondary Surgeon: [BLANK]

Assistants: [BLANK]

Anesthesia: [BLANK]

Indication(s) for Procedure: [**AGE**] year old [**GENDER**] with [**DURATION**] history of [**COMPLIANT**: Exertional chest pain, syncope]. Preoperative cardiac catheterization reveals [**FINDINGS**]. Preoperative cardiac echocardiography demonstrates [**FINDINGS**]. The patient has chosen a [**VALVE CHOICE:** bioprosthetic to avoid lifelong warfarin, or a mechanical prosthetic to reduce risks of future degenerative valve dysfunction].

Description of Procedure: The patient was taken to the operating room on [**DATE**] and was placed upon the operating room table in the supine position.

Swan Ganz catheter and radial artery lines were inserted. General endotracheal anesthesia was administered. Preoperative transesophageal echocardiogram was then performed to evaluate cardiac and valve function. The patient was prepped and draped in the usual sterile fashion.

The saphenous vein was endoscopically harvested from the lower extremity, length sufficient for **X Number** bypass grafts. The tributaries of the vein were controlled with clips and silk ligatures. The access incision was closed in layers.

The chest was opened through a median sternotomy incision. The left pleural cavity was opened and the left internal mammary artery was fully mobilized. The patient was heparinized systemically with 300 IU/kg after which, the internal mammary was transected distally and prepared for anastomosis. The pericardium was opened. Pericardial stays were used for retraction. The space between the aorta and pulmonary artery was exposed. Purse string sutures were placed in the **[LOCATION:** distal ascending aorta or transverse aortic arch], right atrial appendage, and right atrium. A Prolene purse string suture was placed in the right superior pulmonary vein. After ensuring adequate anticoagulation, arterial cannulation and dual-stage venous cannulation was achieved. An antegrade cardioplegia catheter was placed in the ascending aorta. A retrograde cardioplegia catheter was placed via the right atrium into the coronary sinus, positioning confirmed by transesophageal echocardiography and pressure transduction. A left ventricular vent was placed via the right superior pulmonary vein. Cardiopulmonary bypass was initiated. The aortic cross clamp was applied. Cardioplegia was administered in an antegrade fashion followed by retrograde via the coronary sinus [**NOTE:** If there is significant aortic valve insufficiency, then antegrade cardioplegia may not be delivered effectively]. A good diastolic arrest was achieved. The patient was cooled systemically to approximately 32 degrees Celsius.

300-500 ml of retrograde cardioplegia was administered in 20 minute intervals throughout the period of the aortic occlusion. The aorta was then opened revealing a [**DETAILS:** heavily calcified tricuspid valve, with/without fused right and left leaflets]. The aortic valve was then excised, the annulus debrided of any remaining calcium deposits and the left ventricle copiously irrigated with cold saline. The annulus was sized. A **X**mm prosthetic [**IMPLANT type**: Trifecta, MagnaEase, St. Jude mechanical] aortic valve was selected.

The epicardial vessels were identified and incised. The distal anastomoses were accomplished next. Individual segments of reverse saphenous vein were sewn to the [**TARGETS:** diagonal, obtuse marginal, posterolateral branch of the circumflex artery, distal right coronary or posterior descending] artery respectively. Each of these anastomoses were carried out with running sutures of 7-0 Prolene. The anastomoses were tested for patency and hemostasis with gentle syringe infusion. The left internal mammary artery was then brought through a window in the pericardium and was sewn to the left anterior descending vessel with a running suture of 7-0 Prolene. The proximal clamp on the internal mammary was briefly removed to confirm both patency and hemostasis of this anastomosis.

Pledgeted 2-0 Ethibond sutures were placed circumferentially along the aortic valve annulus with pledgets oriented [**DETAILS:** on the ventricular side for bioprosthetics, on the aortic side for mechanical prosthetics]. Sutures were then passed through the sewing ring, the valve lowered into position and tied securely in place. The valve was inspected to be certain it was well seated and the coronary ostia were unobstructed. The aortotomy was closed with a continuous running suture of 5-0 Prolene. The vein grafts were cut to the appropriate length and spatulated. **X number** of aortic tissue buttons were excised and used as **X** proximal anastomoses for the saphenous grafts, which were carried out with running sutures of 5-0 Prolene.

A terminal dose of warm blood cardioplegia (the hot shot) was administered retrograde and the aortic cross clamp was then released. The heart was de-aired using the left ventricular vent and the ascending aortic vent. Temporary pacing wires were placed on the surface of the [**LOCATION:** right atrium, right ventricle].

With the patient fully re-warmed, the heart resumed good contractility and resumed a [**TYPE:** normal spontaneous or paced] rhythm. The lungs were inflated. [**DETAILS:** Inotropes were initiated if the ventricular function was impaired or the cross clamp period was prolonged]. The patient was weaned from cardiopulmonary bypass. Transesophageal echocardiography revealed a well seated valve with no insufficiency and acceptable gradients. The left chest was aspirated. Protamine was administered and decannulation was accomplished. Hemostasis was achieved from all sites, including the skin fat, the mammary bed, cannulation sites, and all proximal and distal anastomotic sites. The entire wound was inspected for hemostasis and was felt to be adequate. [**NUMBER**] mediastinal tube and [**NUMBER**] left pleural tube were placed.

The incision was then closed in layers with #5 stainless steel wires used to approximate the sternum, 2-0 PDS suture used to approximate the fascia, 2-0 monocryl to approximate the subcutaneous tissue, and 4-0 monocryl subcuticular closure used to approximate the skin. Sterile dressings were applied. The patient tolerated the procedure well and transferred to the ICU in stable condition.

All sponge, instrument, and needle counts were correct at the completion of the case.

Dr. [**BLANK**] was present and scrubbed for [**BLANK**] elements of this procedure.

14. Devega Tricuspid Valve Repair

Mathéau A Julien, MD, PhD and Duc Thinh Pham, MD

Tufts Medical Center, Boston, MA

Essential Operative Steps

1. Lines and Monitoring
2. General endotracheal anesthesia
3. Intraoperative transesophageal echocardiogram
4. Median sternotomy
5. Open pericardium, pericardial well, survey ascending aorta for plaque burden
6. Systemic heparinization (400 u/kg)
7. Arterial cannulation
8. Dual stage venous cannulation
9. Restriction of SVC and IVC return into the operative field with Rummels
10. Myocardial protection cannula placement (DLP in aortic root)
11. Check ACT (>400 sec)
12. Initiate CPB
13. Aortic cross clamp (reduce CPB flow rate, apply cross clamp, increase CPB flow to
14. 2.0-2.5L/min/m2)
15. Antegrade cardioplegia (1200 ml) and topical cooling with for cardiac arrest
16. Check for PFO once right atrium opened
17. During suturing, take up a segment of annular tissue with each bite, but leave only a small space between each bite
18. Use of a tricuspid valve annuloplasty calibrator in order to narrow the annulus to the desired size
19. Testing tricuspid valve competence by distending the right ventricle using a Robinson catheter
20. Antegrade warm blood cardioplegia "hot shot" administration for rewarming
21. Remove aortic cross clamp
22. Closure of right atriotomy
23. Check for hemostasis
24. Arterial and ventricular pacer wire placement
25. Drainage tube placement
26. Wean from CPB
27. Venous decannulation
28. Protamine administration for heparin reversal (test dose first)
29. Aortic decannulation
30. Assess hemostasis
31. Sternotomy closure

II. Adult Cardiac Surgery

Potential Complications and Pitfalls

1. Stay midline during sternotomy
2. Avoid injury to innominate vein while making pericardial well
3. Cannulation catastrophe (aortic dissection/ bleeding)
4. Poor choice of location of aortic cannula/ crossclamp (leading to stroke)
5. SA node or right phrenic nerve injury during SVC isolation/cannulation
6. Inadvertent azygous vein rather than SVC cannulation
7. Excessive bleeding or cardiac manipulation during IVC cannulation
8. Inadvertent hepatic vein rather than IVC cannulation
9. Insufficient myocardial protection
10. Insufficient venous drainage
11. Failure to address PFO
12. Injury to tricuspid valve leaflets
13. Failure to improve degree of tricuspid regurgitation
14. Insufficient de-airing prior to removal of aortic root vent
15. Inadequate control of hemostasis prior to sternal closure/ bleeding from one of numerous cardiotomies

Template Dictation

Preoperative Diagnosis: Tricuspid Valve Insufficiency

Postoperative Diagnosis: Same

Procedure(s) Performed: DeVega Tricuspid Valve Repair

Attending Surgeon: [BLANK]

Secondary Surgeon: [BLANK]

Assistants: [BLANK]

Anesthesia: [BLANK]

Indication(s) for Procedure: [AGE] year old [GENDER] mild functional tricuspid regurgitation by echocardiography. While the annular dilatation of moderate to severe tricuspid regurgitation should be managed with a ring-reinforced annuloplasty, the suture annuloplasty technique of DeVega was chosen and has successfully been employed for the repair of mild regurgitation. Of note, this technique is becoming of more historical interest, due to compelling evidence suggesting a higher recurrence rate.

Description of Procedure: After informed consent was obtained, the patient was brought to the operating room and placed in the supine position. General endotracheal anesthesia was induced. A central venous catheter, Swan-Ganz catheter, radial arterial catheter, and Foley catheter were inserted. The patient was prepped and draped in the usual sterile manner. A median sternotomy was performed. The heart was then exposed and marsupialized by supporting the right side of the pericardium. The SVC and IVC were each looped using umbilical tape on a Rummel tourniquet. The patient was systemically heparinized, and cardiopulmonary bypass lines were brought up. Double pursestring sutures were placed in the ascending aorta, and it was cannulated in the usual fashion. The venous line was Y'ed for SVC and IVC cannulation, and after placing single pursestring sutures, these were cannulated as well, using right-angle cannulas. Once a therapeutic ACT was achieved the patient was placed on cardiopulmonary bypass and kept warm.

An aortic root vent / antegrade cardioplegia DLP cannula was placed in the proximal ascending aorta. The aorta was crossclamped, and cardioplegia given antegrade into the aortic root. After there was good cardiac arrest, the superior and inferior vena caval tapes were snared down. The operative field was flooded with carbon dioxide. The right atrium was then opened. No atrial septal defect was identified. Attention was then turned to the tricuspid valve. The valve leaflets were thin and pliable, and the pathology was limited to dilatation of the annulus. To fashion the DeVega annuloplasty, a double-armed 2-0 pledgeted Prolene suture was used. Starting at the commissure between the septal and anterior leaflets of the tricuspid valve, sequential stitches were taken through the tricuspid valve annulus, leaving only a small space between each bite and taking up a segment of annular tissue with each bite. The suture line was completed at the septal-posterior leaflet commissure. The opposite needle was then used to make a second row of suture in the floor of the atrium just outside the annulus of the tricuspid valve. This stitch was also completed at the septal-posterior leaflet commissure. Both needles were passed through a free Teflon pledget. With the aid of a tricuspid valve annuloplasty calibrator, the suture was tightened in order to narrow the annulus to the desired size. Afterwards, tricuspid valve competence was tested by distending the right ventricle using a Robinson catheter. The right atriotomy was then closed with a double-layer running Prolene suture

The patient was successfully weaned off of cardiopulmonary bypass. The heart was deaired and decannulated. The heparin was reversed with protamine. Two temporary right atrial and right ventricular epicardial pacing wires were placed. The pericardial cavity was copiously irrigated, hemostasis was assured, and two mediastinal drainage tubes were placed. The sternum was reapproximated with wires. The rectus and pectoralis fascia were closed with 0 Vicryl. The subcutaneous tissue was closed with 2-0 Vicryl, and the skin was closed with 3-0 Monocryl. All wounds were sterilely dressed. Instrument and sponge counts were correct. The patient tolerated the procedure well and was sent to the critical care unit in stable condition.

Dr. [BLANK] was present and scrubbed for [BLANK] elements of this procedure.

15. Donor Heart Procurement

Alexandra Tuluca, MD and Hari Mallidi, MD, FRCSC

Baylor College of Medicine/ Texas Heart Institute, Houston, TX

Essential Operative Steps

1. Final checklist at the site:
   a. ABO compatibility
   b. Serology (HIV, HCV, HbsAg and CMV)
   c. Laboratory findings (Troponin, Na, ABG)
   d. ECG (look for Atrial fibrillation, bundle or AV blocks and signs of hypertrophy, long QT)
   e. Echocardiography (valvular abnormalities, LV and RV function, wall motion, wall thickness)
   f. Chest X-ray
   g. Coronary angiogram (if performed)
   h. Medications during ICU course (especially catecholamine requirements)
2. Median sternotomy
3. Dissect and remove thymus, open pericardium longitudinally, create pericardial well
4. Expose the great vessels, Aorta with the arch branch vessels
5. Visual inspection and palpation of the heart for injury and lesions; Palpate LM coronary (behind the PA) and branch coronary arteries for evidence of calcification
6. Dissect SVC and IVC circumferentially; Ligate and divide the azygous vein
7. Separate aorta and pulmonary artery
8. Insert cardioplegia cannula in ascending aorta
9. Systemic heparin (300 units/kg)
10. Ligate the SVC above the azygous vein
11. Cross-clamp the aorta
12. Incise IVC supradiaphragmatic - check with liver team
13. Vent the heart (pulmonary vein, main PA or LA appendage - if heart-lung block)
14. Arrest the heart with cardioplegia solution and copious topical cooling
15. Divide SVC and IVC
16. Incise the pulmonary veins/ left atrium
17. Divide the aorta (usually distal arch, with preservation of the arch vessels) and the PA as long as possible; If harvesting for complex congenital transplant divide the PA at branch PA level
18. Remove the heart and inspect again for lesions, contusions, etc.
19. Store in sterile bag (3 bag method, first with cold perfusion solution, outer two with ice water)

Potential Complications and Pitfalls

1. Forgetting to heparinize
2. Allowing ventricular distention
3. Back-walling aorta with cardioplegia needle or angiocath thereby failing to administer cardioplegia
4. Allowing to aortic root pressure to get too high when administering cardioplegia
5. Caution to stay supradiaphragmatic when dividing the IVC
6. Not enough length on the SVC, IVC or the great vessels
7. Injuring RA / Dome of LA when preserving RSPV for lung team
8. Injuring the coronary sinus during IVC transection
9. Failure to identify structural abnormalities
10. Failure to adequately cool and preserve the heart

Template Dictation

Preoperative Diagnosis: N/A

Postoperative Diagnosis: Same

Procedure(s) Performed: Donar heart procurement

Attending Surgeon: [BLANK]

Secondary Surgeon: [BLANK]

Assistants: [BLANK]

Anesthesia: [BLANK]

Indication(s) for Procedure: N/A

Description of Procedure: The donor is positioned supine and prepped and draped in standard sterile fashion from chin to knees. A standard median sternotomy is performed. The thymus is removed and the pericardium is opened longitudinally in a reverse-T along the diaphragm. A pericardial well is created and the great vessels are exposed. The heart is visually inspected and palpated to identify myocardial contusions, coronary atherosclerosis or previous infarction.

The heart mobilization begins by dissecting the SVC from the right atrium to the innominate vein. The azygous vein is ligated in the process and the SVC is encircled with heavy ligature. The IVC is mobilized circumferentially. Next, the aorta is separated from the pulmonary artery and isolated with umbilical tape. A cardioplegia cannula is inserted in the ascending aorta through a purse-string suture and secured with a Rommel tourniquet.

Once the abdominal organs and lungs are mobilized and prepared for explanation, the patient is administered 300 units/kg of heparin intravenously. Anesthesia is asked to pull back any venous neck lines they may have and the SVC is ligated as distal as possible. The IVC is incised and blood allowed to drain into the pericardium. The heart is further vented by incising a pulmonary vein (or alternatively, the left atrial appendage if lungs or a heart-lung block is being harvested). The aortic cross-clamp is applied just proximal to the takeoff of the innominate artery and the heart is arrested with a single flush (1000ml or 10mL/kg for larger donors) of cold crystalloid cardioplegia solution. Watch at this time for appropriate aortic root distention, quick cessation of electrical activity and left ventricular relaxation without distention. Rapid cooling of the heart is achieved with copious topical cold saline solution in the pericardial well. The cardioplegia cannula can now be removed and the purse-string tied.

The IVC is fully transected. The heart is wrapped in an ice-soaked lap pad and the apex of the heart is elevated. The remaining pulmonary veins are divided from inferior to superior, followed by branch pulmonary arteries. If lungs are also harvested, the main PA is divided close to the bifurcation and adequate left atrial cuffs must be negotiated. The aorta and the SVC are divided last with more than adequate length.

The donor heart is then placed in a sterile bag with perfusion solution, then two additional outer bags with sterile ice water. The organ is then placed in a cooler with ice and transported to the recipient hospital.

Dr. [BLANK] was present and scrubbed for [BLANK] elements of this procedure.

16. Hemiarch Replacement with DHCA – Aneurysm

Thomas J Zeyl MD and Tomas D Martin MD

University of Florida, Gainesville, FL

CAVEAT: Aortic surgery, including that of the arch, may vary from institution to institution. Cannulation strategies and cerebral protection can be completed differently. Strategies such as right axillary cannulation for antegrade cerebral protection and bypass, or retrograde cannulation for cerebral protection are both valid methods. The described procedure omits these techniques.

Essential Operative Steps

1. Appropriate patient identification
2. Lines and Monitoring
3. General endotracheal anesthesia
4. Intraoperative transesophageal echocardiogram
5. Median sternotomy
6. Dissect prepericardial fat/thymus to expose innominate vein
7. Open pericardium, pericardial well, survey ascending aorta/arch for pathology and potential cannulation site
8. Systemic heparinization
9. Arterial cannulation
10. Venous cannulation
11. Retrograde cannula in coronary sinus
12. Check ACT (>400 sec)
13. Initiate CPB and cooling
14. LV vent placement
15. Aortic cross clamp
16. Antegrade cardioplegia if no associated AI via a slotted cardioplegia needle, then retrograde cardioplegia
17. Aortotomy with resection of ascending aorta to sinotubular junction.
18. Once electrocerebral silence and adequate temperature, place patient in trendelenberg, turn cardiopulmonary bypass off and remove aortic cannula and cross clamp.
19. Complete resection of aorta into the arch and as far as needed to get to normal aorta, create beveled graft with side-arm
20. Distal anastomosis
21. Reperfusion through side-arm on graft
22. Rewarm
23. Proximal anastomosis to sinotubular junction
24. Dearing via root with slotted needle, retrograde cardioplegia
25. Remove aortic cross clamp
26. Check for hemostasis
27. Atrial and ventricular pacer wire placement
28. Chest tube placement

II. Adult Cardiac Surgery

29. Check for air, remove LV vent, then wean from CPB
30. Remove root vent and venous cannulas
31. Protamine administration for heparin reversal
32. Ligate graft side-arm
33. Assess hemostasis
34. Sternotomy closure

Potential Complications and Pitfalls

1. Stay midline during sternotomy
2. Avoid injury to innominate vein and aneurysmal aorta during initial dissection/creation of pericardial well
3. Cannulation catastrophe (Aortic dissection/ bleeding, Right atrial tear)
4. Coronary sinus injury with retrograde cardioplegia cannulation
5. Poor choice of location of aortic cannula/ crossclamp (leading to stroke)
6. Inadequate cerebral protection (prolonged ischemic time prior to reperfusion)
7. Inadequate deairing prior to removal of aortic root vent
8. Acquired coagulopathy and bleeding

Template Dictation

Preoperative Diagnosis: [INDICATION – e.g. size and extent of aneurysmal disease]

Postoperative Diagnosis: Same

Procedure(s) Performed: Ascending Aorta with Hemiarch Replacement with DHCA using a [DETAILS – Size of Graft]

Attending Surgeon: [BLANK]

Secondary Surgeon: [BLANK]

Assistants: [BLANK]

Anesthesia: [BLANK]

Indication(s) for Procedure: [AGE] year old [GENDER] with a history of [DISEASE – size of aneurysmal disease, and or rate of growth of aneurysm]. Preoperative CT scan revealed [FINDINGS]

Description of Procedure: The patient was taken to the operating room and [HIS/HER] identity and planned procedure verified. The patient was placed on the operating room table in the supine position and general anesthesia was obtained. Hemodynamic catheters were inserted and transesophageal echocardiogram was performed to evaluate cardiac and valve function. The patient was prepped and draped in the usual sterile fashion. The chest was entered via standard median sternotomy. The heart was exposed, and the ascending aorta was inspected and showed [OPERATIVE FINDINGS]. The patient was systemically heparinized with a total of [UNITS] of systemic heparin. Epiaortic ultrasound was performed to assess the aortic wall. The aortic cannulation sutures were then placed in the ascending aorta below the level of the innominate artery take off. The right atrial cannulation sutures were then placed in the right atrium. The retrograde cardioplegia sutures were placed in the right atrium and the left ventricular vent sutures were placed in the right superior pulmonary vein. The ACT and systemic pressure was confirmed and the aortic cannula was then inserted, secured and de-aired. Venous cannula was then placed and secured in the right atrium. A retrograde catheter was placed into the coronary sinus and secured. The patient was placed on cardiopulmonary bypass and eventually cooled to [TEMP] degrees centigrade and electrocerebral silence. Upon fibrillation, a vent was placed in the left ventricle via the right superior pulmonary vein. The aortic cross-clamp was placed and antegrade cardioplegia was administered upon which there was rapid arrest of the heart. This was followed by retrograde cardioplegia. The aorta was opened just proximal to the cross clamp and the ascending aorta was resected to just superior to the sinotubular junction with visualization of the right and left coronary ostia. Once the patient reached approximately [TEMP] degrees centigrade and electrocerebral silence, [HE/SHE] was placed in Trendelenburg position and the pump was turned off. The aortic cannula and cross clamp were removed. The ascending aorta was transected cephalad and the aorta was resected all the way up into the aortic arch, including all diseased aorta in the arch, until there was noted to be relatively normal sized aorta. A [SIZE] side-arm graft was chosen and beveled to fit the transverse arch. The graft was sewn end-to-end to the underneath side of the aortic arch utilizing a running 3-0 Prolene suture. Upon completion of the anastomosis, bioglue was utilized on the graft to cover needle holes. The side-arm was then connected to the arterial line through a regular tubing connector. After de-airing the graft, the graft was clamped and reperfusion was begun. A cross clamp was applied proximal to the joining of the side-arm. Cerebral ischemia time was [TIME] minutes. Rewarming was begun. The graft was cut to the appropriate length and anastomosed end-to-end to the proximal aorta utilizing a running 3-0 Prolene suture. This was done right at the sinotubular junction. Upon completion bioglue was placed on the graft to cover suture holes. The heart was de-aired in the routine fashion utilizing active suction in the aortic root and the left ventricle and retrograde cardioplegia was given. The crossclamp was removed. The patient was rewarmed to [TEMP] degrees.

Atrial and ventricular pacing wires were then inserted and tested for appropriate capture. A [NUMBER] chest tube was placed in the mediastinum and large Blake drains in the [LEFT/RIGHT] pleural space. The heart was de-aired, and the LV vent was removed after minimal air was seen by echo. The patient was weaned from cardiopulmonary bypass. The venous cannula was removed, and the cannulation sutures were secured. Protamine was administered and the patient was monitored for adverse reactions. Coagulopathy was assessed and hemostasis secured. The aortic side-arm was clamped and cut. The remaining stub of the side-arm was closed with a 3-0 Prolene suture and 2 large clips placed at the base.

II. Adult Cardiac Surgery

The operative field was thoroughly inspected for bleeding.

Once adequate hemostasis was achieved, the sternum was closed with a total of [NUMBER] stainless steel sternal wires utilizing a figure of eight interlocking fashion. Vancomycin powder was placed in the wound prior to sternal closure. The fascia was then closed with #1 Vicryl suture in running fashion. The deep dermal layer was then closed with #2- 0 Vicryl suture in running fashion. The skin and subcuticular layer was closed with #4-0 Monocryl in running fashion followed by Dermabond on the skin.

All instrument, sponge and needle counts were confirmed to be correct x 2 at the end of the operation. The patient was subsequently transferred to the postoperative cardiac surgical intensive care unit in critical, but stable condition.

Dr. [BLANK] was present and scrubbed for [BLANK] elements of this procedure.

17. Aortic Root Replacement with Homograft For Aortic Root Abscess (Native And Or Prior Bentall)

Muhammad Aftab, MD, Ourania Preventza, MD

Baylor College of Medicine/Texas Heart Institute, Houston, TX

Essential Operative Steps

1. Lines and monitoring
2. General endotracheal anesthesia
3. Intraoperative transesophageal echocardiogram
4. Right infraclavicular incision for Right axillary cannulation (consider in cases of redo sternotomies)
5. Dacron graft anastomosis to right axillary artery (alternative an innominate artery cannulation can be performed after the chest is opened)
6. Femoral venous cannulation for cardiopulmonary bypass (CPB) (optional)
7. Redo sternotomy
8. Systemic heparinization (400 U/kg). Ensure that activated clotting time (ACT) is >450 seconds
9. CO_2 in the operative field
10. Distal ascending aortic cannulation (alternative to axillary artery graft or to innominate artery cannulation)
11. Dual-stage venous cannulation of right atrium
12. Initiate CPB (2-2.5 L/min/m^2)
13. Systemic hypothermia (28-32°C)
14. Lysis of adhesions
15. Left ventricular sump via right superior pulmonary vein
16. Retrograde cardioplegia cannula in coronary sinus
17. Distal ascending aorta cross-clamped
18. Antegrade cold blood cardioplegia, except in severe aortic insufficiency
19. Combination of antegrade and retrograde cold blood cardioplegia (every 10-15 min during the operation)
20. Divide the native ascending aorta distal to previous graft anastomosis
21. Excise the infected composite valved graft
22. Wide local debridement
23. Mobilize the right and left main coronary buttons
24. Sharp debridement of the infected annular and sub annular region, if necessary
25. Reconstruct the tissue defect with autologous pericardium, bovine pericardium or the mitral leaflet of the valved homograft as needed
26. Completely remove all prosthetic material, previous pledgets, and sutures
27. Aortic annular sizing and selection of homograft
28. Thawing of cryopreserved aortic root homograft as per protocol
29. Trim the proximal end of homograft with 3- to 4-mm myocardial cuff

30. Homograft to aortic annulus/left ventricular outflow tract anastomosis
31. Left main coronary button anastomosis
32. In case of inadequate mobilization of the left main coronary button, an 8- or 10-mm rifampin soaked Dacron graft or SVG as an alternative is used as hemi-Cabrol
33. Distal trimming of homograft
34. Distal anastomosis of homograft to ascending aorta
35. Ensure excellent hemostasis along all the anastomoses
36. Additional interrupted sutures for anastomotic reinforcement, as needed
37. Verify right coronary artery (RCA) button alignment and mobility
38. Start rewarming slowly when the RCA button anastomosis starts
39. RCA button reimplantation to the homograft
40. In case of inadequate mobilization of RCA button, place a saphenous vein graft as an interposition graft between the origin of the RCA button and the homograft (hemi-Cabrol). If hemi-Cabrol (after completion) not satisfactory, perform coronary artery bypass grafting (CABG) to the RCA
41. Place patient in Trendelenburg position, perform deairing maneuvers, and remove the aortic cross-clamp
42. Confirm spontaneous cardiac rhythm, place pacing wires
43. Continue deairing
44. Once patient is rewarmed (36.5°C), resume ventilation
45. Fill the heart with blood and allow the heart to eject
46. Wean from CPB
47. Protamine and sequential decannulation
48. Ensure hemostasis
49. Mediastinal irrigation with antibiotics
50. Residual mediastinal abscess cavity debridement. In an event of a large non collapsible periaortic cavity, omentum can be mobilized to fill mediastinal cavity
51. Place mediastinal drains
52. Sternotomy closure

Potential Complications and Pitfalls

1. The primary indication for aortic root replacement with a cryopreserved homograft is endocarditis of the native or prosthetic aortic valve or composite valved graft with extensive periannular involvement.
2. A safe redo sternotomy is an important initial step in successful reoperative aortic root surgery.

Considerations for a safe sternal reentry include:

   a. Careful evaluation of preoperative imaging to assess the proximity of vital structures to the sternum
   b. Use of an oscillating saw for the anterior table, initially leaving the untwisted sternal wires in place, lifting the sternal edges and incising

the posterior table under direct vision, removing the sternal wires after incising the posterior table

OR

- c. Lifting the sternal edges of the xiphoid process dissect the periaortic tissue and cardiac structures under direct vision from the back of the sternum and then use of regular vertical saw for the sternotomy
- d. Use of peripheral cannulation (femoral-femoral bypass, or femoral to axillary bypass before sternal entry in high-risk situations where the right ventricle or the aorta is adherent at the back of the sternum. In these cases placement of the patient on CPB prior to sternal entry is advisable

3. Dual-stage right atrial venous cannulation is standard. Femoral venous cannulation can be performed in high-risk cases.
4. Complete debridement of all the infected necrotic tissue and removal of any foreign material from the previous operation, including sutures, pledgets, and graft material, is paramount in homograft aortic root replacement for aortic root infection.
5. Coronary buttons are prepared and mobilized. In redo root operations, their mobilization becomes increasingly difficult.
6. Preoperative planning also includes ensuring that the local tissue bank contains the sizes of aortic homografts within your desired annulus diameter range, based on the preoperative echocardiograms and preoperative computed tomography (CT) scan.
7. The aortic annulus is sized by using the standard Freestyle valve sizer or Hagar dilators.
8. A properly matching homograft with an annular (internal) diameter of equal size or a size difference of no more than 2 mm is ideal.
9. The homograft should be carefully evaluated for valve morphology and integrity, as well as for any injuries sustained during the processes of procurement, preservation, and thawing.
10. The proximal end of the homograft is trimmed such that a 3- to 4-mm cuff of myocardium is left below the nadir of the cusps. The anterior mitral leaflet is initially retained during the trimming to repair any annular or periannular defect, if needed.
11. Allograft implantation in anatomic orientation is fairly straightforward, especially when the native aortic valve is tricuspid and both annuli match closely.
12. All the anastomoses are performed with monofilament sutures (eg, polypropylene) in a running fashion. Using foreign material to reinforce the anastomoses is avoided, but if it is necessary, autologous (or bovine) pericardium is the material of choice.
13. Constant tension on the suture line should be maintained by the assistant during the anastomosis; tightening the loose suture line with nerve hooks ensures a hemostatic anastomosis.

II. Adult Cardiac Surgery

14. Any kinking or overstretching of the main coronary arteries during the reimplantation of coronary buttons into the homograft root should be avoided.
15. In reoperative situations, when significant scarring around the root or heavy calcification around the coronary ostia precludes the safe direct coronary button re-implantation, an interposition saphenous vein grafts (SVG) between the origin of the RCA button and the homograft (a hemi-Cabrol) can be used. SVG to RCA can be used as an alternative and the RCA button is oversewn
    a. .For the left coronary button we prefer Dacron graft (8 or 10 mm) soaked in rifampin as the alignment is better than the SVG but SVG can be also used. Ideally any prosthetic material should be avoided.
16. Postoperative bleeding due to coagulopathy should be addressed with targeted blood-product transfusion guided by the laboratory results.
17. Postoperative hypertension should be avoided to prevent any suture line disruption.

Template Dictation

Preoperative Diagnosis:

1. Group B streptococcal endocarditis of composite (mechanical) valved graft.
2. Post resection and replacement of aortic root (Bentall procedure) for annuloaortic ectasia and aortic valve insufficiency.
3. Periannular abscess.
4. New York Heart Association classification III.

Postoperative Diagnosis: Same

Procedure(s) Performed:

1. Redo median sternotomy.
2. Right axillary artery or innominate artery cannulation with an [BLANK]-mm Dacron end-to-side graft for pump return.
3. Total cardiopulmonary bypass.
4. Resection of previous composite valve graft (Bentall) prosthesis and wide debridement of infected tissue.
5. Extensive debridement of mediastinal abscess cavity.
6. Replacement of aortic root with [BLANK]-mm × [BLANK]-cm valved homograft root.
7. Bypass to the right coronary artery with reverse autologous saphenous vein graft.

Drainage: Two 36 Fr Argyle chest tubes were placed in the mediastinum for the drainage.

Fluids and Products: x crystalloid, x colloid, x PRBC, x FFP, x Platelets, x cell saver

Urine output: [BLANK]

CPB time: [BLANK]

Cardiac ischemia time: [BLANK] (cardiac ischemia and aortic x clamp are the same in cases that circulatory arrest is not performed)

Attending Surgeon: [BLANK]

Secondary Surgeon: [BLANK]

Assistants: [BLANK]

Anesthesia: [BLANK]

Indication(s) for Procedure: [AGE] year old [GENDER] who had undergone aortic root replacement with a composite mechanical valve graft 3 years earlier. He initially developed a right eye and sinus infection. Two weeks later, he presented to the hospital with a high-grade fever and dyspnea on exertion. He was febrile and in respiratory distress. Empiric antibiotics were immediately started. Computed tomography showed abnormal fluid collection around the graft. Group B streptococcus was identified in the blood culture. Transthoracic echocardiography revealed mechanical aortic valve stenosis with a 16×6-mm mass at the aortic annulus and a fluid collection around the graft, consistent with the infective endocarditis of previous composite valve graft and perigraft abscess. Consequently, it was decided that operative intervention was indicated, with resection of composite valve graft and replacement with a homograft.

Description of Procedure: After informed consent was obtained and the patient's identity and the surgical site were confirmed, the patient was brought to the operating room and positioned supine on the operating table. Adequate general anesthesia was induced, and all the necessary monitoring lines were placed. Bilateral cerebral near-infrared spectroscopy sensors were placed to monitor brain oxygenation throughout the procedure. A transesophageal echocardiography (TEE) probe was inserted by the anesthesia team. The chest, abdomen, and legs were prepped and draped in sterile surgical fashion. An incision was made under the right clavicle in the deltopectoral groove. The right axillary artery was exposed after the pectoralis major muscle fibers were separated and the pectoralis minor muscle was divided. Adjacent veins were carefully mobilized. We do not touch the cord of the brachial plexus. Intravenous heparin (5000 U) was administered by anesthesia, and a partial occluding clamp was placed on the axillary artery. A [BLANK] mm Dacron graft was anastomosed end-to-side with 6-0 polypropylene and connected to the arterial line of the cardiopulmonary bypass circuit for pump return. [For innominate artery cannulation: The innominate artery is exposed. Intravenous heparin (5000 U) was administered by anesthesia, and a partial occluding clamp was placed on the innominate artery. A [BLANK] mm Dacron graft was anastomosed end-to-side with 6-0 polypropylene and connected to the arterial line of the cardiopulmonary bypass circuit for pump return. During the innominate artery cannulation we keep the MAP 90 mmHg]. [For femoral venous cannulation: A vertical curvilinear incision was made in the inguinal region anterior to the femoral vessels and deepened through the subcutaneous tissue, exposing the fascia. The left/right common femoral vein was exposed. Venous cannulation was done using the standard Seldinger technique through a purse string of 5/0 polypropylene. A 23/25 Fr dual-stage venous cannula was inserted into the right atrium with TEE guidance, and satisfactory venous drainage was achieved.] A midline incision was made over the sternum and carried down to the presternal fascia with electrocautery. The chest was entered through the previous median sternotomy (**with an oscillating sternal saw** initially leaving the untwisted sternal wires in place, lifting the sternal edges and incising the posterior table under direct vision, removing the sternal wires after incising the posterior table, **or with the regular, vertical saw by** lifting initially the sternal edges of the xiphoid and dissecting the perioartic tissue and cardiac structures under direct vision from the back of the sternum) and hemostasis was achieved with electrocautery. Adhesions from the previous operation were taken down with careful sharp dissection.

The patient was then systemically heparinized to keep the ACT>450 seconds. A dual-stage venous cannula was introduced though a purse string in the right atrium with the tip directed into the inferior vena cava and secured with a Rummel tourniquet [Optional: Alternative to femoral venous cannulation]. Cardiopulmonary bypass was initiated. A retrograde cardioplegia cannula was inserted into the coronary sinus, and its position was confirmed by palpation, pressure transduction and or TEE guidance. A left ventricular sump was inserted via the right superior pulmonary vein and the patient was cooled to 32°C.

The distal ascending aorta was cross-clamped. Antegrade and retrograde cardioplegia was given intermittently and generously for myocardial protection. The native ascending aorta was divided distal to the previous anastomosis, and stay suture was placed for retraction. Significant edema and purulent material were encountered as the infected composite valve graft was sharply excised. Portions of the graft were noted to be densely adhered to the surrounding tissue, and some portions were easily separated. The adhesions were taken down with a careful sharp dissection. The right and left main coronary artery buttons were mobilized. The prosthetic aortic valve was sharply excised from the aortic annulus. The annulus was decalcified, and stay sutures were placed over the site of commissures for optimal exposure. The aortic annulus and sub annular region were carefully evaluated for any evidence of aortoventricular or periannular abscess or infected granulation tissue. All the infected annular and sub annular tissue was sharply debrided with a wide local excision. A periannaulr abscess was encountered and debrided of necrotic tissue. The tissue defect was reconstructed with autologous pericardium (or with bovine pericardium_ which was secured to the firm, healthy myocardial tissue by using 3/0 polypropylene in continuous fashion). All the previous pledgets and sutures were carefully and completely removed. Wherever possible, the surrounding tissue was also completely debrided.

To select a homograft of appropriate diameter, the aortic annulus was sized with standard valve sizers. The homograft was thawed as per protocol and trimmed. The homograft was sutured to the aortic valve annulus and left ventricular outflow tract with 2/0 polypropylene in a running fashion. The proximal suture line was reinforced with simple interrupted 3/0 polypropylene. Next, after adequate mobilization of the left coronary button, the left coronary button's alignment with the respective homograft coronary ostium was ensured. The coronary ostium of the graft was enlarged. With continuous 5/0 polypropylene, the left main coronary button was attached to the posterior aspect of the homograft and reinforced with 6/0 polypropylene.[If mobilization of the left coronary button is inadequate due to previous surgery, an 8 or 10 mm Dacron graft soaked in rifampin or a SVG, is used as hemi-Cabrol]. The homograft was then cut to length and anastomosed to the ascending aorta with continuous 4/0 polypropylene in an end-to-end fashion. The anastomosis was reinforced with additional 5/0 polypropylene suture. Similarly, the correct positioning of the right coronary artery to the homograft ostium was verified. The right coronary artery could not be adequately mobilized for a safe coronary button reattachment. A saphenous vein graft was harvested and placed as an interposition graft (reversed saphenous vein graft) between the origin of the right coronary button and the homograft (hemi-Cabrol). At the completion of the anastomosis, the right coronary artery was not aligned to our satisfaction. A coronary artery bypass using SVG to the Right coronary artery was performed. A #11 blade was used to create an aortotomy in the homograft for proximal vein graft anastomosis, and an aortic punch was then used to enlarge the aortotomy. The proximal anastomosis was performed with running 6/0 polypropylene.

Patient was placed in the Trendeleburg position, and after de-airing maneuvers, the cross-clamp was removed. The patient was rewarmed to 36.5°C. Temporary epicardial pacing wires were placed. The patient was weaned from cardiopulmonary bypass without difficulty. Protamine was administered to reverse the heparin, and all cannulas were sequentially removed. All the suture lines and surgical sites were confirmed to be hemostatic. The mediastinum was copiously irrigated with antibiotics, and the abscess cavity was thoroughly and completely debrided. Two 36 Fr Argyle chest tubes were placed in the mediastinum for drainage. The sternum was closed with stainless steel wires. The presternal fascia and subcutaneous and subcuticular tissues were closed in layers with absorbable sutures. Sterile dressings were applied, and the chest tubes were connected to drainage reservoirs. Sponge, needle, and instrument counts were correct. The patient, intubated, was transferred to the intensive care unit in a stable hemodynamic condition.

Dr. [BLANK] was present and scrubbed for [BLANK] elements of this procedure.

18. Unexpected Intraoperative Complications

George Makdisi, MD, John M. Stulak, MD

Mayo Clinic, Rochester, MN

Massive Air Embolism

Essential Operative Steps

1. Perfusionist
   a. Discontinue cardiopulmonary bypass, clamp arterial and venous lines
   b. De-air bypass circuit
   c. Add necessary volume to the reservoir if needed
   d. Cool the perfusate to 20 degrees Celsius
2. Anesthesia
   a. Position table in steep Trendelenburg position
   b. Administer 100% Oxygen
   c. Resuscitate with volume and pressors (keep MAP>60 mmHg)
   d. Can consider administration of steroids/barbiturates/mannitol
3. Surgeon
   a. Disconnect the arterial line from the aortic cannula
   b. Disconnect the venous line from the SVC cannula
   c. Connect the arterial line to:
      i. SVC cannula if bicaval cannulation was performed
      ii. Single two-stage venous cannula can be withdrawn slightly so as to direct it from the RA into the SVC first
   d. Initiate retrograde cerebral perfusion
      i. Can consider cooling to 32 °C (temperature is per surgeon's discretion)
      ii. Flow: 300 ml/min
      iii. For 2-5 minutes (until all air is vented back through aortic cannula/root vent site)
      iv. Bilateral carotid compression by anesthesia team
      v. Keep retrograde cerebral perfusion pressure < 25 mmHg
      vi. Retrograde cerebral perfusion can be repeated
   e. Discontinue perfusion and reconnect the arterial and venous lines back to aortic and SVC cannulae respectively
   f. If single atrial cannula that was in SVC, withdraw it back to the RA
      i. Initiate normal cardiopulmonary bypass
4. Cool for 28 ° C (surgeon discretion based on clinical scenario)
5. Maintain mild hypothermia for approximately 30-40 minutes
   a. Massage coronary arteries
   b. De-air the heart as usual (needle aspiration of the left ventricular apex, left ventricular vent placed through the right superior pulmonary vein, or aortic root vent)
6. Anesthesia/Perfusionist:

a. Ensure normoglycemia
   b. Diuretics if needed
   c. Cardiologist/anesthesia perform TEE to look for presence of air in the heart
   d. Consider hyperbaric oxygen postoperatively
   e. Proceed with planned case if patient condition allows

Potential Complications and Pitfalls
1. Delayed response and recognition
2. Maneuvers to prevent significant brain injury
   a. Cooling the patient expeditiously
   b. Immediate carotid artery compression
   c. Avoid excessively high perfusion pressure during retrograde cerebral perfusion (Goal: < 25mm Hg)
   d. Administer 100% inhaled oxygen
   e. Consider steroids/ barbiturates, and mannitol
3. Consider hyperbaric oxygen postoperatively
   a. Hypothermia offers several advantages, including protection of cerebral metabolism during the period of ischemia, reduction of cerebral edema that follows cerebral air embolism and increased solubility of gas in blood and tissues, thereby decreasing the size of emboli.

Template Dictation

Preoperative Diagnosis: severe aortic stenosis

Postoperative Diagnosis: severe massive air embolism

Procedure(s) Performed: [BLANK] (Example) Bioprosthetic aortic valve replacement, establishment of temporary retrograde cerebral perfusion, management of massif air embolism.

Attending Surgeon: [BLANK]

Secondary Surgeon: [BLANK]

Assistants: [BLANK]

Anesthesia: [BLANK]

Indication(s) for Procedure: [AGE] year old [GENDER] who presented [BLANK] Workup included [CXR, cardiac angiography, TTE], [Mr/ Mrs.] [BLANK] is brought now for surgical intervention.

Description of Procedure: The patient underwent general anesthesia in the supine position, and the monitoring lines were placed. The patient was prepped and draped in the usual sterile fashion. A primary sternotomy was completed without incident. The heart was dissected from adhesions. Heparin was administered. A

22-French straight aortic cannula was placed through two concentric pursestring sutures in the ascending aorta. A 28-French a right-angle venous cannula was placed in the superior vena cava and a 32-French right-angle venous cannula was placed in the inferior vena cava. An aortic root vent was placed. The patient was placed on cardiopulmonary bypass at 2.4 L/min per m2 for [Blank] minutes. An aortic cross-clamp was applied and cold blood cardioplegia given in the antegrade catheter establishing adequate rapid diastolic arrest of the heart. The case was started as planned. We were notified by the perfusionist that there were difficulties in maintaining bypass flow. Air bubbles were seen in the aortic cannula, and a diagnosis of massive air embolism was suspected. The perfusionist was asked to cease cardiopulmonary bypass and a clamp was placed on the aortic cannula. The patient was placed in steep Trendelenburg position. The perfusionist clamped both the arterial and venous lines, and the bypass circuit was de-aired. The arterial line was disconnected from the aortic cannula, and then connected to the SVC cannula. Retrograde cerebral perfusion was started at a flow of 300 ml/min for 3 minutes with perfusion pressure < 25 mmHg. During this time, the anesthesia team was repeating bilateral carotid compression, and retrograde cerebral perfusion was repeated once, as all air was cleared from the bypass tubing. Then the arterial and venous lines were connected back to normal aortic and SVC cannulae respectively and started normal cardiopulmonary bypass the patient was cooled to 28° C for 30 minutes with repeated massage coronary arteries, the heart was de-aired as usual. During the case the patient received steroids, barbiturates, and Mannitol. The patient remained normoglycemic, and transesophageal was done to look for any gross air in the heart. The case was then undertaken as planned [**check dictation from other chapter of the book**]. After completion of the procedure, the aortic-cross clamp was removed. Atrial and ventricular pacing wires were placed. The patient as mechanically ventilated at this point. The patient was weaned off of cardiopulmonary bypass and the venous cannulae were removed. The cardiologist performed TEE to look for presence of air in the heart, and condition of the [BLANK procedure]. Once there was no air in the heart, the aortic root vent was removed and the site repaired with an interrupted Prolene suture. Protamine was administered and hemostasis was obtained. Chest tubes were placed in the mediastinum. The aortic cannula was removed and site repaired with pledgeted Prolene sutures. The mediastinum was irrigated. The sternum was reapproximated with interrupted #6 stainless steel wires. The fascia was sutured with interrupted #1 Absorbable suture. The subcutaneous tissues were sutured with continuous #2-0 Absorbable sutures. The skin was sutured with continuous #4-0 Absorbable sutures. The patient tolerated the procedure well. All needle, sponge, and instrument counts were correct on two occasions. The patient was taken to the hyperbaric oxygen postoperatively.

Dr. [BLANK] was present and scrubbed for [BLANK] elements of this procedure.

Intraoperative Aortic Dissection

Essential Operative Steps

ESS After/During cannulation (Prior to Initiation of Cardiopulmonary Bypass)

1. Suspicion of ascending aorta dissection
   a. Bluish discoloration or hematoma in the ascending aorta
   b. High arterial line pressure
2. Do not go on bypass
3. Perform TEE to visualize intimal flap and extent of the dissection
   a. Confirm patient stability with anesthesia
   b. Cannulate right femoral artery if dissection is identified in ascending aorta
   c. Confirm the wire is in the true lumen
   d. RA for venous cannulation
   e. Cardioplegia: retrograde and through the coronary ostia
   f. CPB
   g. Confirm flow in the true lumen, carotid and coronary artery (TEE)
   h. Cool to circulatory arrest, ice on head, Trendelenburg position
   i. Perform the planned procedure
   j. Replace the ascending aorta and resect the dissection entry site
   k. If the patient is unstable, then expeditious groin cannulation is necessary
4. Option if the dissection is limited to the ascending aorta
   a. TEE-guided direct cannulation of the ascending aorta true lumen (Seldinger technique), recommended only in experienced hands
5. While on bypass
   a. Sudden increase in the arterial line pressure
   b. Evaluate the ascending aorta/TEE
   c. Discontinue CPB immediately
   d. Cannulate the groin
   e. Proceed as outlined above

Potential Complications and Pitfalls

1. The dissection could start at the site of aortic cannulation, the proximal vein graft anastomosis after CABG, aortic root vent and an aortotomy after aortic valve replacement. The main preventive measure is awareness of a possibility of dissection and meticulous surgical technique in handling the tissue
2. Have high suspicion when there is bluish discoloration or hematoma in the proximity of the aortic cannulation site expanding to the aorta, high arterial pressure when you insert and test your aortic cannula, sudden increase in the arterial line pressure during bypass, or unexplained bleeding from the aortic root vent or proximal anastomotic sites.

3. Perfusion the false lumen? Check with TEE and do Seldinger technique to cannulate the true lumen, if not go to the groin for femoral cannulation (recommended)
4. Femoral cannulation be aware of the extent of dissection, be sure that you cannulating and perfusing the true lumen, can consider right axillary artery cannulation for arterial inflow
5. Localized dissection can be fixed with a side bite clamp and strips of Teflon felt (in very select circumstances)
6. If extensive, deep hypothermic circulatory arrest and hemiarch replacement under direct vision is necessary
7. Check for the aortic valve condition if you have moderate or severe regurgitation, commissural resuspension may be required. If not durable, then consider aortic valve or root replacement
8. Check for coronary dissection and consider bypass grafting if needed
9. Reinforce the distal and proximal aorta with double layer of Teflon felt before doing the distal anastomosis
10. Careful hemostasis, good chest tube drainage, and correction of any coagulopathy are critical components
11. Be aware of all complication of Aortic root replacement and dissection pitfalls described in other chapters
12. Don't hesitate to add other cardiac support like ECMO, RVAD or LVAD, IABP could be used carefully because of the distal dissection.
13. Be aware of Lower extremity compartment syndrome if femoral cannulation

Template Dictation

Preoperative Diagnosis: Aortic Dissection

Postoperative Diagnosis: Same

Procedure(s) Performed:

Attending Surgeon: [BLANK]

Secondary Surgeon: [BLANK]

Assistants: [BLANK]

Anesthesia: [BLANK]

Indication(s) for Procedure: [AGE] year old [GENDER] who developed an aortic dissection intraoperatively, [Mr/ Mrs.] [BLANK] is brought now for surgical intervention.

Description of Procedure: The patient underwent general anesthesia in the supine position and the monitoring lines were placed. The patient was prepped and draped in the usual sterile fashion. A primary sternotomy was completed without incident. The heart was dissected from adhesions. Heparin was administered. A

22-French straight aortic cannula was placed through two concentric pursestring sutures in the ascending aorta. A 20-French a right-angle venous cannula was placed in the superior vena cava, a right-angle venous cannula was placed in the inferior vena cava. An aortic root vent was placed. The patient was placed on cardiopulmonary bypass at 2.4 L/min per m2 at 32 degrees centigrade for [Blank] minutes. An aortic cross-clamp was applied and cold blood cardioplegia given in the antegrade catheter establishing adequate rapid diastolic arrest of the heart. The case [Blank] was started and performed as planned.

Dissection from aortic root vent site at the end of the case with aortic valve damage and RCA dissection/ECMO

After removing the aortic root vent there was a bleeding from this site, and a reinforcing suture of 4-0 Prolene backed with felt pledgets was placed.

However, upon tying the sutures, there was an aortic dissection that developed immediately and involved the entire ascending aorta and aortic arch. There was massive bleeding from the very proximal portion of the aorta, and it turns out that the dissection had sheared the right coronary orifice. There was also aortic regurgitation. We had to quickly recannulate the right atrium and institute bypass. I then cooled the patient to 20 degrees centigrade, and we manually compressed the heart to prevent distension. When an adequate level of hypothermia was achieved, we used an [Blank minute] period of circulatory arrest. I transected the aorta obliquely beneath the arch. We excised the aorta above the sinotubular ridge and infused cardioplegia into the left coronary ostium. Repeat infusions of 400 cc were given at 20-minute intervals during the [Blank minute] cross-clamp period. I repaired the distal aorta using two strips of felt, one inside and one outside. These were tacked together, and then we used fibrin glue between the adventitial layer and the media. A 26-mm Hemashield graft was beveled and sewn to the distal aorta with continuous 4-0 Prolene. I switched our cannulae to a femoral artery cannula. This was placed through the right femoral artery, and we resumed flow. I de-aired the graft and the brachiocephalic arteries and then applied an aortic cross-clamp just proximal to our anastomosis. Hemostasis was satisfactory. I then inspected the proximal aorta, and it was clear that the aortic tissues were so friable that we would not be able to preserve the valve. The dissection extended into the noncoronary sinus and completely dehisced the right coronary artery and the right aortic sinus. The left coronary ostium was intact, but the valve was severely damaged, and because the tissues were so friable, I did not think I could repair this. Therefore, I excised the aortic valve and the proximal aorta, leaving only the button around the left coronary ostium. We selected a [Blank Valve]. This was placed inside a tube graft and tacked with 4-0 Prolene sutures. We then sewed this composite prosthesis to the aortic valve annulus with interrupted mattress suture of 2-0 Ethibond backed with felt pledgets. The felt pledgets were on the ventricular side of the valve annulus. After tying the sutures securely, we reinforced the initial layer with over-and-over 3-0 Prolene suture. Next, the graft was trimmed, and we made a button opposite the left coronary ostium. The left coronary ostium was sewn to the graft with 5-0 Prolene. We then trimmed the distal graft to the right and sewed the distal graft to the proximal graft. This was accomplished with 4-0 Prolene. I dissected in the right AV groove and identified the right coronary artery. During a period of cooling, we harvested a segment of saphenous vein from the left thigh. This reverse saphenous vein was sewn to the right coronary artery with 7-0 Prolene. We had released the aortic cross-clamp prior to doing this anastomosis. I put a partial occlusion clamp on the graft in the ascending aorta and excised a small button. The vein graft was beveled and sewn to the aorta with continuous 5-0 Prolene suture. At this point, we released bulldog clamps on the vein graft, and we had re-established blow in the right coronary artery. Flow in the right coronary graft was **[Blank mL/min]**. The cardiac contractions were feeble, but the bleeding seemed to be coming under control. TEE showed aortic dissection in the distal aorta with a double lumen. It was clear that the patient would require hemodynamic support, and I initially planned to insert an intra-aortic balloon. However, because of the fragility of the tissue and the potential difficulty with the dissected descending aorta, I felt it was safer to use extracorporeal membrane oxygenation. We had switched our cannula back from the groin to the ascending aortic graft, and we left this in place. We then placed a second cannula in the right atrium. These two cannulae were connected to the ECMO circuit, and we discontinued regular bypass and began ECMO support. Protamine was administered. There was a great deal of bleeding from all cut surfaces.

The patient had very feeble contraction but did have right ventricular function and some left ventricular contraction when the heart was decompressed. It is our hope that with time his ventricular function will improve. We removed the first venous cannula and repaired the atrial appendage with 2-0 nonabsorbable suture. Considerable time was taken to try to improve hemostasis, although the patient had continued bleeding.

Flow through the ECMO circuit was 2.2 to 2.6 L/min per m2, and we had excellent perfusion. The patient made urine throughout the procedure. When the bleeding seemed better, I felt we should move back to the intensive care unit. Therefore, we packed the anterior mediastinum and placed drainage tubes in both pleural spaces and in the mediastinum. A surgical pause confirmed that all needle, sponge, and instrument counts were correct. The patient was in critical condition but did exit the operating room and was returned to the intensive care unit.

Dr. **[BLANK]** was present and scrubbed for **[BLANK]** elements of this procedure.

19. LVAD – Heartware

Michael Tong MD, MBA

Cleveland Clinic, Cleveland, OH

Essential Operative Steps

1. Lines and monitoring
2. General endotracheal tube anesthesia
3. Intraop TEE
4. Consider inhaled prostacyclin for prophylaxis against RV failure
5. Median Sternotomy
6. Open pericardium
7. Create tunnel for driveline with endoscopic tunneler
8. Systemic heparin
9. Arterial cannulation
10. 2 stage single venous cannulation
11. Check ACT (>480)
12. Initiate CPB (CI 2.2)
13. Lift the apex of heart and identify the apex
14. Sew the HVAD ring into place with 12 pledgeted 2-0 Ethibond sutures
15. Perform ventriculotomy with coring knife
16. Bring a primed pump onto the table and place the inflow cannula through the HVAD ring
17. Externalize the driveline
18. Size the outflow cannula
19. Place a partial cross clamp on the ascending aorta and sew on the outflow graft.
20. Place a deairing vent in the aorta and deair the heart
21. Come off bypass and turn on pump and titrate to appropriate flows
22. Decannulate
23. Give protamine and assure hemostasis.
24. Close chest.

Potential Complications and Pitfalls

1. Stay midline during sternotomy
2. The tunneler for the driveline has potential to hit bowel, liver, vessels, etc.
3. Fragile LV apex that can tear
4. Outflow graft too long/short
5. Pump sitting in a poor position
6. Cannot adequately deair the pump
7. Bleeding
8. RV failure
9. Suction event

II. Adult Cardiac Surgery

Template Dictation

Preoperative diagnosis: [Indication: e.g. ischemic cardiomyopathy]

Postoperative diagnosis: same

Procedure(s) Performed: Implantation of HeartMate II left ventricular assist device as (INDICATION: destination therapy or bridge to transplant)

Attending Surgeon: [BLANK]

Secondary Surgeon: [BLANK]

Assistants: [BLANK]

Anesthesia: [BLANK]

Drains: [BLANK]

Estimated blood loss: [BLANK]

Specimen: [LV core]

Indication(s) for Procedure: [AGE] year old [GENDER] with [DURATION] history of [COMPLAINT]. Preoperative workup showed severe cardiomyopathy and end-stage systolic and diastolic congestive heart failure. Patient is status [INTERMACS LEVEL] with [JUSTIFICATION OF STATUS]. Patient taken to the OR today for implantation of LVAD.

Description of Procedure: The patient was taken to the operating room on [DATE]. Preoperative huddle and preincision timeout was performed. Patient was in supine position. General anesthesia was obtained. A right internal jugular central venous line, pulmonary artery catheter and radial arterial line were inserted. Transesophageal echocardiogram was performed. Patient was prepped and draped in normal fashion.

A midline sternotomy was performed and the pericardium was opened and mobilized all the way to the left to create space for the HVAD device. The patient was heparinized and arterial cannula was placed in the ascending aorta and 2-stage venous cannula was inserted in the right atrial appendage. Once ACT was >480, patient was placed on cardiopulmonary bypass and normothermia was maintained.

The HVAD ring was then sewn on to this region with a 12 pledgeted 2-0 Ethibond sutures. Subsequently, a circular ventriculotomy was performed. Within the ventricle, all scarring and fibrosis and thickened trabecula were resected to ensure that our inflow cannula would be unobstructed. At this time, the LVAD pump was placed in and secured. The heart was then placed back into the pericardium and the driveline of the device was brought out through the right upper quadrant of the abdomen. At this time, we checked the inflow cannula position and it was positioned perfectly, directed toward the mitral. Subsequently, the outflow graft was measured to the ascending aorta and cut to length. A partial cross-clamp was placed over the ascending aorta and after aortotomy was created, the graft was sewn on with 4-0 Prolene suture in an end-to-side fashion. A deairing vent was placed in the ascending aorta. The partial cross-clamp was then removed. The heart was gradually de-aired. We gradually increased the flow on the HVAD and came off cardiopulmonary bypass.

We were able to achieve flows of over 5 L/min and the right ventricular function was excellent. Postop TEE demonstrated no residual TR or MR and no PFO. The patient continued to remain stable. At this time, we decannulated the patient and administered protamine. Subsequently, chest tubes were placed and the sternum, subcutaneous tissue, and skin were closed in the usual fashion. The patient continued to remain well and was taken to the ICU in stable condition.

All instruments, sponges and needles counts were confirmed to be correct x 2 at the end of the case.

Dr. [BLANK] was present and scrubbed for [BLANK] elements of this procedure.

20. LVAD – Heart Mate II

Michael Tong MD, MBA

Cleveland Clinic, Cleveland, OH

Essential Operative Steps

1. Lines and monitoring
2. General endotracheal tube anesthesia
3. Intraop TEE
4. Consider inhaled prostacyclin for prophylaxis against RV failure
5. Median Sternotomy
6. Pump pocket creation in the preperitoneal space
7. Open pericardium
8. Create tunnel for driveline with endoscopic tunneler
9. Systemic heparin
10. Arterial cannulation
11. 2 stage single venous cannulation
12. Check ACT (>480)
13. Initiate CPB (CI 2.2)
14. Lift the apex of heart and identify the apex
15. Core the LV apex and place basket vent into the LV
16. Sew a strip of felt along anterolateral apex of the LV
17. Place a circular strip of felt on the apex and place annuloplasty sutures circumferentially along the LV cavity.
18. Place the annuloplasty stitches through the sewing ring
19. Bring a primed pump onto the table and place the inflow cannula through the sewing ring and secure.
20. Place the pump in the pump pocket and externalize the driveline
21. Size the outflow cannula
22. Place a partial cross clamp on the ascending aorta and sew on the outflow graft.
23. Connect the outflow graft to the pump
24. Place a deairing vent in the ascending aorta and deair the heart
25. Come off bypass and turn on pump and titrate to appropriate flows
26. Decannulate
27. Give protamine and assure hemostasis.
28. Close chest.

Potential Complications and Pitfalls

1. Stay midline during sternotomy
2. The tunneler for the driveline has potential to hit bowel, liver, vessels, etc.
3. Need to create pocket large enough and lateral enough to sit properly
4. Fragile LV apex that can tear
5. Bleeding from the pump pocket

6. Outflow graft too long/short
7. Pump sitting in a poor position. Inflow cannula not directing towards the mitral valve
8. Cannot adequately deair the pump
9. Bleeding
10. RV failure
11. Suction event

Template Dictation

Preoperative Diagnosis: [Indication: e.g. Ischemic cardiomyopathy]

Postoperative Diagnosis: Same

Procedure(s) Performed: Implantation of HeartMate II left ventricular assist device as **(INDICATION: destination therapy or bridge to transplant)**

Attending Surgeon: [BLANK]

Secondary Surgeon: [BLANK]

Assistants: [BLANK]

Anesthesia: [BLANK]

Drains: [BLANK]

Estimated blood loss: [BLANK]

Specimen: [LV core]

Indication(s) for Procedure: [AGE] year old [GENDER] with [DURATION] history of [COMPLAINT]. Preoperative workup showed severe cardiomyopathy and end-stage systolic and diastolic congestive heart failure. Patient is status [INTERMACS LEVEL] with [JUSTIFICATION OF STATUS]. Patient taken to the OR today for implantation of LVAD

Description of Procedure: The patient was taken to the operating room on [DATE]. Preoperative huddle and preincision timeout was performed. Patient was in supine position. General anesthesia was obtained. A right internal jugular central venous line, pulmonary artery catheter and radial arterial line were inserted. Transesophageal echocardiogram was performed. Patient was prepped and draped in normal fashion.

A midline sternotomy was performed and a pocket was created in the left upper quadrant of the abdomen in the preperitoneal space for the HeartMate II LVAD. At this time, the pericardium was opened. The patient was heparinized and arterial cannula was placed in the ascending aorta and 2-stage venous cannula was inserted in the right atrial appendage. Once ACT was >480, patient was placed on cardiopulmonary bypass and normothermia was maintained.

The apex of the heart was subsequently elevated and a core ventriculotomy was performed. A basket sucker was placed in the LV cavity and any residual obstructing bands of muscle within the LV were resected. Subsequently, a strip of felt was sewn onto the anterolateral apex of the heart with a running Prolene suture. A strip of doughnut shaped felt was then placed on top of this and twelve 2-0 Ethibond mattress sutures were placed circumferentially. The annuloplasty sutures were then placed through the inflow cannula and then sewn in. The pump was brought to the table and connected to the inflow cannula and secured with plastic tapes. The body of the pump was then placed in the previously created pump pocket. The driveline was exited initially through a right upper quadrant and subsequently into the left upper quadrant in a double tunneling technique. The VAD was then placed in the proper position and the inflow cannula position was excellent. Hemostasis at the inflow cannula was assured. At this time, the outflow graft was measured to the mid ascending aorta. A partial cross-clamp was placed and the aortotomy was performed. The outflow graft was sewn in an end-to-side fashion with 4-0 Prolene suture. Subsequently, a vent was placed in the aorta, and after the de-airing procedure was done under TEE guidance, the patient was gradually separated from cardiopulmonary bypass and went onto the HeartMate II LVAD support. We were able to achieve flows of over 5 L/min and the right ventricular function was excellent. Postop TEE demonstrated no residual TR or MR and no PFO. The patient continued to remain stable. At this time, we decannulated the patient and administered protamine. Subsequently, chest tubes were placed and the sternum, subcutaneous tissue, and skin were closed in the usual fashion. The patient continued to remain well and was taken to the ICU in stable condition.

All instruments, sponges and needles counts were confirmed to be correct x 2 at the end of the case.

Dr. [BLANK] was present and scrubbed for [BLANK] elements of this procedure.

21. Minimally Invasive Directed Coronary Artery Bypass

M. Scott Halbreiner MD and Joseph Sabik MD

Cleveland Clinic, Cleveland, OH

Essential Operative Steps

1. Lines and monitoring
2. Selective right lung ventilation
3. Intraoperative transesophageal echocardiogram
4. left anterolateral thoracotomy
5. LIMA takedown
6. Systemic heparinization (ACT > 400)
7. Opening pericardium
8. Placement of stabilizers
9. Proximal LAD occlusion or shunt placement
10. Perform anastamosis
11. Securing LIMA pedicle
12. Protamine administration
13. Doppler flow check of anastamosis
14. Chest tube placement
15. Assess hemostasis
16. Reinflation of left lung (assess tension of graft with inflation)
17. Rib reapproximation and soft tissue/skin closure

Potential Complications and Pitfalls

1. Incorrect rib space for entry
2. Injury to LIMA
3. Inadequate right lung isolation
4. Phrenic nerve injury when opening pericardium
5. Insufficient graft length
6. Subclavian vein injury
7. Kinking of graft
8. Fibrillation
9. Need to go on CPB

Template Dictation

Preoperative Diagnosis: [INDICATION – e.g. isolated single coronary artery disease of LAD]

Postoperative Diagnosis: Same

Procedure(s) Performed: Minimally invasive directed coronary artery bypass [DETAILS – e.g. LIMA to LAD]

Attending Surgeon: [BLANK]

II. Adult Cardiac Surgery

Secondary Surgeon: [BLANK]

Assistants: [BLANK]

Anesthesia: [BLANK]

Indication(s) for Procedure: [AGE] year old [GENDER] with [DURATION] history of symptomatic coronary artery disease and [COMPLAINT] – e.g. increasing shortness of breath, angina, etc]. Preoperative coronary angiography reveals [FINDINGS – e.g. 90% stenosis of mid-LAD and ejection fraction of 50%].

Description of Procedure: The patient was taken to the operating room on [DATE]. An appropriate review was performed verifying the patient's identity and planned procedure. While supine on the operating room table, general endotracheal anesthesia was administered without difficult. Single right-sided lung ventilation was achieved with a [double-lumen tube or bronchial blocker] and confirmed by bronchoscopy. A [right/left] internal jugular central line and a [right/left] [radial/axillary/femoral/brachial] arterial line were placed. A pulmonary artery catheter [was/was not] placed. Preoperative transesophageal echocardiogram was performed to evaluate cardiac and valvular function. The patient was then prepped and draped in a sterile fashion including the chest, abdomen, groins and bilateral lower extremities. A time-out was performed. A [BLANK] cm anterolateral skin incision was made in the [4th/5th] intercostal space at the inframammary fold. Dissection was carried down to the intercostal space with minimal division of the pectoralis muscle. The thoracic cavity was then entered in the standard fashion with care to avoid injury to the left internal mammary artery (LIMA). The patient was heparinized with [BLANK] units and ACT verified. The LIMA was then divided distally and carefully dissected from the intrathoracic fascia up to the level of the subclavian vein. The pericardium was then opened. The diseased left anterior descending artery was identified and location of acceptable target was decided upon. There was adequate length of the LIMA. A coronary artery stabilizing device was then placed through a small port incision in the chest to stabilize the LAD target. **[Proximal LAD occlusion was achieved with a 4-0 felt-pledgeted suture / An arteriotomy was performed in the LAD and an intravascular shunt was used to prevent ischemia and]** to achieve hemostasis. The LIMA was then anastamosed to the LAD in an end-to-side fashion with a running 7-0 Prolene suture. Prior to completing the anastamosis the [occlusion suture / intravascular shunt] was removed. At the completion of the anastamosis the pedicled LIMA was suture fixated to the epicardium with interrupted sutures. Protamine was administered to reverse the heparin effects. The flow down the bypass graft was checked and confirmed using a doppler flow probe. The coronary stabilizing device was removed and hemostasis was achieved. A total of [BLANK] chest tubes were placed in the left pleural space and [BLANK] chest tube(s) were placed in the mediastinum. [Atrial/Ventricular] pacing wires were placed in the standard fashion. The thoracotomy was reapproximated with rib sutures and prior to closure the left lung was observed to reinflate completely and imposed minimal tension on the LIMA graft. The subcutaneous tissues and skin were closed in the standard fashion and sterile dressings were applied. The patient tolerated the procedure well and was **[extubated in the operating room and then]** brought to the intensive care unit in stable condition.

All instrument, sponge and needle counts were confirmed to be correct following skin closure.

Dr. **[BLANK]** was present and scrubbed for **[BLANK]** elements of this procedure.

22. Aortic Valve Surgery with Upper Hemisternotomy Approach

Narongrit Kantathut, MD and Stephanie Mick, MD

Cleveland clinic, Cleveland, OH

Essential Operative Steps

1. Lines and Monitoring, external defibrillator pads
2. General endotracheal anesthesia
3. Intraoperative transesophageal echocardiogram
4. Upper hemisternotomy (to level of right 4th intercostal space and taken transversely through this space)
5. Open pericardium, pericardial well, survey ascending aorta for plaque burden (consider epiaortic ultrasound)
6. Systemic heparinization
7. Arterial cannulation (Ascending aorta or femoral artery)
8. Venous cannulation (Right atrial appendage, SVC or Femoral vein)
9. Myocardial protection cannula placement (antegrade cannula in ascending aorta +/-retrograde cannula in coronary sinus)
10. Check ACT (>400 sec)
11. Initiate CPB
12. Aortic cross clamp (reduce CPB flow rate, apply cross clamp, return to full CPB flow)
13. Antegrade cardioplegia +/- topical cooling with ice for cardiac arrest (+/-
14. retrograde cardioplegia)
15. Aortotomy (transverse, oblique)
16. Excision of aortic valve cusps and decalcification
17. Aortic valve replacement
18. Aortotomy closure
19. Warm blood cardioplegia "hot shot" administration for rewarming
20. Remove aortic cross clamp
21. Deairing
22. Placement of pacing wires (ventricular +/- atrial)
23. Chest tube placement while on CPB
24. Wean from CPB
25. Venous decannulation
26. Protamine test and administration for heparin reversal
27. Aortic decannulation
28. Assess hemostasis
29. Sternotomy closure

Potential Complications and Pitfalls

1. Make sure that the sternotomy is absolutely midline and that the midline sternotomy is not carried beyond the level of the transverse part. Otherwise it will result in a lateral fracture, resulting in three sternal fragments, or a continued lower extension of the midline fracture with

retraction that produces severe intraoperative bleeding and difficulty in closure.
2. Care must be taken not to cut too deeply when the sternotomy is continued into the right fourth intercostal space to avoid injury to mediastinal pleura, right internal mammary artery and pericardium
3. Care must be taken when bringing up the pericardium and reopening the retractor, as sudden retraction with elevated cardiac structures could impede venous return causing a sudden drop in cardiac output.
4. Cannulation catastrophe (Aortic dissection/bleeding, Right atrial tear)
5. Insufficient myocardial protection and cardiac arrest (cross clamp not across, aortic insufficiency, insufficient venous drainage)
6. Coronary sinus injury with retrograde cardioplegia cannulation
7. Incomplete decalcification of the aortic valve and annulus resulting in paravalvular leak and dehiscence
8. Perforation of the aorta and anterior leaflet of Mitral valve while calcific deposits are debrided
9. Deep debridement in the area below the junction of the right and non-coronary cusps in the membranous septum or deeply placed valve sutures in this region, resulting in permanent heart block (bundle of His injury)
10. Not capturing debris during procedure or forcing debris into the left ventricle while the aortic root is flushed with saline, this debris may embolize and lead to stroke
11. Incomplete deairing prior to removal of aortic root vent
12. Not recognizing bleeding from aortotomy (particularly at extremes of aortotomy)
13. Inadequate control of hemostasis prior to sternal closure/ bleeding from cannulation sites.
14. Placement of the drains while the heart is full; this must be done on bypass with the heart decompressed or injury to the heart can occur.

Template Dictation

Preoperative Diagnosis: [INDICATION – e.g. Severe AR, Severe AS]

Postoperative Diagnosis: Same

Procedure(s) Performed: Upper hemisternotomy and AVR (**DETAILS** – e.g. Tissue valve or Mechanical valve)

Attending Surgeon: [BLANK]

Secondary Surgeon: [BLANK]

Assistants: [BLANK]

Anesthesia: [BLANK]

Indication(s) for Procedure: [AGE] year old [GENDER] with [DURATION] history of [COMPLAINT – e.g. chest pain, syncope and shortness of breath].

The preoperative echocardiography revealed [**FINDINGS** - e.g. severe AS, mean gradient across aortic valve(mmHg), peak jet velocity(m/s), Aortic valve area (cm^2), severe AR , LV end-diastolic diameter(mm) , LV end-systolic diameter(mm), estimated ejection fraction, morphology of aortic valve – bi-leaflet or tri-leaflet , calcified]. The preoperative coronary catheterization revealed [**FINDINGS** - e.g. No significant coronary artery disease].

Description of Procedure: The patient was taken to the operating room on [DATE]. The patient's identity and planned procedure verified, and the patient was placed on the operating room table in the supine position. General anesthesia was obtained. A right internal jugular central venous line and pulmonary artery catheter and radial arterial line were inserted. External defibrillator pads were attached. Preoperative transesophageal echocardiogram was performed to evaluate cardiac function and valve function. The patient's chest, abdomen, groins, and lower extremities were prepped and draped in standard sterile fashion. A time out was performed.

A 8-10 cm. vertical midline incision was made [Potential additional details: starting at 2-3 cm. inferior to sternal notch or just above the level of the manubriosternal angle]. An upper hemisternotomy was performed from the sternal notch to the level of fourth intercostal space with the standard sternal saw and continued into the right fourth intercostal space using a narrow blade oscillating saw. The sternal retractor was inserted, the thymus divided and the pericardium opened. Pericardial stay sutures were placed and the retractor was removed. The stays were tacked to the subcutaneous tissues and the retractor replaced. [Note: This facilitates exposure by elevating the pericardial contents forward to the operative field.]

The ascending aorta was palpated [and/or epiaortic ultrasound was used] and found to be free of calcification. The patient was heparinized. The [ascending aorta or proximal aortic arch] was cannulated. [Alternative cannulation site for the arterial line is the femoral artery by a small incision at the groin. The arterial cannula can be place via femoral artery by Seldinger technique.] A two stage venous cannula was inserted via the [**right atrial appendage/superior vena cava**]. [Alternatively, a peripheral venous cannula can be placed via the femoral vein by Seldinger technique and under TEE guidance. The cannula is guided into the right atrium and the tip is placed in the superior vena cava.] Cardiopulmonary bypass was initiated.

An antegrade cardioplegia/vent cannula was placed in ascending aorta and a retrograde cardioplegia catheter was placed in the coronary sinus via the right atrium under TEE guidance. [Alternative: this catheter can be placed by the anesthesiologists via the transjugular route prior to the incision). [A right superior pulmonary vein or a left atrial dome vent can be placed.]

The aorta was crossclamped and and the heart arrested with first antegrade and then retrograde cardioplegia. During the remainder of the surgery, cardioplegia was given every 15-20 minutes.

[**Oblique /Transverse**] aortotomy was performed 10-15 mm above the origin of right coronary artery and extended anteriorly and posteriorly. [Additional [ml] of cardioplegia was delivered directly into the [right and/or the left] coronary arteries.] The aortic valve was exposed, examined and found to be [trileaflet, bileaflet, heavily calcified, etc.]. The valve was excised and the annulus decalcified. The [valve company] sizer was used and the outflow tract/annulus found to accommodate a [size] valve. A series of [2-0, type of suture] pledgetted valve sutures were placed around the annulus with the pledgets on the [aortic or ventricular] side. The valve sutures were taken sequentially around the sewing ring of the [company name] valve and the valve was seated, then tied in place. The valve was seated and the sutures tied. The left and right coronary ostia were visualized to be [e.g., well away] from the valve annulus and posts. The aortic root and aorta were again irrigated with normal saline. The aortotomy was closed with two layers of running 4-0 prolene and the aorta was deaired.

The heart and ascending aorta were deaired and aortic cross-clamp was removed. Pacing wires [can specify type] and chest drains [specify site – mediastinal/pleural] were placed. When the patient's heart was adequately recovered and thoroughly deaired, [s/he] was weaned from cardiopulmonary bypass without difficulty. Intraoperative transesophageal echo demonstrated [e.g. a well seated valve with no paravalvular leaks]. All cannulas were removed and the heparin effect was reversed with protamine. Hemostasis was obtained and the wounds were closed in standard fashion. The patient tolerated the procedure well and was brought to the Intensive Care Unit in [e.g. stable] condition.

Dr. [**BLANK**] was present and scrubbed for [**BLANK**] elements of this procedure.

23. Mitral Valve Replacement

Franjo Siric, MD and A. Marc Gillinov, MD

Cleveland Clinic, Cleveland, OH

Essential Operative Steps

1. Lines and Monitoring
2. General endotracheal anesthesia
3. Intraoperative transesophageal echocardiogram
4. Median sternotomy
5. Open pericardium, elevation of the right side of the pericardium with stay sutures, survey ascending aorta for plaque burden and cannulation site
6. Systemic heparinization (400 U/Kg)
7. Aortic cannulation
8. Venous cannulation- Bicaval
9. Aortic root vent
10. Check ACT (>480 sec)
11. Initiate cardiopulmonary bypass
12. Maintain normothermia
13. Aortic cross clamp
14. Antegrade cold blood cardioplegia (1000-1200 ml)
15. Dissect Sondergaard's groove
16. Standard left atriotomy
17. Expose and assess the mitral valve (fill left ventricle with cold saline to identify the mechanism of regurgitation)
18. Excise portion of anterior leaflet, preserving subvalvular apparatus
19. Size valve
20. Place annular valve sutures (pledgits on the left atrial side)
21. Implant valve
22. Check valve struts with a dental mirror
23. Left atriotomy closure
24. De-airing maneuvers
25. Remove aortic cross clamp
26. Check for hemostasis
27. Place epicardial atrial and ventricular pacing wires
28. Wean from cardiopulmonary bypass
29. Evaluate mitral valve with transesophageal echocardiogram
30. Venous decannulation
31. Ensure adequate de-airing of the heart prior to removal of aortic root vent
32. Protamine administration for heparin reversal
33. Aortic decannulation
34. Assess hemostasis
35. Sternotomy closure

Potential Complications and Pitfalls

1. Stay midline during sternotomy
2. Avoid injury to the innominate vein while making pericardial well
3. Cannulation catastrophe (aortic dissection/hematoma, right atrial tear)
4. Poor choice of location of aortic cannula/cross clamp (risk of stroke)
5. Injury of the pulmonary artery during cross clamp application
6. Insufficient myocardial protection and cardiac arrest (cross clamp not across, aortic regurgitation with secondary ventricular distension)
7. Feel the left ventricle during administration of antegrade cardioplegia to ensure absence of ventricular distension and uniform cooling of the ventricle with cardioplegia
8. Poor venous drainage (incorrect choice of cannula size, advancing the two-stage cannula too far in so it is obstructing hepatic veins)
9. Failure to dissect Sondergaard's groove
10. Improper dissection of the Sondergaard's groove with inadvertent opening of the right atrium close to the inferior vena cava
11. Opening the left atrium close to the right superior pulmonary vein with subsequent difficulty in exposing the mitral valve
12. Retractor injury with subsequent shearing tear of the left atrial wall edges which complicates closure
13. Failure to recognize important vital structures in relation to the mitral valve: atrioventricular node, coronary sinus, aortic valve and circumflex coronary artery
14. Improper placement of the annular sutures with misidentification of the mitral annulus and subsequent placement of the sutures in the left atrial wall
15. Deep placement of annular sutures with subsequent injury to the circumflex coronary artery in a left dominant system
16. LVOT obstruction by the valve strut
17. Improper de-airing prior to removal of aortic root vent
18. Lifting the heart with the prosthesis in place causing AV disruption
19. Inadequate control of hemostasis prior to sternal closure/bleeding from cannulation sites
20. Improper closure of sternotomy

Template Dictation

Preoperative Diagnosis: Severe mitral valve regurgitation/stenosis

Postoperative Diagnosis: Same

Procedure(s) Performed:

1. Intraoperative transesophageal echocardiography
2. Mitral valve replacement

Attending Surgeon: [BLANK]

II. Adult Cardiac Surgery

Secondary Surgeon: [BLANK]

Assistants: [BLANK]

Anesthesia: [BLANK]

Indication(s) for Procedure: [AGE] year old [GENDER] with [DURATION] history of [COMPLAINT –e.g. increasingly shortness of breath]. Preoperative transthoracic echocardiography reveals [FINDINGS - e.g. severe mitral valve regurgitation and stenosis due to advanced rheumatic disease].

Description of the Procedure: After satisfactory general endotracheal anesthesia was induced, a right internal jugular central venous line, pulmonary artery catheter and brachial arterial lines were inserted. Transesophageal echocardiogram was performed to evaluate the mitral valve and cardiac function. The patient was prepped and draped in the supine position.

A standard median sternotomy was performed and sternal retractor was placed. We opened the pericardium in an inverted T-shape fashion and pericardial stay sutures were placed on the right side. Heparin was given systemically and an aortic cannula was inserted through two pursestring sutures in the distal ascending aorta, secured and de-aired. Bicaval cannulation. An aortic root cardioplegia/vent was then inserted. After confirming ACT of more than 480 seconds, cardiopulmonary bypass was commenced at 2.4 L/min per m^2. We maintained normothermia during perfusion. The aorta was cross clamped. After administering 750ml of Buckberg cardioplegia antegrade we administered 500ml of cardioplegia in the retrograde fashion. Thereafter cold blood cardioplegia was given retrograde very 15 to 20 minutes. Simultaneously we developed Sondergaard's groove between left and right atrium and opened the left atrium about 1-2cm away from the orifice of right upper pulmonary vein to decompress it. A self-retracting Cosgrove retractor was applied to sternal retractor. Once cardioplegia was given, the self-retracting arms of Cosgrove retractor were placed starting cranially to visualize the mitral valve. Once we confirmed that the valve could not be repaired we incised the anterior leaflet in its mid-portion. Before we cut it all out we started placing everting, interrupted #2-0 ethibond pledgeted stitches on anterior annulus gently lifting the anterior leaflet to facilitate visualization. We made our way to both commissures, detached the remainder of the anterior mitral leaflet and divided it in the middle and brought the segments to the left and right to preserve chordae. Preserved portions of the anterior leaflet were sewn to the annulus towards the left and right commissures, away from central portion of the inflow, with double armed interrupted #2-0 ethibond pledgeted mattress stitches. Appropriately sized **[Valve type and size]** valve was selected and sutures were placed through sewing cuff orienting the struts in a way to avoid obstructing the left ventricular outflow tract. Atrial closure was completed after deairing. Retrograde and antegrade hot-shot was given and the aortic crossclamp was released. Following thorough deairing we removed the aortic vent. The IVC cannula was removed while still on partial bypass, the cannulation site was reinforced and CPB weaned off. Ventricular and atrial pacing wires were placed. Every attempt was made not to lift the heart with the bioprosthesis in place given the possibility of posterior LV wall rupture. A test dose of protamine was administered and the patient was monitored for adverse reaction before the protamine was resumed. The aortic cannula was then removed. Adequate hemostasis was then confirmed within the mediastinum. The sternum was then closed with a total of [NUMBER] stainless steel sternal wires. The wound was irrigated with antibiotic solution. The fascia was then closed with #1 Vicryl suture in running fashion. The deep dermal layer was then closed with #2-0 Vicryl suture in running fashion. The skin and subcuticular layer was closed with #3-0 Monocryl in running fashion. The skin of the wound was cleansed with sterile saline and dressed with antibiotic ointment and a Primapore dressing.

All instrument, sponge and needle counts were confirmed to be correct x 2 at the end of the operation. The patient was subsequently transferred to the postoperative cardiac surgical intensive care unit in critical condition."

Dr. [BLANK] was present and scrubbed for [BLANK] elements of this procedure.

24. Minimally Invasive Mitral Surgery

Brian Solomon, MD and Eugene Grossi, MD

New York University Langone Medical Center, New York, NY

Essential Operative Steps

1. Lines and Monitoring
2. General endotracheal anesthesia +/- Right Lung Isolation
3. Intraoperative trans-esophageal echocardiogram (Evaluation of Aortic atherosclerotic disease)
4. Femoral vessel dissection and palpation of cannulation sites
5. Purse-string of femoral artery and vein
6. Right anterior thoracotomy – 4th intercostal space
7. Chest wall retraction, soft tissue retractor, and exposure
8. Open pericardium, survey ascending aorta and right atrium
9. Carbon dioxide line
10. Systemic heparinization (100 u/kg)
11. Femoral arterial cannulation
12. Long venous cannulation through femoral vein – placement under TEE guidance
13. Lines tested
14. Check ACT (>450 sec)
15. Initiate CPB
16. Myocardial protection cannula placement (DLP in aortic root, +/- retrograde cannula in coronary sinus)
17. Flexible aortic cross clamp placed (reduce CPB flow rate, apply cross clamp, increase CPB flow to 2.0-2.5L/min/m2)
18. Antegrade cardioplegia (20 cc/kg initial dose) and (+/- retrogrograde cardioplegia)
19. Incision in Sondergaard's groove. Intra-atrial septal retractor blade and handle placed.
20. Valve inspected. Saline distention test. Reconciliation with TEE pathology
21. Triangular resection of posterior leaflet, re-approximation with primary sutures
22. Valve measured along base and size of anterior leaflet
23. Ethibond sutures placed in posterior annulus from anterior to posterior trigone
24. Sutures passed through annuloplasty band
25. Annuloplasty band seated along annulus and secured
26. Saline distention test
27. Left ventricular vent placed
28. Closure of atriotomy – 2 rows running 4-0 prolene
29. Cross-clamp removed with root and LV vents on suction
30. Heart defibrillated

31. De-airing confirmed with TEE
32. Removal of vents and over-sewing of vent sites, tying LA closure sutures
33. Temporary epicardial pacer wire placement
34. Removal of arterial and venous cannulae
35. Reversal of heparinization
36. Hemostasis obtained
37. Blake drain placed in pericardium
38. Loose closure of pericardium
39. Pleural chest tube placement
40. Intercostal block
41. Closure of thoracotomy and groin incision

Potential Complications and Pitfalls

1. Entering incorrect intercostal space – resulting in poor exposure
2. Avoid injury to IMA when performing thoractomy
3. Avoid damage to femoral vessels or profunda when dissection groin vessels
4. Cannulation catastrophe (Aortic dissection/ bleeding, Right atrial tear)
5. Poor choice of location of aortic cannula/ crossclamp (leading to stroke)
6. Insufficient myocardial protection and cardiac arrest (cross clamp not completely across aorta, unrecognized aortic insufficiency, insufficient venous drainage)
7. Coronary sinus injury with retrograde cardioplegia cannulation – if used
8. AV groove dissociation if dissecting posterior annulus
9. Incomplete coaptation of valve with residual mitral insufficiency
10. Valve sutures placed excessively deep, risking damage to circumflex artery
11. Valve sutures placed excessively deep, risking damage to conduction system / AV block
12. Valve sutures placed too deep causing injury to left cusp aortic valve – resultant aortic insufficiency
13. Mitral annular calcification with resultant annular disruption for valve sutures
14. Postoperative systolic anterior motion of the anterior mitral leaflet.
15. Bleeding

Template Dictation

Preoperative Diagnosis: [INDICATION – e.g. Mitral Valve Insufficiency, Mitral Valve Prolapse, Ischemic Mitral Valve Disease]

Postoperative Diagnosis: Same

Procedure(s) Performed: Minimally invasive mitral valve repair (**DETAILS – e.g.** resection of posterior leaflet prolapse, suture valvuloplasty, annuloplasty with #30 Medtronic Future band).

II. Adult Cardiac Surgery

Attending Surgeon: [BLANK]

Secondary Surgeon: [BLANK]

Assistants: [BLANK]

Anesthesia: [BLANK]

Indication(s) for Procedure: [AGE] year old [GENDER] with [DURATION] history of [COMPLAINT –e.g. congestive heart failure and shortness of breath]. Preoperative evaluation revealed [PRE-OPERATIVE FINDINGS - e.g. torn chordae in the posterior mitral valve leaflet and severe mitral valve insufficiency with normal ventricular size and function, but pulmonary hypertension in response to exercise].

Operative Findings: Fibroelastic deficiency of the valve with ruptured chordae in the P2 segment of the posterior leaflet. Left ventricular systolic function was normal.

Wound Classification: Clean.

Specimens: Segment of posterior mitral valve leaflet was sent to Pathology.

Implant: Mitral valve annuloplasty – [Make, Model, Size, Serial Number]

Pump Data:

Cross-clamp time: [TIME]

Bypass time: [TIME]

Blood: None

Description of Procedure: The patient was taken to the operating room and general anesthesia was induced without hemodynamic change. A central venous catheter and an arterial pressure measuring lines were placed. Trans-esophageal echocardiography was performed and pre-operative pathology was confirmed. TEE was used to monitor throughout the case. Patient was prepped and draped in the usual sterile fashion. Evaluation confirmed that patient was good candidate for retrograde arterial perfusion. A 4 cm transverse small incision was made in the right groin, inferior to the inguinal ligament. The common femoral artery and vein were exposed. The artery was palpated. It was noted to be soft, without visible or palpable calcifications. A purse-string suture was then placed in the anterior wall of the femoral vein. An 8 cm right anterior thoracotomy incision was performed at the level of the 4th intercostal space, adjacent to the right sternal border. The fourth intercostal space was entered using electrocautery. A skin retractor was secured within the incision and a soft tissue retractor placed in the intercostal space using the [Color] blades, to expose the underlying pericardium. The pericardium was visualized and opened, exposing the lower ascending aorta and right-sided cardiac structures. The field was flooded with carbon dioxide throughout the case to minimize intracardiac air.

The patient was systemically heparinized. Next, an arterial cannula was placed in the right common femoral artery over a guidewire, using the modified Seldinger technique, within the arterial purse-string. A long venous cannula was placed through a purse-string suture in the right common femoral vein, also using the modified Seldinger technique. The long venous cannula was positioned in the right atrium with the tip in the superior vena cava, confirmed by echocardiography. The cannulae were attached to cardiopulmonary bypass and the lines tested. Cardiopulmonary bypass was begun and the patient was systemically cooled to 32 degrees centigrade. A cardioplegia catheter was placed into the aortic root. The ascending aorta was occluded with a flexible cross-clamp through the thoracotomy. Cardioplegia was then re-injected part way through the cross-clamp time and myocardial protection was excellent.

In the event of concurrent aortic insufficiency: The heart became somewhat distended, due to a degree of aortic insufficiency. A small atriotomy incision was made and under direct vision, a retrograde cardioplegia catheter was placed in the coronary sinus. The atriotomy was closed and cardioplegia was reinitiated with retrograde cardioplegia.

An incision was made in the left atrium posterior to the interatrial septum in Sondergaard's groove. Septal retractor blade was placed nicely exposing the mitral valve. It was secured to a "iron intern" retractor through a 0.5 cm separate incision placed just medial to the thoracotomy. The valve was carefully inspected, comparing all leaflet to P1. Valve were inspected for deformity, coaptation, ruptured chordae, and prolapse. Cold saline was gently instilled into the left ventricle and the valve was assessed for regurgitation. The following findings were observed: [**Findings** - e.g. - P2 segment of the posterior leaflet had several ruptured chordae and was flail in its midportion, with intact chordae on each side]. The decision was made to repair the mitral valve.

In the event of a mitral valve repair: The flail leaflet was excised in a triangular V-type fashion. A primary repair was performed with figure-of-eight 4-0 Ethibond sutures. The mitral valve was measured using mitral valve sizing tools. It was measured from along the anterior leaflet from anterior to posterior commissure and a [**size**] annuloplasty ring was selected. Next, 2-0 Ethibond sutures were placed in each trigone. Additional 2-0 Ethibond sutures were placed along the annulus posteriorly. The sutures were placed through the sewing ring of the annuloplasty. The annuloplasty device was seated on the mitral valve annulus and each suture was tied using [**extracorporeal knot pusher or Core Knot**] and cut.

In the event of a mitral valve replacement: The mitral valve was measured using mitral valve sizing tools. It was measured from along the anterior leaflet from anterior to posterior commissure and a [**size**] mitral valve prosthesis was selected. The anterior leaflet of the mitral valve was excised sharply from the posterior to

II. Adult Cardiac Surgery

anterior commissure. The posterior leaflet was left in situ to protect the AV groove. Next, 2-0 Ethibond sutures were placed in each trigone. Additional 2-0 Ethibond sutures were placed along the annulus posteriorly. Finally 2-0 Ethibond sutures were placed along anterior annulus. The sutures were placed through the sewing ring of the valve prosthesis. The prosthesis was seated on the mitral valve annulus and each suture was tied using **[extracorporeal knot pusher or Core Knot]** and cut.

Gentle distention of the left ventricle with cold saline revealed a competent valve in all zones. A vent was placed through the atriotomy incision across the valve and the left ventricle. The atriotomy incision was closed with double layer of 4-0 prolene. With the left ventricular vent and the aortic root vent on suction, the cross-clamp was removed and the heart re-perfused. It was subsequently defibrillated and returned to normal sinus rhythm. The vents remained on suction until all micro-bubbles were cleared from the circulation and cardiac tone returned. This was confirmed on echocardiography. The vents were then removed. The vent sites were securely sutured with 4-0 prolene.

Temporary right atrial and right ventricular pacemaker wires were placed on the heart. Left ventricular function was **[description of EF]** and the echocardiogram confirmed no residual mitral valve insufficiency. The venous cannula was removed and bleeding was controlled by tying the purse-string suture in the anterior wall of the femoral vein. It was then oversewn with 5-0 prolene. After obtaining proximal and distal control of the femoral artery with vascular clamps, the arterial cannula was removed. The arteriotomy was then closed with a running 5-0 prolene suture. Distal pulses were confirmed and the femoral artery was palpated to assure no residual thrill in the artery. Heparin was reversed with protamine.

Hemostasis was obtained at all operative site. A 24 Fr Blake drain was placed within the pericardium. The pericardium was partially closed over the ascending aorta and the right atrium. A 28 Fr straight chest tube was placed in the right pleural cavity. An intercostal block was performed using 0.25% Marcaine. The intercostal space was then closed with blunt #2 Vicryl sutures. The fascia was closed in 3 layers with vicryl suture. The skin was then closed with 4-0 monocryl sutures in a running subcuticular fashion. The groin incision was also closed in layers with vircyl and monocryl suture. The patient was brought to the recovery room in stable condition without complication.

Dr. **[BLANK]** was present and scrubbed for **[BLANK]** elements of this procedure.

25. Mitral Valve Repair for Bileaflet Prolapse

Sameh M. Said, MD, and Hartzell V. Schaff, MD

Mayo Clinic, Rochester, MN

Essential Operative Steps

1. Lines and Monitoring
2. General endotracheal anesthesia
3. Intraoperative transesophageal echocardiogram
4. Median sternotomy
5. Open pericardium, elevation of the right side of the pericardium with stay sutures, survey ascending aorta for plaque burden and cannulation site
6. Systemic heparinization (400 U/Kg)
7. Aortic cannulation
8. Venous cannulation-single two-stage right atrial cannula
9. Aortic root vent/cardioplegia needle
10. Check ACT (>400 sec)
11. Initiate cardiopulmonary bypass
12. Maintain normothermia
13. Aortic cross clamp (reduce pump flow rate, apply cross clamp, increase pump flow rate to 2.0-2.5 L/min/m^2)
14. Antegrade cold blood cardioplegia (1000-1200 ml)
15. Dissect Waterston's groove
16. Standard left atriotomy
17. Expose and assess the mitral valve (fill left ventricle with cold saline to identify the mechanism of regurgitation)
18. Triangular excision or plication of the prolapsed posterior leaflet
19. The remaining edges of the posterior leaflets are sewn together in two layers with 4-0 Prolene suture or plication with figure of-eight 4-0 Prolene
20. For anterior leaflet repair, artificial chordae (Gore-Tex) are used to correct prolapse
21. Posterior annuloplasty band (63 mm in length) is placed from trigone-to-trigone secured with interrupted 2-0 Ethibond, usually 7 or 8 sutures
22. The mitral valve is checked with cold saline injection into the left ventricle, ensure aortic root vent is off
23. Left atriotomy closure
24. De-airing maneuvers
25. Lowering pump flow rate and removal of aortic cross clamp
26. Check for hemostasis
27. Placement of epicardial atrial and ventricular pacing wires
28. Chest tube placement
29. Wean from cardiopulmonary bypass
30. Evaluate mitral valve with transesophageal echocardiogram
31. Venous decannulation

32. Ensure adequate de-airing of the heart prior to removal of aortic root vent
33. Protamine administration for heparin reversal
34. Aortic decannulation (systolic blood pressure 90-100 mmHg)
35. Assess hemostasis
36. Sternotomy closure

Potential Complications and Pitfalls

1. Stay midline during sternotomy
2. Avoid injury to the innominate vein while making pericardial well
3. Cannulation catastrophe (aortic dissection/hematoma, right atrial tear)
4. Poor choice of location of aortic cannula/cross clamp (risk of stroke)
5. Injury of the pulmonary artery during cross clamp application
6. Insufficient myocardial protection and cardiac arrest (cross clamp not across, aortic regurgitation with secondary ventricular distension)
7. Feel the left ventricle during administration of antegrade cardioplegia to ensure absence of ventricular distension and uniform cooling of the ventricle with cardioplegia
8. Poor venous drainage (incorrect choice of cannula size, advancing the two-stage cannula too far in so it is obstructing hepatic veins)
9. Failure to dissect Waterston's groove
10. Improper dissection of the Waterston's groove with inadvertent opening of the right atrium close to the inferior vena cava
11. Opening the left atrium close to the right superior pulmonary vein with subsequent difficulty in exposing the mitral valve
12. Retractor injury with subsequent shearing tear of the left atrial wall edges which complicates closure
13. Failure to recognize important vital structures in relation to the mitral valve: atrioventricular node, coronary sinus, aortic valve and circumflex coronary artery
14. Excessive excision of the prolapsed leaflet tissue which may compromise the repair
15. Poor judgement of the neochordal length with either persistence of leaflet prolapse or poor leaflet coaptation
16. Improper placement of the annuloplasty sutures with misidentification of the mitral annulus and subsequent placement of the sutures in the left atrial wall
17. Deep placement of annuloplasty sutures with subsequent injury to the circumflex coronary artery in a left dominant system
18. Improper de-airing prior to removal of aortic root vent
19. Failure to recognize systolic anterior motion (SAM) of the mitral valve anterior leaflet postrepair by transesophageal echocardiogram
20. Inadequate control of hemostasis prior to sternal closure/bleeding from cannulation sites
21. Improper closure of sternotomy

Template Dictation

Preoperative Diagnosis:

1. Severe mitral valve regurgitation
2. NYHA class II
3. Prolapse of the middle scallop of the posterior leaflet
4. Prolapse of the middle segment of the anterior leaflet

Postoperative Diagnosis: Same

Procedure(s) Performed:

1. Mitral valve repair with triangular excision of the unsupported lateral half of the middle scallop of the posterior leaflet
2. Placement of two artificial Gore-Tex chordae to the middle segment of the anterior leaflet
3. Insertion of C-shaped posterior annuloplasty band (63 mm)
4. Establishment of temporary extracorporeal circulation using the FX15 membrane oxygenator with 3000-ml reservoir with 3/8 loop to 37 degrees
5. Cardioplegic arrest (blood) 4:1
6. Intraoperative transesophageal echocardiography

Attending Surgeon: [BLANK]

Secondary Surgeon: [BLANK]

Assistants: [BLANK]

Anesthesia: [BLANK]

Drainage: 2 No. 32 Argyle chest tubes

Indication(s) for Procedure: [AGE] year old [GENDER] with [DURATION] history of [COMPLAINT – e.g. increasingly shortness of breath]. Preoperative transthoracic echocardiography reveals [FINDINGS - e.g. severe mitral valve regurgitation secondary to bileaflet prolapse, rupture chord of the middle scallop of the posterior leaflet with estimated ejection fraction of 50-55%], and preoperative coronary angiography revealed non-significant coronary artery disease.

Description of the Procedure: After satisfactory general endotracheal anesthesia was induced, a right internal jugular central venous line, pulmonary artery catheter and radial arterial line were inserted. Preincision transesophageal echocardiogram was then performed to evaluate the mitral valve and cardiac function. The patient was prepped and draped from chin to knees while in the supine position. A standard median sternotomy was performed and Morse sternal retractor was placed. We opened the pericardium in an inverted T-shape fashion and pericardial stay sutures were placed on the right side. Heparin was given systemically and a 20-French DLP cannula was inserted through two pursestring sutures in the distal ascending aorta, secured and de-aired. A two-stage cannula was placed in the right atrium for venous return and was secured. An aortic root cardioplegia/vent was then inserted. After confirming ACT of more than 400 seconds, cardiopulmonary bypass was commenced at 2.4 L/min per m2 for 41 minutes. We maintained normothermia during perfusion. The aorta was cross clamped and 1 L of antegrade cold blood cardioplegia was administered. Waterston's groove was dissected and an incision was then made posterior to the interatrial groove to expose the mitral valve. There was redundancy of the valve, and the appearance was typical for a myxomatous mitral valve disease. The prolapsing portion of the posterior leaflet was the lateral half of the middle scallop and the medial half of the lateral scallop. We excised this area in a triangular fashion and sewed the middle scallop to the lateral scallop in two layers with 4-0 Prolene. The middle segment of the anterior leaflet was noted to prolapse as well, and we placed two 2/0 Gore-Tex sutures to this prolapsed segment passing each limb of the suture twice through the free edge of the leaflet. One mattress suture was anchored to the anterolateral papillary muscle and one was anchored to the posteromedial papillary muscle. The valve was tested with saline infusion to facilitate adjustment of the Gore-Tex suture length, and the sutures were tied with multiple knots. Next, seven interrupted mattress sutures of 2-0 Ethibond were placed along the posterior circumference of the valve beginning at the right and ending at the left fibrous trigones. These sutures were passed through a 25 Medtronic annuloplasty band (63 mm in length) and tied securely. We tested the valve, and there was no leakage. The left atrial incision was closed with 3-0 Prolene. Air was evacuated from the heart and the aortic cross-clamp was released after 30 minutes. Sinus rhythm was restored with a single countershock. We de-aired the heart thoroughly and discontinued bypass easily. No inotropic agents were required. Postprocedure transesophageal echocardiography confirmed absence of mitral regurgitation, good ventricular function and absence of SAM.

The right atrium was decannulated and confirmation of adequate de-airing of the heart, the aortic root vent was removed. Protamine was administered followed by removal of the aortic cannula. All cannulation sites were reinforced with 3-0 and 4-0 Prolene sutures. Two atrial pacing wires were attached to the heart. Two No. 32 Argyle chest tubes were led into the mediastinum through stab wounds inferior to the incision. After adequate hemostasis was obtained, we closed the chest using interrupted stainless steel wire for the sternum and Vicryl for the subcutaneous and subcuticular layers.

All instrument, sponge and needle counts were confirmed to be correct x 2 at the end of the operation. The patient tolerated the procedure well and was transferred to the intensive care unit in a stable hemodynamic condition.

Intraoperative autotransfusion was present.

Dr. [BLANK] was present and scrubbed for [BLANK] elements of this procedure.

26. Orthotopic Heart Transplantation

Jose P. Garcia, MD and Tae H. Song, MD

Massachusetts General Hospital, MA

Essential Operative Steps

1. Communication with procurement team throughout procedure
2. Lines and monitoring
3. General endotracheal anesthesia
4. Intraoperative transesophageal echocardiogram (TEE)
5. Median sternotomy after confirmation from procurement team
6. Dissection to free up heart / ventricular assist devices if present
7. Creation of pericardial well
8. Proceed with cardiopulmonary bypass once donor heart close to arrival
9. Systemic heparinization 350-400 units/kg
10. Arterial cannulation
11. Bicaval venous cannulation
12. Check activated clotting time (ACT) > 400-450 secs
13. Initiate cardiopulmonary bypass
14. Aortic cross clamp, tighten caval snares
15. Cardiectomy
16. Left atrial anastomosis
17. Inferior vena cava (IVC) anastomosis
18. Superior vena cava (SVC) anastomosis
19. Pulmonary artery (PA) anastomosis
20. Start rewarming
21. Aortic anastomosis
22. Remove aortic cross clamp
23. Wean from cardiopulmonary bypass
24. Venous decannulation
25. Atrial and ventricular epicardial pacing wire placement
26. Protamine administration for heparin reversal
27. Check for hemostasis, inspect suture lines
28. Aortic decannulation
29. Chest tube placement
30. Sternotomy closure

Potential Complications and Pitfalls

1. Difficult redo sternotomy, cardiectomy
2. Inadequate communication with procurement team
3. Prolonged donor heart ischemic time due to above issues
4. Cannulation issues (aortic dissection/bleeding, caval injury)
5. Inadequate cuffs for anastomosis
6. Kinking of anastomoses and/or insufficient length resulting in tension

II. Adult Cardiac Surgery

7. Sinoatrial node injury
8. Improper deairing
9. Bleeding from anastomoses
10. Inadequate control of hemostasis prior to sternal closure / bleeding from cannulation sites
11. Coagulopathy
12. Right heart failure

Template Dictation

Preoperative Diagnosis: [INDICATION – e.g. End-stage heart failure]

Postoperative Diagnosis: Same

Procedure(s) Performed: Orthotopic heart transplantation

Attending Surgeon: [BLANK]

Secondary Surgeon: [BLANK]

Assistants: [BLANK]

Anesthesia: [BLANK]

Indication(s) for Procedure: The patient is a [AGE]-year-old [GENDER] with a [DURATION] history of [COMPLAINT – e.g. ischemic cardiomyopathy, idiopathic dilated cardiomyopathy, end-stage heart failure secondary to amyloid deposition]. The patient had previously undergone placement of a left ventricular assist device (LVAD) as a bridge to transplant, and an organ appropriate for implantation became available.

Description of Procedure: The patient was taken to the operating room on [DATE]. After identification of the patient and verification of informed consent, the patient was placed on the operating room table in supine position. General anesthesia was administered after endotracheal intubation. A right internal jugular central venous line and a PA catheter was placed, and a right radial arterial line was inserted. The chest, abdomen, and groins were prepped and draped in sterile fashion. A timeout was performed, including confirmation that preoperative antibiotics had been given. Aminocaproic acid was also started. A 5 French right femoral artery catheter was then placed to provide quick access if needed during the procedure.

After confirming with the procurement team that the donor organ was suitable for implantation, median sternotomy was performed. Communication with the procurement team was continued throughout the case. The heart and LVAD was dissected free while being careful not to disrupt the conduit from the LVAD to the ascending aorta and avoiding injury to the right ventricle. Careful dissection was continued to free up the native heart and great vessels. Aortic cannulation sutures were then placed in the distal ascending aorta close to the arch. Bicaval cannulation sutures were placed in the SVC and IVC / right atrium junction. With the donor heart near the hospital, intravenous heparin was given. The aortic cannula was then inserted, secured and de-aired. The PA catheter was withdrawn into the sheath. SVC and IVC venous cannulas were then placed and secured. Umbilical tape snares were passed around the SVC and IVC. After verifying adequate ACT, cardiopulmonary bypass was initiated, and the patient was cooled to 28 degrees celsius.

The aortic cross-clamp was applied, and the caval snares were tightened. The proximal aorta and PA was transected, and the left atrium was incised along the atrioventricular groove, leaving an adequate cuff. The SVC and IVC was also divided, leaving sufficient length for anastomosis. The heart and LVAD was explanted. Hemostasis was achieved, and the vessels and atrial cuff were examined and trimmed in preparation for anastomosis. During this time, the donor heart had been brought into the room and was prepared at the back table. This was done by Dr. [BLANK]. A patent foramen ovale was found in the donor heart and was closed. ABO compatibility was verified and documented in the chart. The donor heart was then brought onto the field. We first performed the left atrial anastomosis using a double-armed 3-0 Prolene suture. A catheter was placed in the right superior pulmonary vein and fed into the left ventricle just before closing the anastomosis. After this anastomosis was completed, we then gave 500 mL of cold blood cardioplegia down the cardioplegia catheter in the donor aorta. We then turned our attention to the vena cava. First the IVC, then the SVC anastomosis was performed using 4-0 Prolene suture. We made sure that there was no narrowing at the caval anastomoses, and used locking technique so as not to cause the anastomosis to pursestring. We were also careful not to injure the sinoatrial node during manipulation of the SVC. Another 400 mL of cold blood cardioplegia was given. Next, the PA anastomosis was performed after it had been cut to size. This was done using 4-0 Prolene suture. Rewarming was started, and then the aortic anastomosis was completed using 4-0 Prolene suture.

The aortic cross-clamp was removed after giving 1 gram of Solu-Medrol. The heart was allowed to re-perfuse for an appropriate amount of time before attempting to wean from bypass. The lungs were suctioned and ventilation was started. The caval snares were released. The heart chambers were checked for air on TEE, and deairing maneuvers were performed. Inotropes and pressors were started by anesthesia, and the patient was weaned off cardiopulmonary bypass. TEE showed good biventricular function, and widely patent anastomoses. The venous cannulae were removed, and the PA catheter was re-advanced into the main PA. Protamine was administered and hemostasis was achieved, and the suture lines were inspected carefully. Atrial and ventricular pacing wires were placed, and atrial pacing was started. After ensuring hemodynamic stability, the aortic cannula was removed. Two 28 French chest tubes were placed in the mediastinum, one curved tube at the diaphragm, and one straight tube anteriorly. 19 French Blake drains were placed in the right and left pleural spaces. The sternum was closed with a total of [BLANK #] stainless steel sternal wires. The fascia was closed with number 1 PDS suture in running fashion. The deep dermal layer was then closed with running 2-0 Vicryl suture. The skin was closed with 4-0 Monocryl in running fashion, and sterile dressing was applied. All sponge and needle counts were correct times two. The total cardiopulmonary bypass time was [NUMBER] minutes. The total ischemic time of the donor heart was [NUMBER] minutes. The patient tolerated the procedure well, and was taken to the cardiac intensive care unit in stable condition.

Dr. [BLANK] was present and scrubbed for [BLANK] elements of this procedure.

27. Thoracoabdominal Aneurysm Repair

Zarrish S. Khan, MD and Leonard N. Girardi, MD

New York Presbyterian –Weill Cornell Medical Center

Essential Operative Steps

1. Preoperative workup- CTAngiogram, cardiac catheterization, lung function tests, room air ABG, bowel preparation.
2. Lines and Monitoring
3. General anesthesia, endotracheal intubation with bronchial blocker
4. Spinal drain
5. Right lateral decubitus position
6. Thorocoabdominal incision (5th IC thoracotomy with paramedian extension into abdomen)
7. Take down diaphragm circumferentially.
8. Expose the entire extent of diseased aorta and identify sites for clamping- take down attachments from lung, medial visceral rotation in abdomen.
9. Have a plan for clamping, extent of resection, spinal and visceral protection and monitoring. Be ready to change the plan.
10. Systemic heparinzation
11. Cannulation for left atrial-femoral artery bypass
12. Prioxal and distal clamps
13. Aortotomy
14. Oversew briskly backbleeding intercostals, plan to re-anastomose large intercostals with no back bleeding
15. Transect proximal aorta and end-to-end anastomosis with 3-0 prolene.
16. Move down cross clamp and check hemostasis
17. Come off partial bypass
18. Balloon tip catheters placed in mesenteric and renal arteries and selective perfusion initiated.
19. Reattach intercostals arteries
20. Reattach renal and visceral arteries as an island or individually as buttons.
21. Reclamp below this anastomosis
22. Distal anastomosis
23. Trendelenburg position. Remove clamp
24. Check for backbleeding intercostals
25. Reverse heparin. Assess hemostasis
26. Wrap the graft with native aorta
27. Close diaphragm
28. Place anterior and posterior chest tubes and abdominal closed suction drains
29. Incision closed in layers.

Potenital Complications and Pitfalls

1. Have an efficient team-limit cross clamp time

II. Adult Cardiac Surgery

2. Use systemic cooling if unable to cross clamp or anticipate long cross clamp.
3. Failure to adequately protect spinal cord. Paraplegia/ paraparesis. Strategies to protect include ensuring adequate cerebral perfusion with MAP goal 85-90, CSF drainage at L3-L5 level, distal aortic perfusion, intercostal / lumbar artery re-attachment, intrathecal vasodilator, deep hypothermic circulatory arrest, monitoring including transcranial Doppler ultrasound (TCD), electroencephalogram (EEG) and motor-evoked potentials (MEP).
4. Inability to keep up with hemodynamic and metabolic effects of clamping and blood loss.
5. Inadequate exposure from incision that is placed too low
6. Left vagus, left phrenic and left recurrent nerves injury during placement of proximal clamp
7. Iatrogenic injury –rib fracture, chyle leak, esophageal injury, spleen laceration, bowel/ureter injury
8. Embolization-stroke, visceral , extremity/visceral ischemia
9. Renal failure
10. Failure to leave adequate diaphragmatic cuff for closure-potential for diaphragmatic herniation
11. Inadequate fascia closure-herniation

Template Dication

Preoperative Diagnosis: [Indication eg size and Extent (I/II/III/IV/V) thoracoabdominal aortic aneurysm, dissection, coarctation, traumatic injury].

Postoperative Diagnosis: Same.

Procedure(s) Performed: Repair of thoracoabdominal aortic aneurysm with reimplantation of the visceral and renal vessels utilizing left atrial to distal aortic bypass utilizing a 26 mm(size) woven Dacron graft.

Attending Surgeon: [BLANK]

Secondary Surgeon: [BLANK]

Assistants: [BLANK]

Anesthesia: [BLANK]

Cross clamp time: [NUMBER]

Pump time: [NUMBER]

Renal Ischemia Time: [NUMBER]

Urine Clearance Time: [NUMBER]

Blood Products: [NUMBER] units packed red blood cells, [NUMBER] units FFP, [NUMBER] units platelets.

Pulse Status: 2+ femoral, SMA and celiac axis.

Drains: chest tubes, 36-French times 2, Reliavac in abdomen.

Complications: [BLANK].

Indication(s) for Procedure: [AGE] year old [GENDER] with history of [PMH] who was found to have [SIZE] thoracoabdominal aortic aneurysm extending from the left subclavian artery down to the bifurcation [EXTENT]. It was thrombus filled. His [BRANCH VESEEL STATUS] eg left renal artery was occluded, had stenosis of the celiac axis and and mild stenosis of the right renal artery,iliac arteries were patent and non aneurysmal.

In preparation for surgery, cardiac catheterization was performed which showed [[BLANK] eg no significant coronary disease. PFTs were obtained that showed FEV1 of [BLANK], DLCO of [BLANK]. His kidney function was adequate with baseline Cr [BLANK]. He is able to walk 5 city blocks without any symptoms (Exercise capacity). He was advised to undergo the aforementioned procedure. Risks, benefits and alternatives were explained to the patient and family including the risk of paraplegia, paraparesis, stroke, respiratory failure, renal failure, infection, myocardial infarction, hemorrhage, recurrent nerve palsy and death. He expressed understanding and agreed to proceed.

Description of Procedure: The patient was brought into the operating room and placed on the operating table in supine position. General endotracheal anesthesia was induced without difficulty. Right radial arterial line, right internal jugular Swan-Ganz catheter and foley catheter were placed. Right groin cordis was placed for rapid infusion during operation. Bronchial blocker was placed for single lung ventilation. The patient was placed into the right lateral decubitus position with bean bags and pressure points padded. Spinal drainage catheter was placed in the L3-L4 interspace. Shoulders were supported at 60 degrees. Hips were rotated posteriorly 45 degrees and he was prepped and draped in the usual sterile fashion using betadine solution.

Sigmoid thoracoabdominal incision was made behind scapula to mid-axillary line than angled toward umbilicus. Fifth intercostals space was entered and costal margin divided The 6th rib was excised. Inferior pulmonary ligament was taken down. The diaphragm was taken down circumferentially and a medial and visceral rotation was performed for retroperitoneal approach. Proximal control of the aorta was obtained just beyond the left subclavian artery. The left vagus, left phrenic and left recurrent nerves were identified and preserved. 6000 units of heparin were given. A cannula was placed in the left inferior pulmonary vein (or left atrium) . Return cannula was placed in the aorta at the level of the diaphragm (distal aorta/ femoral artery). Flows were initiated at 3 L/minute at a temperature of 32 degrees Celsius.

II. Adult Cardiac Surgery

The proximal and distal clamps were applied. The aorta was opened longitudinally. A large volume of thrombus was evacuated. Small intercostal arteries were oversewn with 2-0 silk sutures. (plan to reimplant large intercostals without brisk bleeding). The aorta was then transected circumferentially and dissected off the esophagus. End-to-end anastomosis was carried out with a running 3-0 Prolene suture and a 26 mm graft. This was reinforced with pledgeted Prolene sutures. The crossclamp was moved down below this anastomosis which was checked for hemostasis.

Partial bypass was discontinued. The aorta was opened down to just above the bifurcation. If selective perfusion is planned celiac, superior mesenteric and renal arteries are cannulated with balloon perfusion catheters and selective perfusion is initiated. [Number eg two] pairs of intercostal arteries were selected for reattachment and sutured to an opening in the side of the graft.

The right renal artery, superior mesenteric,celiac, left renal arteries were then reattached with running 3-0 Prolene suture as an island. This was reinforced with pledgeted Prolene sutures. Clamp was moved down below this anastomosis. Renal ischemic time 19 minutes. [This can also be done as separate anastomoses by tailoring buttons out of aorta at each vessel orifice, mobilizing proximal portion and anatomizing to an 8mm limbs of a four branch Dacron graft]

The aorta was reconstructed just above the bifurcation with a running 3-0 Prolene suture and a 26 mm graft. The patient was placed in Trendelenburg position. Crossclamp was removed. Graft was de-aired. Crossclamp time was 44 minutes. Methylene blue was administered and appeared in the urine in 10 minutes. There were no other intercostals that were backbleeding.

Protamine sulfate was administered to reverse the heparin. All cannulas were removed. The aneurysm sac was then wrapped around the graft with 3-0 Prolene suture. Diaphragm was reapproximated with running 1-0 Prolene suture.

Relia-Vac drain (closed suction) was placed in the retroperitoneum and the abdomen was closed with running #1 Prolene suture. Two chest tubes were placed one anteriorly and one posteriorly. The chest was reapproximated with interrupted #2 pericostal Vicryl sutures. Chest wall musculature was closed with PDS sutures and the skin with skin staples. Sterile dressing was applied.

The patient was placed back in the supine position. All instrument, sponge and needle counts were confirmed to be correct x 2 at the end of the operation. The patient was subsequently transferred to the postoperative cardiac surgical intensive care unit in critical condition.

Dr. [BLANK] was present and scrubbed for [BLANK] elements of this procedure.

28. Permanent Pacemaker Insertion

Jonathan C. Hong, MD and Jamil Bashir, MD

Division of Cardiovascular Surgery, St. Paul's Hospital

University of British Columbia, Vancouver, BC

Essential Operative Steps

1. Peripheral venous access and monitoring
2. Prophylactic antibiotics
3. Local anesthetic +/- conscious sedation
4. Incision along the deltopectoral groove
5. Formation of a subcutaneous pocket
6. Cephalic vein cut down
7. Central venous access
8. Lead placement
9. Pacing parameters testing (sensing, impedance, and pacing threshold)
10. Connect leads to generator and placement of generator into pocket
11. Wound closure

Potential Complications and Pitfalls

1. The pocket is created before lead placement, thus reducing the chance of inadvertently displacing the leads once they are positioned.
2. The usual course of the cephalic vein is in the delto-pectoral groove, penetrating the clavi-pectoral fascia to join the axillary vein medial to the pectoralis minor muscle. A variant of the cephalic vein runs over the superficial surface of the clavicle to join the external jugular vein.
3. When encountering difficulty obtaining central venous access, a venogram can be performed using the peripheral intravenous line in the antecubtial fossa to visualize the course of the vein. Increasing venous filling (intravenous fluids and elevating the legs) may also help.
4. A hydrophilic guide wire can be used when the venous valves obstruct the passage of a lead.
5. If there are poor pacing parameters despite good visual anatomic position, troubleshoot systemically by checking all connections from the analyzer to the lead. If there no correctable problems and the pacing parameters are still poor, then the lead will need to be repositioned.
6. The RV lead can be inadvertently placed into the coronary sinus. Identification of coronary sinus placement includes: the lead coursing more posterior than expected in the LAO projection, lack of ventricular ectopy, and a right bundle branch block pattern when pacing on the lead.
7. If pacing parameters suddenly worsen, perforation may have occurred. Monitor for hemodynamic stability and consider echocardiogram to rule out pericardial effusion.

8. The RA lead in the right atrial appendage should course anteriorly in the LAO projection. The classical "figure-of-eight" movement of the lead tip suggests the lead is in good position in the right atrial appendage.
9. When checking the pacing parameters in bipolar leads, the black clip goes to the distal ring and the red to the proximal. If using monopolar leads (rare, but may be seen in older generator changes), the black clip goes to the ring and the red clip is attached to the subcutaneous tissue.
10. Pacing parameter testing:
    a. **Sensing** (mV) should be P wave > 1.5 mV, R wave > 5.0 mV. If the R wave is too small, there is a risk of R-on-T arrhythmias and inappropriately sensing ventricular artifact as activity. For the RA lead, it is also important to consider the "far field" sensing of ventricular activity at the atrial lead. If the far field activity is high, then the atrial lead may inappropriately sense the ventricular activity as atrial.
    b. **Impedance** (Ω) should 400-1000 Ω.
    c. **Pacing threshold** (V) should be <1 V at 0.5 ms. The lower the value, the less energy is required to pace each beat. Maximal output pacing at 10 V should also be performed to ensure there is no stimulation of the diaphragm or any extra cardiac structures.
11. When securing the cephalic vein to the proximal end of the leads with a silk tie, ensure it is not too tight as to damage the insulation of the lead.
12. Ensure that the correct lead is placed in the correct port by checking serial numbers. Confirm that the lead is placed completely into the generator and that all screws are tightened appropriately.
13. All extra length from the leads are looped and placed posterior to the generator to prevent damage to leads when performing subsequent generator changes.

Template Dictation

Preoperative Diagnosis: [INDICATION – e.g. syncope secondary to sinus bradycardia, etc.]

Postoperative Diagnosis: Same

Procedure(s) Performed: Permanent pacemaker insertion [DETAILS – e.g. programmed mode of pacemaker at the time of insertion, manufacturer/model of leads and generator]

Attending Surgeon: [BLANK]

Secondary Surgeon: [BLANK]

Assistants: [BLANK]

Anesthesia: [BLANK]

Indication(s) for Procedure: [AGE] year old [GENDER] with [COMPLAINT

– e.g. syncope] and electrocardiographic evidence of [**FINDINGS** – e.g. sinus bradycardia < 40 beats/minute].

Leads Implanted: [Manufacturer/Model/Serial number] of right atrial and right ventricular leads

Device Implanted: [Manufacturer/Model/Serial number]

Fluoroscopy Time: [Minutes]

Pacing parameter characteristics: [Sensing (mV), Impendence (Ω), and Threshold (V) of RA and RV leads]

Description of Procedure: The patient was taken to the operating room/electrophysiology suite on [**Date**]. The patient's identity, consent, and planned procedure were verified. The patient was placed on the operating table in the supine position. A peripheral venous line was obtained in the left antecubital fossa. Prophylactic antibiotics, analgesia and sedation were administrated to the patient as per hospital protocol. We then proceeded to prep and drape the left chest and neck. A time out was performed. [**Amount**] of [**Local anesthetic**] was infiltrated along the planned incision and pocket.

A 5 cm incision along the deltopectoral groove was made. A combination of electrical cautery and blunt dissection was used to create a subcutaneous pocket at the level of the prepectoral fascia. The deltopectoral groove was dissected to identify the cephalic vein and 2 cm of the vein was freed from the surrounding tissue. Distal and proximal control of the vein was obtained with #3-0 silk ties. The distal end of the vein was tied off. A venotomy incision was made with Iris scissors. A vein lifter was used to insert the RV lead and a guide wire for the RA lead. Using fluoroscopy, the RV lead was advanced through the tricuspid valve and positioned in the [**RVOT/high septum or RV apex**] using [**Active/passive**] fixation. Anatomical positioning was confirmed in the LAO projection. Pacing parameters for the RV lead were checked and documented above. An introducer sheath was inserted into the cephalic vein using the guide wire for the RA lead. The introducer and guidewire was removed. The RA lead was inserted through the sheath and was positioned into the right atrial appendage using fluoroscopy. Anatomical positioning was confirmed in the LAO projection. The sheath was peeled away and removed. Pacing parameters for the RA lead were checked and documented as above. The pacing parameters for the RV lead were rechecked. The RA and RV leads were secured to the generator and anchored into place with #0 silk tie around their suture sleeve. The leads were placed in loops underneath the generator in the subcutaneous pocket. The subcutaneous tissue was closed with two layers of running #2-0 Vicryl. The subcuticular layer was closed with #4-0 Monocryl in running fashion. The patient was transferred to the post anesthetic care unit in stable condition.

Dr. [**BLANK**] was present and scrubbed for [**BLANK**] elements of this procedure.

29. Repair of Post-Infarction Ventricular Septal Defect

Amit Pawale, MD, FRCS, Anelechi Anyanwu, MD, MSc, FRCS

Mount Sinai Medical Center, New York, NY

Essential Operative Steps

(This patient already had a pulmonary artery catheter, radial arterial line, intra-aortic balloon pump, and Foley catheter with temperature probe)

1. General endotracheal anesthesia
2. Median Sternotomy
3. Opening pericardium, pericardial well, epiaortic ultrasound
4. Systemic heparinization
5. Aortic cannulation
6. Right atrial cannulation
7. Checking ACT (>480 seconds)
8. Initiation of cardiopulmonary bypass
9. Aortic root vent and cardioplegia cannula
10. Systemic hypothermia 30 degree Celsius
11. Right ventriculotomy
12. Ventricular septal defect closure with two patch technique
13. Ventriculotomy closure
14. Rewarming
15. Deairing
16. Weaning from cardiopulmonary bypass
17. Venous decannulation
18. Protamine administration
19. Aortic decannulation
20. Hemostasis
21. Sternotomy closure

Potential Complications and Pitfalls

1. In this technique left ventriculotomy is avoided to preserve as much left ventricular ejection fraction as possible.
2. Care should be taken not to make the right ventriculotomy too close to the left anterior descending (LAD) artery
3. The right ventriculotomy should also not be made far from the LAD so there is minimal compromise of right ventricular function.
4. Adequate distance from the ventricular septal defect is very critical while taking the sutures to avoid bites through fragile necrotic tissue.
5. Care must be taken to retrieve fragments of muscle and BioGlue from the ventricle to prevent embolization.
6. The LAD must not be compromised during closure of the ventriculotomy.

Template Dictation

Preoperative Diagnosis: Post myocardial infarction ventricular septal defect, cardiogenic Shock and multi-organ failure

Postoperative Diagnosis: Same

Procedure(s) Performed: Repair of post-infarct ventricular septal defect

Attending Surgeon: [BLANK]

Secondary Surgeon: [BLANK]

Assistants: [BLANK]

Anesthesia: [BLANK]

Indication(s) for Procedure: [AGE] year old [GENDER] with [COMPLAINT – e.g. syncope] was transferred from an outside hospital in cardiogenic shock, intubated and mechanically ventilated. He had sustained an acute ST elevation myocardial infarction one-week prior due to occlusion of left anterior descending artery to which a stent had been placed. He developed a ventricular septal defect post myocardial infarction and had initially been supported with a percutaneous impeller ventricular assist device, which stopped functioning yesterday and he progressed into advanced cardiogenic shock. He had evidence of multiorgan dysfunction and his neurologic status was unknown. An intraaortic balloon pump was placed in the intensive care unit. Because of severe shock he was brought to the operating room for emergency closure of his ventricular septal defect and possible ventricular assist device placement. Because of the patent recent stent, no coronary bypass surgery was planned. Prior to taking him to the operating room, we made a check to confirm his readiness for surgery.

Description of Procedure: The patient was taken to the operating room on [DATE]. The patient's identity and planned procedure was verified, and the patient was placed on the operating room table in the supine position. Patient already had arterial monitoring line, pulmonary artery catheter. Preoperative trans esophageal echocardiogram was performed. It showed severe biventricular dysfunction, an anterior ventricular septal defect with a large left to right shunt.

Median sternotomy was performed, the pericardium was opened. The right ventricle was distended and there was poor biventricular contraction. There was also fibrinous pericarditis. Epiaortic ultrasound of the ascending aorta was performed. [BLANK] units of heparin were administered intravenously. Ascending aorta and right atrium were cannulated. Cardiopulmonary bypass was initiated when ACT was above 480. An aortic root vent was placed. Systemic cooling was started aiming systemic temperature 30 degree Celsius. The aorta was cross-clamped and the heart was protected with cold blood cardioplegia given in the antegrade route, this was repeated every 20 minutes.

We decided to close the VSD via right ventricular approach and two-patch technique with one patch on either side of the ventricular septum. With a number 11 blade a longitudinal right ventriculotomy was performed about one cm away from and parallel to the left anterior descending artery, going from the apex of the right ventricle toward the right ventricular outflow tract, adequate enough to expose the septum. Two 2-0 Ethibond pledgeted stay sutures were placed in horizontal mattress fashion without tying on each lip of the ventriculotomy and clipped to the drapes for better visualization of the cavity and the defect. The right ventricular trabeculations were excised as needed to expose the interventricular septum, a thrombus was removed. A 3 cm diameter ventricular septal defect in the mid-anterior septum was identified. The edges were friable and the septum was thinned out with recent infarct. The friable edges were trimmed. Two large bovine pericardial patches (A and B) were rinsed in normal saline and trimmed to the size of about 6 cm diameter. A series of interrupted 3'0 prolene sutures with SH needle were placed through the patch 'A' in horizontal mattress fashion, about 1-1.5 cm from the edge of the patch along its circumference. These were passed through the interventricular septum about 2 cm from the margin of the defect from left ventricular side coming out into the right ventricle. Same sutures were then passed through another bovine pericardial patch 'B' in a manner similar to patch 'A'. Anteriorly, rather than passing sutures through the rim of the defect, plegeted sutures were passed through the Left ventricle just to the left of the left anterior descending artery then thorough the Patches as previously. Patch 'A' was placed into the left ventricle through the defect and these sutures were pulled so that the patch 'A' lies on the left ventricular side of the defect, covering it nicely. The patch 'B" was parachuted down and covered the right ventricular side of the defect. All sutures were tied but the last two. The aortic root vent was switched off and the cardiopulmonary bypass flow was lowered, BioGlue was placed within the space between these two patches to add some strength and hemostasis to the suture line, and the last two sutures were tied. The root vent and full flow was resumed. The ventricular septum was therefore sandwiched between two bovine pericardial patches.

The right ventriculotomy was closed with a double layer of 3-0 Prolene sutures (first layer horizontal mattress and second layer running) with a strip of Teflon felt reinforcement on either side of the ventriculotomy, taking care to avoid compromising the left anterior descending artery.

The heart was reperfused and the cross-clamp was removed. Pacing wires were placed on the right ventricle and right atrium. Following a period of de-airing and reperfusion, cardiopulmonary bypass was weaned with the aid of high dose inotropes, intra-aortic balloon pump and inhaled nitric oxide. Echocardiography confirmed absence of a residual ventricular septal defect. No step up of oxygen saturation was noticed by direct blood gas sampling of the right atrium and pulmonary artery. Patient was oxygenating well and the left atrial pressure ranged between 15 and 20 mm of Hg., while the right atrial pressure ranged from 10 to 15 mm of Hg. A ventricular assist device was not placed due to stable hemodynamics.

Venous decannulation was performed, the heparin was reversed and the aortic cannula was removed. Hemostasis was secured from all the surgical sites. There were bilateral straw-colored pleural effusions, which were drained. Drains were placed within the mediastinum and both pleural cavities. The sternum was reapproximated with stainless steel wires and the soft tissues were closed with absorbable sutures.

All instrument, sponge and needle counts were confirmed to be correct twice at the end of the operation. The patient was subsequently transferred to the postoperative cardiac surgical intensive care unit in stable but critical condition.

Dr. [BLANK] was present and scrubbed for [BLANK] elements of this procedure.

30. Repair of Post-Infarction Ventricular Aneurysm (Dor Endoventricular Circular Patch Plasty (EVCPP))

James H. Neel, MD and Mark S. Slaughter, MD

University of Louisville; Louisville, KY

Essential Operative Steps

(Steps 1-14 are part of CABG portion of procedure)

1. Lines and monitoring
2. General endotracheal anesthesia
3. Intraoperative TEE
4. Median sternotomy
5. Conduit choice
6. Pericardiotomy, pericardial well creation, assess ascending aorta for cannulation, anastomotic sites, etc.
7. Heparinization (400 U/kg)
8. Arterial/Venous cannulation (+/- LV vent)
9. Cardioplegia cannula placement (antegrade +/- retrograde)
10. Confirmation of ACT (> 400 sec)
11. Commencement of CPB
12. Aortic cross clamp
13. Cardioplegia (antegrade, topical, retrograde)
14. Distal anastomoses (proximal anastomoses to be performed after EVCPP)
15. (Proceeding w/ Dor procedure)
16. Ventriculotomy (into depressed aneurysmal portion of ventricular wall)
17. Removal of thrombus
18. +/- cryotherapy for VT therapy (if indicated)
19. Mitral repair/replacement (if indicated)
20. Purse string suture at margin of normal-fibrous muscle (2-0 non-absorbable monofilament)
21. LV sizing w/ balloon device (approximately 40-50 ml/kg)
22. Placement of patch (Gore-tex, Dacron, autologous, heterologous) at "neck", secured with running 3-0 or 4-0 monofilament
23. Oversewing/resection of excess aneurysmal ventricular free wall
24. (Back to CABG procedure)
25. LIMA-LAD anastomosis
26. Proximal anastomoses
27. Warm antegrade blood cardioplegia ("Hot Shot")
28. De-airing maneuvers
29. Removal of aortic cross clamp
30. Assessment of hemostasis
31. CPB weaning
32. Protamine administration
33. Placement of A/V wires

34. Chest tube placement
35. Venous decannulation
36. Aortic decannulation
37. Repeated hemostasis assessment
38. Sternotomy closure

Potential Complications and Pitfalls

1. Paramedian sternotomy
2. Innominate vein injury
3. IMA injury
4. Problems with cannulation (bleeding, iatrogenic dissection, atrial tear)
5. Poor myocardial protection (malpositioned aortic cross clamp, AI, poor venous drainage)
6. Coronary sinus injury (retrograde)
7. Intramyocardial coronary arteries
8. Injury to coronary arteries (dissection, back wall puncture)
9. SVG length problems (too short = tension, too long = kinking)
10. Air embolism (ineffective/inadequate de-airing maneuvers)
11. Anastomotic bleeding
12. Poor hemostasis (anastomoses, LIMA bed, cannulation sites, ventriculotomy repair)
13. Arrhythmias
14. Dehiscence or bleeding from ventriculotomy repair
15. Low cardiac output from small residual LV volume

Template Dictation

Preoperative Diagnosis: [INDICATION: CAD with Post-infarction LV aneurysm, ventricular akinesia]

Postoperative diagnosis: Same

Procedure(s) Performed: Coronary artery bypass grafting [DETAILS: LIMA-LAD, SVG targets, etc.] with endoventricular circular patch plasty (EVCPP) and EVH

Attending Surgeon: [BLANK]

Secondary Surgeon: [BLANK]

Assistants: [BLANK]

Anesthesia: [BLANK]

Indication(s) for Procedure: [AGE] year old [GENDER] with [DURATION] history of [COMPLAINT]. Patient was found on preoperative echocardiography to have a left ventricular aneurysm, specifically [DETAILS]. Preoperative angiography revealed [FINDINGS].

II. Adult Cardiac Surgery

Description of Procedure: The patient was taken to the operating room on **[DATE]**. The patient's identity and planned procedure were confirmed. The patient was placed on the operating room table in the supine position. General endotracheal anesthesia was induced per the anesthesia team. Arterial line(s) and central venous access were obtained **[DETAILS: location, type of access, etc.]**. Pulmonary artery catheter was also placed. Preoperative TEE was performed to evaluate cardiac function, valve function, as well as aneurysmal dimensions/characteristics. The patient was then prepped and draped in the standard surgical fashion with all bony prominences padded appropriately. A pre-incisional time-out was performed.

Median sternotomy was performed. Simultaneously to this, saphenous vein conduit was harvested from the **[Right/left leg]** utilizing **[Open/Endoscopic]** technique. Upon gaining entrance into the chest, the IMA retractor was placed in the chest and the LIMA was harvested utilizing a pedicled technique. Once LIMA was dissected, 5000U Heparin was administered by anesthesia prior to distal division. LIMA bed was then examined and confirmed to be hemostatic. The LIMA was then wrapped in a papaverine soaked gauze sponge and placed back into the chest. CPB tubing was brought up onto the field and passed off to perfusion in the standard fashion. At this point, the pericardial well was established by incising the anterior pericardium utilizing electrocautery and tacking the pericardial edges up to the chest wall. Care was taken to avoid injury to the innominate vein. Aortic cannulation stitches were placed in the ascending aorta below the innominate artery takeoff. Right atrial cannulation stitches were next placed. The patient was then fully heparinized per anesthesia staff. The aortic cannula was inserted into the aorta, secured, de-aired, and attached to the CPB arterial tubing. Venous cannula was inserted into the right atrium, secured, and attached to the venous CPB tubing in the standard fashion. An aortic root vent was then placed into the ascending aorta below the level of the proposed site of cross clamp application. The vent was secured with monofilament suture and connected to the vent/cardioplegia tubing. SVG conduit was then checked for appropriateness and any needed repairs made. CPB was initiated and proper flows confirmed with perfusion team. Aortic cross clamp was placed and **[Total volume]** ml antegrade cardioplegia was administered causing rapid arrest of cardiac function.

Next, attention was turned to identifying suitable targets on distal coronary arteries **[Specify sites/targets]**. Arteriotomy was performed in the standard fashion. SVG was trimmed, spatulated to the appropriate size to match the arteriotomy. The SVG graft anastomosis was performed with running 7-0 Prolene suture in the standard end-to-side fashion. Antegrade flow through the anastomosis was checked and hemostasis was confirmed. **[Repeat for subsequent SVG target sites.]** Following SVG anastomoses, a suitable site on the LAD **[Specify target site]** was confirmed and the artery opened. Again, care was taken to avoid injury to the back wall of the vessel.

Following completion of the distal anastomoses, attention was turned to the ventricular aneurysm. The heart was decompressed and the area of ventricular wall defect was confirmed. A longitudinal ventriculotomy was performed utilizing a #11 scalpel blade and lengthened encompassing the full extent of the defect. Care was taken to avoid injury to the surrounding coronary vessels. All visualized thrombus was removed from the left ventricle. The endocardial scar was resected sharply. A 2-0 Prolene purse string suture was passed along the surrounding border of the defect at the level of the junction of normal and fibrous ventricular muscle. [May or may not measure appropriate ventricular volume with balloon-type device] Next, a piece of [Specify graft material used] was selected and trimmed to appropriate size. The graft was secured in place over the defect utilizing a running 2-0 Prolene suture. The extraneous ventricular free wall musculature was then re-approximated and oversewn covering the defect utilizing pledgeted 2-0 Prolene suture.

Next, the LIMA was prepared, trimmed to appropriate length, and spatulated to match the arteriotomy on the LAD. The anastomosis was performed in the usual end-to-side manner utilizing a running 7-0 Prolene. The bulldog clamp was removed briefly to ensure forward flow through the anastomosis and check for hemostasis.

Attention was then turned to the proximal aorta. The [Specify graft target] SVG was brought up to the proposed site of proximal anastomosis and measured to ensure appropriate length. The vein graft was then trimmed to correct length and the end spatulated in the standard fashion. The site for proximal anastomosis was selected and an aortotomy was performed using a #11 scalpel and enlarged utilizing a 4mm aortic punch. The proximal anastomosis was performed utilizing a running 6-0 Prolene in the standard end-to-side fashion. [Repeat for each proximal SVG anastomosis.]

Upon completion of the proximal anastomoses, a dose of warm blood (Hot Shot) cardioplegia was administered and the patient was rewarmed. De-airing maneuvers were performed. The bulldog clamp was removed from the LIMA and the LIMA-LAD anastomosis was re-checked to ensure adequate flow and hemostasis. The aortic cross clamp was removed and the aorta was further de-aired utilizing the aortic root vent. Chest tubes were then placed [Specify number and location]. Pacing wires were then inserted, secured, and tested for appropriate capture. TEE was utilized to confirm adequateness of de-airing and the aortic root vent was removed and sutures secured. The patient was weaned from cardiopulmonary bypass. Aortic cannula was removed and sutures secured. Protamine was administered. Venous cannula was next removed and sutures secured. Hemostasis was ensured at all sites within the mediastinum as well as the LIMA bed. The sternum was then re-approximated utilizing #7 stainless steel wires [Specify number and type of wire sutures]. The incision was then irrigated copiously with antibiotic saline solution. The fascia was then closed with running 0 Vicryl followed by running 2-0 Vicryl for the deep dermal layer. Skin was approximated with running 3-0 Monocryl suture. Sterile dressings were applied. Chest tubes were connected to drainage canisters.

All sponge, instrument, and needle counts were correct x 2 at the completion of the case. The patient was then transferred to the Cardiac ICU in critical but stable condition.

Dr. [BLANK] was present and scrubbed for [BLANK] elements of this procedure.

31. Pulmonary Embolectomy

Amit Pawale, MD, FRCS, Ramachandra Reddy, MD, MBA

Mount Sinai Medical Center, New York, NY, 10029

Essential Operative Steps

1. Internal Jugular triple lumen catheter, Radial arterial line, Foley catheter with temperature probe

   (No pulmonary artery catheter)
2. General endotracheal anesthesia
3. Median Sternotomy
4. Pericardiotomy, creation of pericardial well, epiaortic ultrasound
5. Systemic heparinization
6. Aortic cannulation
7. Bicaval venous cannulation
8. Initiation of cardiopulmonary bypass
9. Aortic root vent, Right superior pulmonary vein vent
10. Systemic hypothermia 30 degree Celsius
11. Pulmonary arteriotomy
12. Removal of saddle
13. Removal of segmental thrombi under direct vision using gall stone forceps
14. Caval tapes
15. Right atrial and right ventricular exploration
16. Rewarming
17. Closure of Pulmonary artery and right atrium
18. Inferior Vena Cava filter insertion
19. Careful de-airing
20. Weaning from cardiopulmonary bypass
21. Decannulation and heparin reversal
22. Hemostasis
23. Sternotomy closure

Potential Complications and Pitfalls

1. Left ventricular distension can occur if heart fibrillates before left ventricular vent is introduced.
2. Pulmonary valve can be injured during pulmonary arteriotomy
3. Inadvertent branch pulmonary artery tear can occur during selective removal of segmental emboli
4. Since pulmonary artery is open and the left ventricular vent is in place, air can be sucked from pulmonary vasculature into the left ventricular

II. Adult Cardiac Surgery

5. Right atrium and right ventricle should be explored before closing the pulmonary artery as clots missed and left in these chambers can lead to further pulmonary emboli
6. IVC filter should be placed during the same operative intervention, as further embolization to pulmonary artery from lower extremities is possible awaiting IVC filter insertion.

Template Dictation

Preoperative Diagnosis: Acute pulmonary embolism with right ventricular strain

Postoperative Diagnosis: Same + transit thrombus in the right ventricle

Procedure(s) Performed: Pulmonary embolectomy, exploration of right atrium and right ventricle, removal of right ventricular thrombus, insertion of IVC filter

Attending Surgeon: [BLANK]

Secondary Surgeon: [BLANK]

Assistants: [BLANK]

Anesthesia: [BLANK]

Indication(s) for Procedure: [AGE] year old [GENDER] who presented relatively bedridden due to gastrointestinal bleeding for the last 2 weeks with progressive shortness of breath over the last week and a syncopal episode immediately prior to admission. She was tachycardiac, tachypneic and hypotensive with systemic blood pressure 90 mm of Hg systolic. The CT pulmonary angiogram showed a saddle pulmonary embolus with bilateral large emboli occluding 2/3 of segmental branches, Echocardiogram showed evidence of right ventricular strain and troponins were elevated. Based on her presentation and investigation findings, decision was made to proceed with a pulmonary embolectomy.

Description of Procedure: The patient was taken to the operating room on [DATE]. The patient's identity and planned procedure were verified. The patient was placed on the operating room table in the supine position. A left radial arterial line was inserted. General anesthesia was initiated. A right internal jugular central venous line and Foley catheter were inserted.

Preoperative trans esophageal echocardiogram was performed. It showed large embolus in distal main pulmonary artery and right pulmonary artery, a clot in the right ventricle and severe right ventricular dysfunction. The left ventricular function was preserved. Patient's chest, abdomen, groins were prepped and draped in sterile fashion. A time out was performed.

Median sternotomy was performed, the pericardium was opened.

The right ventricle was found to be distended. Heparin was administered intravenously. Ascending aorta and both cavae were cannulated. Cardiopulmonary bypass was initiated when ACT was above 480. A left ventricular vent via right superior pulmonary vein was placed. An aortic root vent was placed at a level higher than the superior border of right pulmonary artery (to avoid it getting in the way while retracting open the right pulmonary artery later). Systemic cooling to 30 degree Celsius was initiated.

4'0 prolene stay sutures were placed on either side of the main pulmonary artery. The pulmonary artery was opened longitudinally. The stay sutures were clipped to the drape with adequate tension to aid the visualization. A large thrombus was seen in the main pulmonary artery. With a sponge holding forceps and a stone forceps the clot was pulled out as much intact as possible like a rope pulling. Making sure the systemic temperature is at 30 degree Celsius; systemic flow was reduced to 500 cc/ minute. Two nerve root retractors were placed in the left main pulmonary artery and the walls retracted to expose all the segmental artery origins. With a cell saver suction and gall stone forceps, clots from each segmental artery were removed under direct vision. Guessing is strictly avoided as grabbing and injuring the pulmonary artery endothelium can lead to pulmonary artery dissection or rupture. The low flow state is terminated in 2-3 minutes and repeated if necessary after 5 minutes of full flow. No clot was left in any segmental or sub-segmental branches.

Same procedure was repeated in the right pulmonary artery and the retraction was provided by long blade of army- navy retractor lifting the anterior wall of right main pulmonary artery lifting partly along with it, the ascending aorta. A nerve root retractor is placed in the right pulmonary artery to retract the inferior wall down.

After clearing both sides of clot, the caval tapes are passed around the cavae and snared. The right atrium was opened parallel to the atrioventricular groove and inspected for any thrombus or patent foramen ovale. The right ventricle, its apex and the outflow tract were inspected trough the tricuspid valve. A large thrombus was found in the right ventricular trabeculations and was extracted. The main pulmonary artery incision was closed with 4'0 prolene, running suture, over and over, in two layers. The right atrium was closed with double-layered running 4'0 prolene sutures. The caval tapes were then released. Systemic rewarming was started. (The heart is defibrillated if fibrillating).

A purse string suture was applied to the right atrial appendage. A guide wire was introduced through the right atrium into the inferior vena cava and passed distally into the left common iliac vein. A cavogram was performed. A 'Cook' IVC filter was deployed below the renal veins in the inferior vena cava.

Milrinone infusion was initiated. Atrial and Ventricular pacing wires were placed. Ventilation was initiated and careful sequential de-airing from right superior pulmonary vein vent and aortic root vent was performed. When rewarmed completely, patient was weaned off the cardiopulmonary bypass. Venous decannulation was performed. Protamine was administered. Aortic cannula was removed. Cannulation sites were reinforced. Hemostasis of the entire mediastinum was performed. Two mediastinal chest tubes were placed. The sternum was approximated with four figure of eight sternal wires. Subcutaneous tissue and skin was closed in layers.

All instrument, sponge and needle counts were confirmed to be correct twice at the end of the operation. The patient was subsequently transferred to the postoperative cardiac surgical intensive care unit in stable but critical condition.

Dr. [BLANK] was present and scrubbed for [BLANK] elements of this procedure.

32. Redo Sternotomy and Difficult Sternal Closure

George Makdisi, MD, Leker Locker, Chaim MD.

Mayo Clinic, Rochester, MN

Essential Operative Steps

Redo Sternotomy:

1. Check preoperative imaging, including CXR PA & lateral (evaluate space between heart and sternum, and number of wires), Chest CT and coronary angiogram (patent grafts, IMA position related to sternum, sternal adhesions), evaluate also the patency of the femoral vessels for femoral cannulation if needed.
2. Defibrillation pads/external defibrillator in the room.
3. Excise previous scar, and expose well the sternal wires on both sides for the whole width of the wire.
4. Mark your definite midline with cautery! If needed undermine fascial tissue towards the intercostal spaces on both sides.
5. Cut the wires at midline, and keep sternal wires in situ, apply 4 perforating towel clips; 2 on each side.
6. Prepare your plane at the xiphoid level under the sternum with gentle manual digital palpation and sharp dissection with cautery and heavy scissors with the help of 2 racks one on each side of the xiphoid. Feel the RV with your finger tip (risk of arrhythmias and RV perforation).
7. Start sawing the anterior plate at the level of the xiphoid with oscillating saw (very superficial at the xiphoid as usually there is no wire protecting you!), with slight careful forward biting movement of the tip of the saw. When you reach to the level above the very lowest wire, you can safely dig further into the bone until you feel the wire. (Stop and knock with the tip of the saw on the wire, you know you're at the right level when you get the definite metal sound). Keep moving towards the next wire but more superficially. Complete the whole length of the anterior plate up to the suprasternal notch level.
8. Start to dissect and divide the posterior sternal plate adhesions from the level of the Xiphoid by using heavy Metzenbaum scissors, and remove wires as you advance. Your assistant needs to pull on the perforating towel clips upward and lateral, keep the field dry by the tip of your scissors (don't cut blindly!) Keep the lower half part of the scissors always in parallel to the heart and sternum with the tip pointing upwards.
9. Be sure you're not cutting any previous patent grafts, if any, with your scissors.
10. If the space between bones is very narrow, you can open it a bit more by moving your closed scissors right to left in between the two sternal bone edges at horizontal plane.
11. Complete the whole length of the sternum.

II. Adult Cardiac Surgery

12. Sometimes the area of the suprasternal notch is very stubborn adhesed, use you saw very superficially and carefully or use heavy scissors to cut the bone or the thick band holding both sides. Make sure not to cut into the innominate vein.
13. Apply hemostasis with electrocautery to the periosteum all around the sternal bone bilaterally and use bone wax if needed.
14. When the sternum is completely opened and dry, lower cautery power to 30-40 at early dissection to avoid fibrillation/perforation. Start always at the level of the xiphoid towards the left pleura. Your assistant needs to pull up the left sternal edge with 2 racks/ hook (careful with this pulling, you may perforate the RV if too excessive).
15. Develop the plane underneath the sternum, stay just 1 millimeter below the sternal bone. Use your other hand to gently press on the heart with a sponge at the point where you cauterize. Your goal is to reach and open the lower part of the left pleura.
16. Keep moving upwards by sharp or electrocautery dissection. (Be careful as the LIMA, if patent, at the upper part of your track of dissection. Keep opening to a point where you suspect the LIMA to be close. At this point, if you are unable to dissect and discover it safely, leave it alone, and get back to it later after completing the rest of the steps (you might need to go on bypass).
17. Open the right pleura all the way up starting at the xiphoid level. Be aware that the IMA bundle is crossing on the right side more medially. Sometimes you have to further dissect above the innominate vein in order to be able to open the sternum safely with the retractor.
18. Place the sternal retractor. Make sure not to disrupt the innominate vein.
19. Your first step in the dissection of the structures would be to free the aorta to be able to cannulate it in case of emergency (You'll be able to transfuse through the aortic cannulae and use your pump suckers for venous drainage). Next, dissect the right atrium to be able to venous cannulate, and then, follow with complete dissection of the rest of the heart and bypass conduits if applicable.
20. At any point if you're unable to safely continue with your dissection, expose the groin vessels, cannulate and go on bypass, and keep going with your dissection.
21. Injury to the innominate vein or brachiocephalic artery should be avoided by careful pulling the sternum upwards by perforator towel clips or racks, and manual palpation to eliminate traction while spreading the sternal retractor, the innominate vein needs to fall away in the chest as the injury most likely occurs with wide opening of the sternal retractor (patch it if needed to avoid stenosis).
22. If femoral cannulation! Be aware of lower extremity ischemia and compartment syndrome.
23. Once you've completed your intrathoracic dissection on femoral bypass. You can switch to the aorta and right atrial cannulation.
24. Be aware of potential air emboli in case of right to left shunt:

a. If R-sided structure injured use mild hypothermia.
   b. If L-sided structure injured use profound Hypothermia.

Sternal Closure

1. Sternal closure and type of closure should be personalized to every case, evaluate all the risk factors and the situation of the sternum after sternotomy.
2. Careful hemostasis before starting sternal closure.
3. Protect the heart, the vessels and the graft from injury by the wire needle by covering them with a sponge and/or using bands to lift the sternal edges to insert the wire under direct vision.
4. Consider a 6 mm wire for every 10 kg of wight as a rule, put more if long sternum, you might use Myo double sternal wires if indicated.
5. The first 2-3 wires are inserted in the manubrium.
6. The following wires are inserted in the intercostal spaces (enter and exit the intercostal spaces just lateral to the sternal edges to avoid the IMA injury; and on the top of the lower rib to avoid the intercostal vascular bundle injury).
7. Make sure the lower part of the sternum and the xiphoid have enough wires as most of dehiscences start in this area.
8. Check for bleeding from the wire sites.
9. Accurate approximation of the bone edges, to reduce postoperative override and shift of the sternal verges.
10. Start twisting at the bottom wires while your assistant tightens the crossed upper 4 wires.
11. Make sure the wires are tight; you might need to re twist and tighten the previous wire.
12. Make sure the fascia at the very bottom of the sternal wound below the xiphoid, is tightly closed with interrupted absorbable 1-0 sutures.
13. The sternal fascia is closed by interrupted or running absorbable 1-0 sutures.
14. Close the subcutaneous tissue by absorbable 2-0 sutures.
15. Close the skin by running absorbable 4-0 sutures.
16. You might use binder especially in obese patients and females with large breast size to decrease the tension on the wires and suture closure.

Potential Complications and Pitfalls

1. Make every effort to open every patient in the midline of the sternum. Adequate identification of the midline is easy by checking the lateral border by digital palpation or a mosquito (careful with the possibility of IMA injury), or if still unclear; undermine and dissect using electrocautery to identify the edge of the sternum and the beginning of the intercostal space.

II. Adult Cardiac Surgery

2. Cutting the sternochondral cartilage or ribs will be difficult to repair and lead to complex wound complications and inadequate blood supply to the bone for healing.
3. During sternal rewiring, avoid injuring the grafts, myocardium by covering them by sponge or using bands to elevate the sternal edges.
4. Consider a 6 mm wire for every 10 kg of wight as a rule, but even if patient weighs 70kg and the sternum is long and requires 10 wires, obviously put 10. You might use also Myo double wires (Only in very wide and large sternum and in patients with high BMI, where the bone will tolerate and the wire won't cut through the bone).
5. Accurate approximation of the bone edges is essential to minimize sternal dehiscence and postoperative pain. Make sure the edges are fitting each other on both sides so there is no step or override in between the 2 verges. If so, push the bone down to make it fits just after crossing but prior to twisting the wires.
6. Bleeding: When inserting wires in a parasternal fashion, one should be aware of the presence of the internal thoracic pedicle. Any injury must be immediately recognized and controlled to avoid postoperative bleeding and tamponade. Put stiches to the intercostal space or stitch the intrathoracic pedicle directly.
7. Skin erosion: Wires should be deeply embedded into the sternal periosteum to avoid progressive skin erosion, check with your finger by the end of this stage.
8. Dehiscence: Sternal dehiscence is not exclusively the result of poor operative technique! Poor quality of the bone, as with osteoporosis, is a classic cause of dehiscence. In these cases, careful tissue handling and very meticulous closure is mandatory to prevent complications. The twisting of the wires in those cases needs to be very careful and make sure you don't cut into the bone with twisting the wire, on the other hand don't leave it loose!
9. In order to prevent dehiscence in the lower sternum; be generous with the number of your wires, and make sure the very lower part of the xiphoid area is tightly closed.
10. Start twisting at the bottom wires while your assistant tightens the crossed upper 4 wires. This will prevent creating a step. After twisting a wire, go back and check the previous wire; it might need to be tightened a bit further.
11. If the sternum is osteoporotic and friable, the previous sternal closure has disrupted, or you are severely off midline; Robicsek closure is successful in most of these patients.
12. Fracture of the sternum: Approximation of the fractured sternal edges is a difficult task. Wires are passed parasternally above and below the fracture site (in a figure of eight configuration, to include the fracture well in) with the costal margins intervening to stabilize the fracture.
13. After completing the wiring, make sure the fascia at the very bottom of the sternal wound below the xiphoid, is tightly closed with interrupted

sutures. Don't leave any gaps as this may initiate infection and disruption of the wound involving the rest of the wound upwards.
14. Apply generously antibiotic mixed saline solution and irrigate all edges to prevent infection.

Template Dictation

Preoperative Diagnosis: severe aortic stenosis

Postoperative Diagnosis: severe massive air embolism

Procedure(s) Performed: Aortic valve replacement with tissue valve

Attending Surgeon: [BLANK]

Secondary Surgeon: [BLANK]

Assistants: [BLANK]

Anesthesia: [BLANK]

Indication(s) for Procedure: [AGE] year old [GENDER] who presented [BLANK] Workup included [CXR, cardiac angiography, TTE], [Mr/ Mrs.] [BLANK] is brought now for surgical replacement in satisfactory condition

Description of Procedure:

Robicsek technique: The sternum was frail by the repeated sternotomy with some areas were off the midline. We decided to proceed with Robicsek sternal closure to better stabilize the sternum, The mediastinum was washed with copious amount of fluids and antibiotics, the mediastinal chest tubes were positioned correctly, the heart and vessels were protected by a sponge, with the surgical assistant using 2 bands to raise the sternum. A No.6 stainless steel wire was inserted in the manubrium to exit on the top of the 2nd rib just lateral to the sternal edge then we proceeded with parasternal woven running wire, with alternating sutures passed anteriorly and posteriorly to the costal cartilages in a wavy shape, down to the xiphoid process level. The wire was reversed and led in the cranial direction, passing the cartilage posteriorly where it had passed anteriorly and vice versa ending by passing below 2nd rib to exit in the manubrium, the exit and the entrance to intercostal spaces was always lateral to the sternal edges and on the top of the lower rib. Same process was repeated on the right side of the sternum. Then we put our classic sternal closure by 3 wires inserted horizontally in the manubrium, followed by 6-8wiers between intercostal space just lateral to the sternal edge and the top of the inferior rib. Care was taken to avoid the injury of the internal thoracic artery and the intercostal bundle. The sponge was removed. A careful hemostasis was done with Bovie cautery and some absorbable 1-0 suture stitches used to stop bleeding from around the wires. The woven vertical wires of Robicsek technique were tightened first followed by crossing and twisting the vertical wires from the lower end proceeding to the upper end. The sternal repair was satisfactory and the sternum was stable. The abdominal fascia and the sternum were closed by interrupted suture of Absorbable 1-0 suture, followed by absorbable 2-0 suture. The skin was closed by a running subcuticular suture using absorbable 4-0 suture. The patient tolerated the procedure well. No intraoperative complications. All needle, sponge, and instrument counts were correct on two occasions. [Mr/ Mrs.] [BLANK] appeared to tolerate the procedure well and was transferred to the ICU in stable condition.

Dr. [BLANK] was present and scrubbed for [BLANK] elements of this procedure.

Sternal fractures figures of eight: The sternum was frail by the repeated sternotomy with some areas of sternal fractures. The mediastinum was washed with copious amount of fluids and antibiotics, the mediastinal chest tubes were positioned correctly, the heart and the vessels were protected by a sponge. We started our sternal closure using No.6 stainless steel wires. 3 wires were inserted in a transverse fashion in the manubrium, followed by a figure of 8 including the fractured area by and one rib above and below the fractured area, the next wire was in the same intercostal space below the fracture followed by 6-8wiers between intercostal space just lateral to the sternal edge and the top of the inferior rib. Care was taken to avoid the injury of the internal thoracic artery and the intercostal bundle. The sponge was removed and careful hemostasis was achieved with Bovie cautery and absorbable1-0 stitches needed to stop bleeding from around the wires. The wires were crossed and the hemodynamics were stable, we started tightening the wires from lower proceeding to the top ensuring the sternal plates were at the same level. The sternal repair was satisfactory and the sternum was stable. The abdominal fascia and the sternum were closed by interrupted suture of absorbable 1-0 sutures, followed by absorbable 2-0 suture. The skin was closed by a running subcuticular suture using absorbable 4-0 suture. The patient tolerated the procedure well. No intraoperative complications. All needle, sponge, and instrument counts were correct on two occasions. [Mr/ Mrs.] [BLANK] appeared to tolerate the procedure well and was transferred to the ICU in stable condition.

Dr. [BLANK] was present and scrubbed for [BLANK] elements of this procedure.

Sternal fractures plates: The sternum was frail by the repeated sternotomy with some areas of sternal fractures. The mediastinum was washed with copious amount of fluids and antibiotics, the mediastinal chest tubes were positioned correctly, the heart and the vessels were protected by a sponge. We started our slandered sternal closure using No.6 stainless steel wires. 3 wires were inserted transverse way in the manubrium, followed by 4-6 wirers between intercostal space just lateral to the sternal edge and the top of the inferior rib. Care was taken to avoid the injury of the internal thoracic artery and the intercostal bundle. The sponge was removed. Careful hemostasis was done with Bovie cautery and absorbable 1-0 stitches needed to stop bleeding from around the wires. The wires were crossed and the hemodynamics were stable, we started tightening the wires from lower proceeding to the top. The presternal pectoral muscle tissue dissected off the anterior table of the body of the sternum, and then we proceeded with rigid titanium plate fixation by using H shape plates [number of plates], the plates were bent to the appropriate curvature and then secured to the fractures sternum above the fracture using appropriately sized bicortical locking screws with [number of screws]. The sternal repair was satisfactory and the sternum was stable. The abdominal fascia and the sternum were closed by interrupted suture of absorbable 1-0 sutures, followed by absorbable 2-0 suture. The skin was closed by a running subcuticular suture using absorbable 4-0 suture. The patient tolerated the procedure well. No intraoperative complications. All needle, sponge, and instrument counts were correct on two occasions. [Mr/ Mrs.] [BLANK] appeared to tolerate the procedure well and was transferred to the ICU in stable condition.

Dr. [BLANK] was present and scrubbed for [BLANK] elements of this procedure.

Open chest: Considering the long procedure time and the continuous generalized oozing due to coagulopathy a decision was made to keep the chest open.

The mediastinum was washed with copious amount of fluids and antibiotics, the mediastinal chest tubes were positioned correctly. The chest was packed using two rolls of 6-inch Kerlix; the chest was covered with sterile Ioban dressing. The tubes were hooked to suction, the patient tolerated the procedure well, remained intubated and moved to ICU.

Dr. [BLANK] was present and scrubbed for [BLANK] elements of this procedure.

33. Resection of Atrial Myxoma

Paul A. Perry, MD and J. Nilas Young, MD

University of California Davis, Sacramento, CA

Essential Operative Steps

1. Lines and Monitoring
2. General endotracheal anesthesia
3. Intraoperative transesophageal echocardiogram
4. Median sternotomy
5. Open pericardium, pericardial well, survey ascending aorta for plaque burden (consider epiaortic ultrasound)
6. Systemic heparinization (400 u/kg)
7. Arterial cannulation
8. Bicaval cannulation
9. Antegrade (+/- retrograde) cardioplegia catheter
10. Carbon dioxide diffusion into operative field
11. Check ACT (>400 sec)
12. Initiate CPB
13. Aortic cross clamp
14. Cardioplegia and topical cooling for cardiac arrest
15. Atriotomy. For left atrial masses usually open right atrium and divide atrial septum at fossa ovalis (most tumors will be located in left atrium along septum); alternatively, can expose and incise left atrium
16. Expose base of mass
17. Sharply excise mass off atrial wall en bloc with 1 cm margin
18. Irrigation of atrium/ventricle to remove any debris
19. Repair atrium. Patch closure of septum
20. Close right atrium with pledgeted running prolene suture (allow heart to fill with blood prior to completing suture line)
21. Remove aortic cross clamp
22. Atrial and ventricular pacer wire placement
23. Vigorous deairing under TEE guidance
24. Wean from CPB
25. Check for normal sinus rhythm
26. Venous decannulation
27. Protamine
28. Aortic decannulation
29. Meticulous hemostasis
30. Chest tube placement
31. Sternotomy closure

Potential Complications and Pitfalls

1. Tumor embolization due to manipulation of the heart before cross-clamp
2. Phrenic nerve injury during dissection of SVC

3. Atrial incision site selection should be specified to the location of the mass, as indicated by pre-operative imaging
4. SA node, AV node, or conduction system injury during atrial exposure or mass excision
5. Valvular injury during atrial exposure or mass excision
6. Goal is to obtain negative margins
7. Resected tissue should be sent for pathologic evaluation

Template Dictation

Preoperative Diagnosis: [INDICATION – e.g. embolism, arrhythmia, obstruction]

Postoperative Diagnosis: Same

Procedure(s) Performed: Resection of Left/Right Atrial Mass

Attending Surgeon: [BLANK]

Secondary Surgeon: [BLANK]

Assistants: [BLANK]

Anesthesia: [BLANK]

Indication(s) for Procedure: [AGE] year old [GENDER] with [DURATION] history of atrial mass. Preoperative echocardiogram reveals [FINDINGS - e.g. 2 cm pedunculated left atrial myxoma].

Outcome: TEE demonstrated preserved biventricular function and no ASD.

Description of Procedure: The patient was taken to the operating room on [DATE]. Identity and planned procedure were verified, and the patient was placed on the operating room table in the supine position. General anesthesia was obtained. Central venous and radial arterial lines were inserted. Preoperative transesophageal echocardiogram was performed and the mass was identified. The chest, abdomen, groins, and lower extremities were prepped and draped in sterile fashion. A surgical time-out was performed.

Median sternotomy was created and a sternal retractor placed. After identification of the innominate vein, the pericardium was opened and a pericardial well was created. [UNITS] of systemic heparin were administered. The aortic cannulation sutures were placed in the ascending aorta below the level of the innominate artery. The aortic cannula was then inserted, secured, de-aired, and confirmed to have pulsatile flow by the perfusionist. Venous cannulation sutures were then placed and the SVC and IVC cannulas were inserted and secured. The superior and inferior vena cavae were dissected out and encircled with umblical tape. After placing a purse-string suture in the proximal ascending aorta, an aortic root vent needle was inserted for administration of antegrade cardioplegia. Gas diffuser was placed along the wound edge and used to flood the operative field with carbon dioxide. The aortic cross-clamp was placed. Antegrade cardioplegia was administered and there was rapid myocardial arrest. A total of [BLANK] ml of cardioplegia was given. Ice was applied to the heart. For the duration of the procedure, [BLANK] ml of cardioplegia was administered at 15-20 minute intervals.

The right atrium was exposed and atriotomy was made parallel to the atrioventricular groove. The fossa ovalis was identified and atrial septotomy was performed. The atrial retractor was inserted, and the atrial mass was identified along the [BLANK]. A 15 blade scalpel was then used to excise the mass off the atrial wall, taking care to obtain an approximate 1 cm margin of myocardial tissue. The excision site was then over-sewn with multiple interrupted 5-0 prolene sutures, resulting in excellent approximation of endocardium. The left atrium was copiously irrigated with [BLANK] ml of saline. The atrial septotomy was repaired with a patch of bovine pericardium, and the right atriotomy was then closed with pledgeted 4-0 prolene.

Hot shot cardioplegia was administered and the patient was rewarmed. The aortic cross-clamp was removed. Atrial and ventricular pacing wires were inserted and tested for appropriate capture. Vigorous de-airing maneuvers were performed under TEE guidance and the aortic root vent was removed. The patient was weaned from cardiopulmonary bypass. A normal sinus rhythm was noted. The venous cannulae were removed. A test dose of protamine was administered and the patient was monitored for adverse reaction before the protamine was resumed. The aortic cannula was then removed. A total of [NUMBER] chest tubes were placed in the [LEFT/RIGHT] pleural space, and [NUMBER] chest tubes were placed in the mediastinum. Hemostasis was confirmed. The sternum was closed with [NUMBER] stainless steel sternal wires. The wound was irrigated with saline. The soft tissue was closed in layers and the skin approximated with staples. The wounds were dressed.

All instrument, sponge and needle counts were confirmed to be correct x 2 at the end of the operation. The patient was subsequently transferred to the postoperative cardiac surgical intensive care unit with stable hemodynamics and [BLANK] inotropic support.

Dr. [BLANK] was present and scrubbed for [BLANK] elements of this procedure.

34. Septal Myectomy

Michael P. Robich, MD and Nicholas Smedira, MD

Cleveland Clinic, Cleveland, OH

Essential Operative Steps

1. TEE- have a clear understanding of septal thickness and length of hypertrophy toward apex
2. Median sternotomy
3. Pericardial cradle sutures only on the right
4. Standard aortic and single 2-stage venous cannulation
5. Left atrial vent
6. Transverse aortotomy- oblique, slightly closer to the sinotubular ridge than for aortic valve replacement, staying above the sinotubular junction
7. Complete septal myectomy from trigone to trigone, excise hypertrophied septum beyond endocardial scar to mid-papillary muscles (if there is not a proximal bulge)
8. Post TEE (off bypass) to assess adequacy of myectomy and residual mitral regurgitation (provocation with Isuprel to ensure that outflow tract gradient is minimal and no SAM).

Potential Complications and Pitfalls

1. Damage to aortic valve
2. Damage to mitral valve, papillary muscles or chordea
3. Creation of VSD
4. Inadequate myectomy. You have to go deeper toward the apex than you think.
5. Overlooking abnormal papillary muscles or chordae
6. Post operative atrial fibrillation can look like ventricular tachycardia due to left bundle branch block

Template Dictation

Preoperative Diagnosis: [INDICATION – e.g. Hypertrophic Obstructive Cardiomyopathy (HOCM)]

Postoperative Diagnosis: Same

Procedure(s) Performed: Septal Myectomy (**DETAILS** – e.g. Tissue valve or Mechanical valve)

Attending Surgeon: [BLANK]

Secondary Surgeon: [BLANK]

Assistants: [BLANK]

Anesthesia: [BLANK]

II. Adult Cardiac Surgery

Specimen: septal muscle

Counts: sponge, instrument, and needle counts correct

Drains: mediastinal x2

Skin incision: [TIME]

Closure: [TIME]

Complications: [BLANK]

Indication(s) for Procedure: [AGE] year old [GENDER] with [DURATION] history of [COMPLAINT – e.g. chest pain, syncope and/or shortness of breath].

Patient presented with frequent syncopal episodes. There is no family history of HOCM or sudden cardiac death. The SBP dropped during exercise. Preoperative echocardiogram demonstrated a 28mm septum (normal <13 mm). The resting gradient was 36mm Hg, gradient on valsalva was 64mm Hg. With amyl nitrate the gradient increased to 110mm Hg. Systolic anterior motion of the anterior mitral leaflet with septal contact was noted at rest with trivial mitral regurgitation and there was no AS/AR. Preoperative cardiac MRI revealed asymmetric (basal and mid) septal hypertrophy (28mm) with a preserved EF (65%). The papillary muscles are multiheaded without thickening. There appears to be an abnormal chordal attachment of an accessory head of the anterolateral papillary muscle to the septum. Coronary arteries were free of disease.

Description of Procedure: After induction of general anesthesia and central line placement the patient was prepped and draped. TEE was used to confirm the preoperative findings. Median sternotomy was made, heparin was given, and standard aortic and a single 2-stage right atrial venous cannulation performed. A left atrial vent was placed in the left atrium just beyond the entry of the right superior pulmonary vein. The heart was arrested with one liter of antegrade del Nido cardioplegia. A transverse aortotomy was made and 2-0 silk retraction sutures x3 were placed in the aortic wall (one on the superior and 2 on the inferior aspect of the aortotomy) and the aortic valve leaflets gently retracted to reveal the left ventricular outflow tract (LVOT). A hand-held ribbon retractor was placed in the LV and upward traction applied. A sponge on a stick was used to depress the left ventricle and to rotate the septum posteriorly.

Fibrosis from the contact of the anterior mitral valve leaflet septum was evident and the myectomy was initiated here. An angled #10 scalpel was used to make a two incisions 5mm apart, 8mm in depth creating a strip of myocardium 2.5cm below the nadir of the right cusp that was extended toward the level of the papillary muscles. The resection with the scalpel was continued from the medial to lateral commissures of mitral valve taking segments of myocardium approximately 5mm thick, 10mm wide and 15mm deep. These two incisions were connected using a #15 blade, excising a 5mm x8mm x1.5- 3cm strip of myocardium. Two similar strips of muscle were then excised; one medially to the right fibrous trigone and the next laterally to the left trigone. These three resections have excised the basal portion of the septum, exposing the septum over the papillary muscle heads. To treat concentric hypertrophy the myectomy continues into the ventricle to excise septum over the distal, mid, and sometimes basal portions of the papillary muscle. Care was taken to avoid creating a VSD and the RV was observed for dimpling to suggest collapse of the septum into the LV cavity. The accessory head of the anterolateral papillary muscle was resected. The LV cavity was then irrigated with cold saline.

Once the resection was thought to be adequate the aortic valve leaflets were examined for any damage and the aortotomy was closed with a running 4-0 prolene in the standard fashion. The LA vent was removed, but the pursestring left loose to allow deairing. The pursestring was then tightened, the cross clamp removed, and TEE used to assess for intracardiac air. The patient was separated from CPB. TEE was used to assess the adequacy of resection, presence of SAM and MR. Isuprel drip (10-20 mcg/min) was started and LVOT gradient was reassessed. The gradient was less than 15mmHg. The heart was decannulated. Protamine was given and the chest closed in the usual fashion. The weight of the removed septum was 8 grams (normal 3-12 grams). The patient left the OR in stable condition with the expected left bundle branch block.

Dr. [BLANK] was present and scrubbed for [BLANK] elements of this procedure.

35. Endovascular Repair of Descending Thoracic Aortic Aneurysm (Tevar)

Mohiuddin Cheema, MD and Ali Khoynezhad, MD, PhD

Cedars Sinai Medical Center, Los Angeles, CA

Essential Operative Steps

1. Lines and Monitoring (make sure radial aline on right if left subclavian artery being covered)
2. Lumbar drain if high risk for spinal cord ischemia
3. General Anesthesia
4. TEE to make sure no aortic valve or root pathology and good LV function
5. Access artery exposure for delivery of stentgraft (open surgical cutdown of CFA vs iliac artery vs percutaneous perclose technique)
6. Percutaneous access of brachial or contralateral femoral artery for diagnostic angiography
7. Systemic heparin bolus (100units/KG) to keep ACT above 250
8. IVUS (intravascular US) evaluation of aorta and iliac arteries to map out landing zones and assess diameters
9. Measure the aortic diameter at both proximal and distal intended landing zones (IVUS and CTA)
10. Measure the length of aorta that needs to be covered using sizing pigtail catheter
11. Choose the appropriate stentgrafts based on above measurements (refer to company's sizing guidelines for different stentgrafts)
12. Perform left carotid subclavian bypass if indicated for intentional coverage of left subclavian artery (consult vascular surgery if needed)
13. Access the femoral artery using seldinger technique and exchange soft wire for a stiff guide wire parked in ascending aorta
14. Advanced an appropriately sized large bore delivery sheath into the abdominal aorta for delivery of endoprosthesis (be careful not to push too aggressively if iliac artery is tortuous or calcified)
15. Advance a sizing pigtail catheter from contralateral femoral artery for angiogram
16. Obtain thoracic arch aortogram in steep left anterior oblique projection (45 degrees or more) to splay open the arch and brachiocephalic vessels.
17. Advance endograft to appropriate location over stiff wire after device flushing to evacuate air from delivery system (air embolism is a major cause for stroke).
18. Reimage with IVUS or angiogram to confirm location before final deployment
19. Deploy stentgraft per company's guidelines with brief period of asystole (adenosine 12-24mg IV bolus) or with very low systolic BP to avoid graft migration or wind socking effect.

20. Deploy additional stentgrafts as needed with adequate overlap (generally 3-5cm overlap recommended for most stentgrafts) to coverage aortic pathology (up to the Celiac artery if necessary).
21. Ensure spinal drain pressure below 10cm H2O (drain additional fluid if necessary upto 20cc max/hr) and MAP above 75-80 for adequate spinal cord perfusion
22. Balloon the proximal and distal attachment sites as well as stentgraft overlap sites with appropriate compliant balloons as recommended by the manufacturers.
23. Final angiogram and IVUS to ensure no endoleak or migration
24. Remove all the wires, catheters and sheaths and close arteriortomies surgically or percutaneously as planned.
25. Reverse anticoagulation with protamine

Potential Complications and Pitfalls

1. Avoid accessing small and calcified ileofemoral arteries. Access iliac arteries directly or sew a conduit if necessary for large bore sheaths (iliac artery rupture carries high morbidity and mortality and sometimes presents in delayed fashion)
2. Size the aorta and pick stentgrafts appropriately using preop CTA and IVUS
3. Avoid left subclavian artery coverage if patent LIMA to LAD graft or if patient has large dominant left vertebral artery with small or absent right vertebral (perform left CCA to SCA bypass preoperatively if necessary)
4. Use lumbar drain Judiciously in cases where the risk of spinal cord ischemia is high
5. Avoid deployment of stentgrafts at the distal curvature of the aortic arch as it bends into descending aorta to avoid bird beaking and collapse of the stentgraft especially in younger patients with tighter aortic curvatures
6. Ensure at least 2 cm of normal healthy parallel aorta at the proximal and distal landing zones to avoid Type 1 endoleaks
7. Ensure at least 3-5 cm of overlap between stentgrafts to avoid graft separation and type 3 endoleaks
8. Choose the stentgrafts with 10-20% oversizing for native aorta
9. Inadvertent coverage of left carotid or subclavian artery requires urgent bypass or retrograde stenting to avoid cerebral ischemia
10. Acute drop in BP after removal of a large bore sheath is concerning for iliac artery rupture and requires urgent endovascular or surgical repairs to avoid catastrophe (so called "iliac on the stick")

Template Dictation

Preoperative Diagnosis: Descending thoracic aortic aneurysm status post previous aortic valve replacement, ascending aortic enlargement.

Postoperative Diagnosis: Same

II. Adult Cardiac Surgery

Procedure(s) Performed:

1. Endovascular repair of descending thoracic aortic aneurysm.
2. Percutaneous access of right femoral artery with iliac and femoral artery angiogram.
3. Intravascular ultrasound (IVUS) before and after stent grafting.
4. Angiogram before and after stent grafting.
5. Radiology interpretation and supervision of above-mentioned procedure.
6. Transcranial Doppler monitoring throughout the entire case.

Attending Surgeon: [BLANK]

Secondary Surgeon: [BLANK]

Assistants: [BLANK]

Anesthesia: [BLANK]

Indication(s) for Procedure: [AGE] year old [GENDER] with history of aortic aneurysm pathology. He had an aortic valve replacement in the past due to bicuspid aortic valve and came in with back pain to the emergency room over the weekend. Evaluation of the descending thoracic aorta using an MRA revealed a 5.6 cm descending thoracic aneurysm. After discussing risks and benefits, he wanted to proceed with endovascular repair.

Operative Findings: Enlarged aortic root. Descending thoracic aortic aneurysm from distal to the left subclavian artery extending upto the mid descending aorta with at least 2 cm of normal aorta at proximal and distal attachment sites. Completion angiogram revealed no evidence of endoleak.

Description of Procedure: After informed consent was obtained, the patient was taken to the operating room and placed supine on the table. Groin was prepped and draped in standard sterile fashion. Percutaneous access using ultrasound guidance was performed in the right femoral artery. This was confirmed using angiogram of the distal iliofemoral artery. Next, percutaneous ProGlide was deployed and dilators used to increase the size of the femoral arteriotomy. Next, an 8-French sheath was placed and the wire was advanced under fluoroscopic guidance into the ascending aorta. It was exchanged for a stiff wire and intravascular ultrasound (IVUS) catheter was advanced. The evaluation of entire thoracic aorta and iliac arteries was performed using IVUS. The sizing was confirmed, which was a **[BLANK]** (eg. Medtronic Valiant stent graft 46 x 46x 157 mm graft). An angiogram was performed to confirm the location of the aneurysm. The Medtronic Valiant stent graft was advanced to the desired location and deployed without any problems. Subsequently, a 16-French sheath was placed in the groin after removal of the delivery catheter and intravascular ultrasound confirmed a good location of the stentgraft. The completion angiogram also confirmed no evidence of any endoleak. At this time, the catheter and the wires were all removed. The femoral arteriotomy was percutaneously closed. Please note that the patient was heparinized prior to the intervention and we confirmed the ACT to be above 250 throughout the case. The anticoagulant was reversed using protamine at the end of the case.

CONTRAST USED: (Visipaque 320) 55 mL.

FLUOROSCOPY TIME: 5 minutes.

TOTAL RADIATION DOSE: -------mSV

Dr. [**BLANK**] was present and scrubbed for [**BLANK**] elements of this operation.

36. Total Arch Replacement with Deep Hypothermic Circulatory Arrest For Aneurysm

Sanford Zeigler, MD

Stanford University, Stanford, CA

Essential Operative Steps

1. Preoperative planning for CPB cannulation
2. Induction, intubation, lines, and monitoring
3. Right radial arterial pressure line
4. Neuromonitoring (cerebral oximetry, transcranial Doppler, EEG)
5. Intraoperative transesophageal echocardiogram
6. Median Sternotomy
7. Divide thymus, encircle innominate vein
8. Dissect out innominate artery, encircle with silastic
9. Open pericardium, create pericardial well
10. 5000 IU IV Heparin
11. Satinski or dual Novare clamps on proximal innominate artery
12. 5-0 Prolene to sew 6-8mm knitted Dacron graft to proximal innominate in end to side fashion
13. De-air and connect arterial cannula
14. Dissect out Left Carotid, Left subclavian, and encircle with silastic
15. Mobilize PA from Aorta for cross clamp; completely encircle ascending aorta
16. Full heparinization (400 IU/kg)
17. 4-0 Prolene pursestring to RA; venous cannulation with two stage cannula; connect to circuit
18. Place cardioplegia cannulae – root vent to ascending, retrograde through coronary sinus
19. Confirm ACT >480sec
20. Initiate CPB
21. Initiate systemic hypothermia to 24 degrees Celsius (cooler depending on more distal work, degree of difficulty)
22. Place Right Superior Pulmonary Vein Vent
23. Aortic cross clamp, antegrade cardioplegic arrest with ~1L cold blood cardioplegia
24. CPB Flows 2-2.5L/min/m2
25. Insert temperature probe into RV free wall
26. Insert cooling jacket or apply topical cold
27. Maintain myocardial temp <10 deg C with retrograde cardioplegia through case
28. Resect diseased ascending aorta to crossclamp
29. Give Hydrocortisone, Phenobarbital, Mannitol, Lasix
30. Drop flow to 10mL/kg/min
31. Clamp innominate proximal to graft

32. Remove aortic crossclamp
33. Ensure back flow from Left carotid, clamp if adequate
34. Add arterial perfusion balloon (pediatric retrograde) to L carotid if inadequate flow
35. Check for L Subclavian backflow, clamp; Keep R arm MAP ~40
36. Resect aortic arch, leaving 1cm Carrel buttons around arch vessels
37. Size proximal descending aorta; open and prepare multi-branch Dacron graft
38. Running 5-0 Prolene for open distal anastomosis
39. Attach Y'ed arterial cannula to grafts' perfusion sidelimb; clamp graft, resume full flow through body and innominate
40. Reimplant L subclavian with running 5-0 Prolene, deair, move distal clamp proximal to this anastomosis
41. Reimplant L common carotid, deair, move distal clamp proximal to this anastomosis
42. Reimplant Innominate, deair, move clamp proximal to innominate
43. Remove Innominate clamp (end SACP)
44. Begin rewarming (no greater than 2 degrees C temperature gradient)
45. Clamp, cut, and oversew perfusion sidelimb of graft
46. Check and repair anastomoses
47. Graft to Ascending aorta anastomosis with running 3-0 Prolene
48. Deair (pump down, clamp off); tie
49. Remove cooling jacket and temp probe
50. "Hot Shot" – Retrograde warm blood cardioplegia
51. Place ventricular pacing wires
52. Deep Trendelenberg position
53. Remove crossclamp
54. Check for hemostasis
55. Place chest tube
56. Engage root vent as rhythm returns
57. Wean from CPB
58. Deair heart and aorta through root vent
59. Remove LV vent
60. Remove Retrograde and Venous cannulae
61. Give Protamine
62. Remove arterial cannula
63. Reinspect for bleeding, achieve hemostasis
64. Pack chest
65. Place Sternal Wires
66. Check wires for bleeding
67. close sternum
68. Close Skin
69. (close axillary incision)

II. Adult Cardiac Surgery

Potential Complications and Pitfalls

1. Stay midline during sternotomy
2. Innominate vein injury
3. Brachial plexus injury during axillary exposure
4. Injury/delamination of arch vessels during dissection
5. Failure to protect recurrent laryngeal nerves
6. Failure of left arm arterial line
7. Tracheal injury during arch dissection
8. Failure to insulate phrenic nerves from cold
9. Innominate/axillary dissection or bleeding from perfusion limb graft
10. Improper Venous cannula positioning (hepatic vein, RV)
11. Bleeding complications from venous cannulation
12. Coronary Sinus Perforation
13. Poor right heart protection (poor retro position)
14. Air embolism from improper deairing of any arterial graft segment
15. Poor LV venting
16. Low outflow from perfusion graft
17. Air embolism during open distal
18. Unilateral cerebral perfusion 2/2 unrecognized Circle of Willis obstruction
19. Excessive or inadequate flow during SACP
20. Failure to recognize bleeding from distal anastomoses prior to proximal anastomosis
21. Reperfusion injury from excessively fast rewarming
22. Coronary air embolism during dearing
23. Unrecognized bleeding from sternal wires

Template Dictation

Preoperative Diagnosis:

1. [**expanding, symptomatic**] Aortic Arch Aneurysm of [**cm**]
2. [**connective tissue disorder**]

Postoperative Diagnosis: Same

Procedure(s) Performed:

1. Total Aortic Arch Repair with deep hypothermic circulatory arrest and selective antegrade cerebral perfusion
2. [**axillary artery cutdown**]

Attending Surgeon: [BLANK]

Secondary Surgeon: [BLANK]

Assistants: [BLANK]

Anesthesia: [BLANK]

Indication(s) for Procedure: [AGE] year old [GENDER] with [DURATION] history of [relevant connective disorder, autoimmune disease, or infection] presented with an aortic arch aneurysm that was [size] [+/- growth rate].

Description of Procedure: The patient was taken to the operating room on [DATE]. The patient's identity and planned procedure verified, and the patient was placed on the operating room table in the supine position. General anesthesia was induced. Neurologic monitoring was set up using [BLANK]. A left radial arterial line was placed, as were right right internal jugular central venous line. A transesophageal echo probe was placed and formal evaluation of the cardiac function was performed. The patient was prepped and draped in the usual fashion, leaving both groins exposed. A time out was performed to confirm the correct patient, site, and procedure. Prophylactic antibiotics were given.

[A right axillary artery cutdown was performed taking care not to damage the trunks of the brachial plexus. The axillary artery was isolated and proximal and distal control were obtained with silastic loops. 5000 Units of IV Heparin were administered and allowed to circulate for 3 minutes. An 8mm Dacron graft was sewed end to side onto the artery using 5-0 Prolene in a running fashion. The graft was deaired as the vascular clamps were removed. A tubing connector was secured to the graft.]

Median sternotomy was then performed. The thymus was divided and a pericardial well was created. The innominate vein was encircled with a silastic and the arch vessels were dissected free, taking care to protect the left recurrent laryngeal nerve around the distal arch. The ascending aorta and arch were dissected free. [An 8mm Dacron graft was sewn to the proximal innominate artery taking care to avoid the right recurrent laryngeal nerve near the takeoff of the right sublavian].[**Total Units**] of IV heparin were administered and allowed to circulate.

A purestring suture was placed in the right atrial appendage and a [**size**] two stage venous cannula was placed into the IVC through the right atrium and secured. The perfusion graft was deaired and connected to the CPB circuit. A small pursestring was placed on the right atrium and a retrograde cardioplegia cannula was inserted into the coronary sinus. After confirmation of proper ACT, cardiopulmonary bypass was initiated. A left ventricular vent was placed through the right superior pulmonary vein through a pursestring and position confirmed with TEE. Retrograde cold blood cardioplegia were administered with the heart vented. The aortic crossclamp was placed. After diastolic arrest was achieved, a cooling jacket and RV temperature probe were inserted. Systemic hypothermia was initiated to [**degrees**] Celsius.

As the patient was cooled, the diseased ascending aorta was resected up to the crossclamp. The healthy ascending aorta was sized at [**cm**] and the appropriate Dacron graft opened. The proximal graft to aorta anastomosis was constructed using two running 3-0 prolene sutures. When systemic hypothermia was achieved, Mannitol, propofol, and hydrocortisone were administered. CPB flow was stopped and the aortic crossclamp was removed. Flow was then increased to [**10 mL/kg/min**]. The innominate artery was clamped after backbleeding to deair. [Good retrograde flow was seen from the left common carotid artery, and the artery was clamped.] [Poor retrograde flow was seen from the left common carotid artery, and a pediatric retrograde cannula that was hooked to the arterial circuit was placed into its ostium. The artery was then clamped]. The left subclavian artery [**was/was not**] clamped.

Carrel patches were fashioned out of each arch vessel. The aortic arch was resected to just past the left subclavian. The proximal descending aorta was sized at [**cm**] and the appropriate multibranch arch graft was opened and trimmed. The distal graft to aorta anastomosis was constructed with 3-0 prolene in a running fashion. The graft was deaired and clamped, and an aortic cannula was placed in the graft's perfusion sidelimb. Hemostasis was achieved. Normal CPB flow was reestablished and circulatory arrest terminated. Anastomoses were then constructed to the left subclavian, the left common carotid, and the innominate artery, in that order, using 5-0 Prolene in a running fashion. Hemostasis was assured each anastomosis appropriately deaired. As each anastomosis was completed, vascular clamps were removed restoring flow to the respective territory in a sequential matter. After the innominate anastomosis was complete, the aortic crossclamp was placed on the proximal arch graft, and the small [**innominate/axillary**] perfusion graft was doubly clamped and divided. It was oversewn with 3-0 Prolene in two layers, obliterating dead space.

Systemic rewarming was then begun. The proximal graft to graft anastomosis was completed using 5-0 Prolene in a running fashion. The ascending aorta was deaired and a retrograde hotshot was administered. The crossclamp was removed and ventricular pacing wires placed. Normal sinus rhythm was restored and the patient weaned from CPB. Ventilation was restarted. The heart was deaired through a Cooley needle in the ascending aorta. The retrograde cardioplegia catheter was removed.

Protamine was administered and the venous cannula was removed. The graft's perfusion sidelimb was clamped, divided, and oversewn with 5-0 prolene in two layers. All suture lines were inspected and hemostasis achieved. [**# of chest tubes**] were placed. The sternum was then reapproximated with eight #6 steel sutures. The wound was irrigated and closed using 0 Vicryl for the periosteal fascia, 3-0 Vicryl for the deep dermal layer, and 4-0 monocryl for the subcuticular layer. [The axillary incision was closed in two layers].

At the end of the case all sponge and needle counts were correct. The patient was then transferred to the CVICU in stable but critical condition. There were no complications.

CPB Time: [**minutes**]

Crossclamp Time: [**minutes**]

SACP Time: [**minutes**]

Lowest Temperature reached: [**minutes**]

Dr. [**BLANK**] was present and scrubbed for [**BLANK**] elements of this operation.

37. Total Artificial Heart

Michael Tong MD, MBA

Cleveland Clinic, Cleveland, OH

Essential Operative Steps

1. Lines and monitoring
2. General endotracheal tube anesthesia
3. Intraop TEE
4. Median Sternotomy
5. Open pericardium
6. Systemic heparin
7. Arterial cannulation
8. Bicaval venous cannulation
9. Check ACT (>480)
10. Initiate CPB (CI 2.2)
11. Insert aortic vent
12. Clamp the aorta and snare the cava
13. Perform the cardiectomy leaving the aorta, pulmonary artery and a 1cm cuff of LV and RV and 1cm of TV and mitral valve.
14. Buttress the rims of the LV and RV +/- a strip of felt
15. Sew the inflow cuffs onto the LV and RV.
16. Set the outflow grafts on the aorta and PA
17. Tunnel the driveline and connect the main body of the pump to the inflow cuffs and outflow grafts.
18. Connect the left pump and then the right pump
19. Deair
20. Start the left pump and then the right pump
21. Come off bypass
22. Decannulate
23. Give protamine and assure hemostasis.
24. Wrap the pump with Gore-Tex
25. Close chest.

Potential Complications and Pitfalls

1. Stay midline during sternotomy
2. Patient's chest cavity too small to accommodate the TAH
3. Not enough valvular tissue resected which leads to inflow obstruction
4. Atrial cuffs too large or too small leaving gaps or dog-ears.
5. Drivelines externalized too medially causing the pump to be medial and compressing the IVC.
6. RV turned on first, causing pulmonary edema.
7. Cannot adequately deair the pump
8. Bleeding

Template Dictation

Preoperative diagnosis: [Indication: e.g. Ischemic cardiomyopathy]

Postoperative diagnosis: same

Procedure(s) performed: Implantation of Total artificial heart as a bridge to transplant

Attending Surgeon: [BLANK]

Secondary Surgeon: [BLANK]

Assistants: [BLANK]

Anesthesia: [BLANK]

Indication(s) for Procedure: [AGE] year old [GENDER] with [DURATION] history of [COMPLAINT]. Preoperative workup showed severe cardiomyopathy and end-stage systolic and diastolic congestive heart failure. Patient is status [INTERMACS LEVEL] with [JUSTIFICATION OF STATUS]. Patient taken to the OR today for implantation of Total artificial heart

Drains: [BLANK]

Estimated Blood Loss: [BLANK]

Specimen: [LV core]

Description of Procedure: The patient was taken to the operating room on [DATE]. Preoperative huddle and pre-incision timeout was performed. Patient was in supine position. General anesthesia was obtained. A right internal jugular central venous line, pulmonary artery catheter and radial arterial line were inserted. Transesophageal echocardiogram was performed. Patient was prepped and draped in normal fashion.

A midline sternotomy was performed and the pericardium was opened. The patient was heparinized and arterial cannula was placed in the ascending aorta and bicaval venous cannula was inserted. Once ACT was >480, patient was placed on cardiopulmonary bypass and normothermia was maintained. A vent was inserted on the aorta to be used later for deairing.

The heart was mobilized, encircling the superior, inferior vena cava. The aorta and pulmonary artery were also mobilized. We then performed the cardiectomy specifically designed for the insertion of the total artificial heart. Starting from the RV, an incision was made 1-2 cm below the AV groove. The Tricuspid valve was cut 1 cm below the annulus. The incision was carried through the base of the RV, into the septum and the LV and the Mitral valve was cut 1 cm below the annulus. The aorta and pulmonary artery are then cut at the level of the commissural attachments. The remaining attachments of the ventricles were then excised. The left atrium and left atrial appendage was examined for thrombus and the left atrial

II. Adult Cardiac Surgery

appendage was oversewn from within the right atrium. The coronary sinus was oversewn. This leaves us with the left atrium with a rim of left ventricle, right atrium with a rim of right ventricle, aorta and pulmonary artery.

Then, the rim of right ventricle and left ventricles were buttressed with 1 cm of felt around the free edge of both ventricles using 3-0 prolene. [If the ventricles are thick, the felt doesn't have to be used but the edge of the ventricles should still be buttressed with 3-0 prolene]

The quick connect atrial cuffs of the TAH were trimmed and inverted and sewn onto the rims of the left and right ventricles. The atria were then pressure tested to ensure there were no leaks from the cuffs. The cuffs were then everted.

The outflow grafts were pre-sprayed with co-seal as the graft material is not impermeable to blood. We measured our outflow graft 3 cm for the aorta, 6 cm through the pulmonary artery and sewed these to the respective great vessels. Prior to connecting the bodies of the pump, a sheet of Gore-Tex is sewn to the posterior pericardium and was used later for wrapping of the device.

We then tunneled our driveline in a left subcostal position to make sure the pump was on the left hand side of the pericardial space. The left pump was inserted into the inflow cuff and outflow graft, trying to deair along the way. The right pump was attached in similar manner. We then further de-aired the pump and then as soon as we removed the cross-clamp, we began pumping the left ventricle followed by the right ventricle.

We were able to easily ramp up of the flow and then separate from bypass. Cannulas were removed, cannulation sites oversewn. Once we were satisfied with the hemodynamics and hemostasis, the remainder of the Gore-Tex was wrapped around the pumping chambers in the great vessel. Two chest tubes were inserted and then closure was commenced in usual fashion. The patient was then transported to the Intensive Care Unit in stable condition.

All instruments, sponges and needles counts were confirmed to be correct x 2 at the end of the case.

Dr. [BLANK] was present and scrubbed for [BLANK] elements of this operation.

38. Transcatheter Aortic Valve Implantation (TAVI): (Transfemoral-Transapical Approach)

Dimitrios Topalidis, MD and Gabriel Loor, MD

University of Minnesota, Minneapolis, MN

Essential Operative Steps

1. Lines and Monitoring
2. General endotracheal anesthesia
3. Intraoperative transesophageal echocardiogram
4. Unilateral arterial and bilateral venous groin access
5. Pigtail catheter placement/advancement to the aortic root
6. Temporary pacemaker placement in the RV
7. Aortogram to determine optimal radiographic angles during valve deployment
8. Left anterior thoracotomy (5th-6th space depending on 3D CT and spot fluoroscopy)
9. Pericardial stay sutures and exposure of the LV apex (for redos the pericardium can be left intact with creation of separate small slits for drainage later)
10. Radiographic and TEE confirmation of optimal LV puncture site
11. Systemic heparinization (400 u/kg)
12. Check ACT (>400 sec)
13. Double pursetring suture on the LV apex with pledgets
14. LV apex puncture with a guide needle and advancement of a soft access guide wire across the aortic valve and into the descending aorta under fluoroscopic guidance
15. 12fr Sheath advancement into the LV
16. Float the Berman PA catheter through the aortic valve and into the descending aorta.
17. Amplatz wire through the Berman
18. Delivery of the device introducer sheath over the wire
19. Balloon aortic valvuloplasty with rapid ventricular pacing
20. Removal of the balloon and advancement of the deployment system with the valve across the annulus (50% above, 50% below)
21. Actual valve deployment under apnea, rapid RV pacing with simultaneous retrieval of the pigtail aortogram catheter
22. TEE confirmation of appropriate valve deployment and lack of significant AI.
23. Retrieval of the valve deployment system and guide wire.
24. Removal of the deployment sheath
25. Surgical hemostasis of the LV puncture site using rapid pacing
26. Administration of protamine for heparin reversal
27. Retrieval of the venous pacemaker and closure of the groin puncture sites
28. Thoracotomy closure

II. Adult Cardiac Surgery

Potential Complications and Pitfalls

1. Vascular arterial and/or venous groin injury during access
2. Performance of thoracotomy at a level and position away from the LV apex
3. Lung Injury/ LV Injury during initial entry in the thoracic cavity
4. LAD injury during placement of puersetring sutures on the LV
5. Poor Choice of valve size resulting in aortic annulus disruption/VSD formation during valve deployment in case of an oversized valve
6. Significant paravalvular AI after valve deployment
7. Valve dislodgement into the LV or distally
8. Obstruction/dissection of Coronary Ostia
9. Heart block
10. Bleeding at LV puncture site

Template Dictation

Preoperative Diagnosis: [INDICATION – e.g. Severe Aortic Stenosis]

Postoperative Diagnosis: Same

Procedure(s) Performed: Transapical aortic valve Implantation

Attending Surgeon: [BLANK]

Secondary Surgeon: [BLANK]

Assistants: [BLANK]

Anesthesia: [BLANK]

Indication(s) for Procedure: [AGE] year old [GENDER] with [DURATION] history of [COMPLAINT – e.g. , [FINDINGS -].

Description of Procedure: Patient was taken to the hybrid operating room /cardiac catheterization lab. Patient was placed on the fluoroscopy table in the supine position. After induction of general anesthesia, patient was intubated with a double lumen endotracheal tube. Arterial, central venous, and pulmonary artery catheters were placed by anesthesia without difficulty. Transesophageal echo probe was placed. The patient was positioned in the supine position with a bump under the left chest. Chest and bilateral groin areas were prepped and draped in the usual sterile fashion.

Under direct fluoroscopic guidance, and using the micro puncture kit, 7F arterial and venous sheaths were placed into the right common femoral artery and vein. A pigtail catheter was advanced into the aortic root and a trans venous pacemaker was placed into the right ventricle. A contralateral 7F venous sheath was placed for possible CPB.

Next, a small left anterior thoracotomy through the fifth intercostal space was carried out. The wound protector was inserted. The pericardium over the ventricular apex was incised and the adhesions were lysed. Pericardial stay sutures were placed. Systemic heparinization was initiated. Double purse string sutures of 3-0 Prolene with pledgets were placed in the appropriate site on the left ventricle apex. Next, the left ventricular apex was punctured with a needle and a soft guide wire was advanced into the LV cavity towards the aortic valve. Over this guide wire, a 7 French sheath was placed. The wire was then exchanged through the sheath with a Berman PA catheter to cross the aortic valve. An Amplatz wire was advanced through the Berman into the descending aorta. The Edwards transapical deployment sheath was advanced over the Amplatz. Through this, a BAV was performed under apnea and rapid ventricular pacing. The BAV balloon was withdrawn and a prepared Edwards Sapien [BLANK] 26 or 23 mm valve oriented in the correct manner on its Ascendra deployment system was introduced. Under radiological and TEE guidance the device was positioned across the aortic annulus. When the positioning of the valve was found to be satisfactory, the valve was deployed under apnea and rapid ventricular pacing with balloon expansion. Echo and fluoroscopy were used to document any AI or other valve-related issues. Next, the deployment system and guide wire were removed. With rapid pacing the left ventricle sheath was removed and the purse string sutures were tied.

Heparin was reversed with protamine. General hemostasis was achieved. A #28 right angle chest tube was left in the pleural cavity and a Blake drain in the anterior pericardium.

The ribs were re-approximated with a heavy Vicryl suture and the thoracotomy was closed in layers with running absorbable sutures.

The patient tolerated the procedure well and was returned to the intensive care unit in stable condition. Sponge, needle and instrument counts were correct prior to closing.

Dr. [BLANK] was present and scrubbed for [BLANK] elements of this procedure.

39. Valve Sparing Root Replacement

Walter F. DeNino, MD and John S. Ikonomidis, MD, PhD

Medical University of South Carolina, Charleston, SC

Essential Operative Steps

1. Lines and Monitoring
2. Sternotomy and creation of pericardial well
3. Aortic and venous cannulation, placement of ante- and retrograde cardioplegia cannulae, LV vent
4. Antegrade arrest, topical cooling
5. RV/RVOT tacking
6. Coronary buttons, trimming aorta to annulus
7. Hegar sizing of outflow tract, graft size selection
8. Annular suture placement followed by placement through graft
9. Circulatory arrest and selection of distal graft including side branch
10. Distal hemiarch anastomosis performed, return to CPB and cannulation of side graft
11. Rewarming
12. Reimplantation of valve commissures
13. Reimplantation of the coronary arteries
14. Graft-graft anastomosis
15. De-air aortic root, place chest tubes/drains, assess repair by TEE, pacing wires, come off CPB, remove cannulae, close chest

Potential Complications and Pitfalls

1. Thorough inspection of native aortic valve to ensure proper morphology and function adequate for valve-sparing procedure.
2. Proper sizing of the graft utilizing the David Method (based on height of aortic valve leaflets) or that outlined here using a Hegar dilator (Hegar size + 11).
3. Replacement of all ascending aortic tissue to the level of proximal hemiarch to prevent subsequent dilation of the remaining distal ascending aorta and proximal hemiarch, potentially requiring a subsequent aortic replacement.
4. The graft used for the hemiarch replacement is smaller in diameter than the graft used for the valve-sparing aortic root replacement so care must be taken to appropriately adjust the needle bites in the two grafts so that the larger proximal graft will telescope down to create a uniform neo-sinotubular junction.
5. A careful inspection of the suture lines should take place while on CPB to eliminate any surgical causes of bleeding. Following protamine administration, the repair is tightly packed for 5 to 10 minutes. During this time, appropriate blood product infusion should be accomplished. On pack removal, the majority, if not all, of the suture lines should have

ceased bleeding. If the patient is coagulopathic, repacking and infusion of blood products may be appropriate. If the patient is completely warm, if all laboratory values are normalized, if all surgical bleeding is controlled, and if bleeding has still not ceased, it is appropriate at this point to consider infusion of recombinant activated factor VII concentrate.

6. One should aim for a cusp coaptation length of 5 mm or more. When this can be achieved, this operation is likely to be very durable. If any more than trivial insufficiency is encountered, consider re-arresting the heart and inspecting the repair. If the reason for the insufficiency is not identified or not repairable, it may be necessary to excise the leaflets and replace the aortic valve with either a mechanical or tissue prosthesis based on patient preference.

Template Dictation

Preoperative Diagnosis: [INDICATION – e.g. Aortic root dilation and aortic insufficiency, Type A dissection, etc]

Postoperative Diagnosis: Same

Procedure Performed: Valve Sparing Root Replacement (DETAILS – e.g. 34 mm Dacron graft anastomosed to a 26 mm Dacron graft)

Attending Surgeon: [BLANK]

Secondary Surgeon: [BLANK]

Assistants: [BLANK]

Indication(s) for Procedure: [AGE] year old [GENDER] with [DURATION] history of [COMPLAINT – Aortic root aneurysm]. The patient was originally found to have an enlarged aortic root measuring XX cm. The patient's aortic root now measures between XX and XX cm in diameter, depending on the imaging modality. A preoperative echo showed an ejection fraction of XX% with an aortic root diameter of XX cm and moderate aortic insufficiency. Due to the findings of progressive aortic root dilatation and aortic insufficiency, the patient was evaluated by CT Surgery and consented for a valve sparing aortic root replacement.

Estimated Blood Loss: [NUMBER]

Urine Output: [NUMBER]

Total CPB time: [NUMBER]

Cross Clamp time: [NUMBER]

Circulatory Arrest time: [NUMBER]

Specimens: [BLANK]

II. Adult Cardiac Surgery

Complications: [BLANK]

Description of Procedure: Under general anesthesia, the patient was positioned in the supine position with the chest/abdomen/pelvis and lower extremities prepped and draped in sterile fashion. A radial arterial line and central venous line with pulmonary artery catheter were placed by anesthesia. Pre-operative IV antibiotics were administered. A median sternotomy was performed and the pericardium opened widely in the usual fashion. The right portion of the pericardium was suspended, allowing the ventricular mass of the heart to fall downward into the left chest and provide better exposure to the aortic valve. Following systemic heparinization, standard aortic and two-stage right atrial cannulation was undertaken. A [XX F] aortic cannula was used that would later accommodate the Dacron side arm of the graft used for the hemiarch replacement. Both antegrade and retrograde cardioplegic catheters were placed to first arrest the heart antegrade with blood cardioplegia and then switch to retrograde cardioplegia during the remainder of the procedure. This was supplemented with topical iced saline for cooling of the heart. The myocardial temperature was monitored with a probe placed just right of the left anterior descending coronary artery and angled into the interventricular septum. Interventricular septal temperature was maintained between 10 and 15°C for the entire cross-clamp procedure with intermittent 250 to 500 mL retrograde cardioplegic infusions every 20 minutes. For venting, a [14-F] vent is placed directly in the apex of the left ventricle. Once on bypass, the patient was systemically cooled to a bladder temperature of [20°C].

The superior margin of the right ventricle and right ventricular outflow tract were retracted downward and to the left, respectively, using needled silastic sutures anchored under a reasonable amount of tension. Following cardioplegic arrest, the ascending aorta was transected and the aortic valve carefully inspected to ensure that it is a morphologically normal structure with no significant calcifications, fenestrations, or tears.

The left and right coronary buttons were excised and gently retracted with 4-0 polypropylene sutures. Following completion of this, the residual aorta was carefully trimmed, leaving the aortic annulus and valve encircled by approximately 7 to 8 mm of native aorta. Next, careful dissection was completed separating the aortic root from the pulmonary artery, right ventricular outflow tract, and the left atrium. Dissection proceeded down to the level of the aortic annulus circumferentially and slightly below.

Hegar dilators were carefully placed across the aortic valve to a dilator size that fit comfortably in the outflow tract but not tightly. Then 5 mm (accounting for 2.5 mm on either side of the outflow tract) was added to the dilator number and an additional 6 mm to allow for billowing of the graft (11 mm total).

A total of [12 -15] multifilament 2-0 polyester sutures were placed in horizontal mattress fashion under the annulus such that one horizontal mattress suture was placed under each commissure in planar fashion using an equal number of stitches per sinus. Caution was employed to make sure that the sutures did not breach the aortic endothelium but all stay buried beneath it. Next, the previously sized Dacron graft was brought into the operative field and a marking pen was used to mark the graft at approximately 120° intervals. The horizontal mattress sutures were then placed sequentially through the graft. The graft was lowered into position such that the valve and all of the aortic tissues sat firmly within the graft. Care must was taken to make sure that all layers of the aorta were sitting inside the graft before the sutures were tied. The Hegar dilator that was used to size the annulus was placed across the valve before tying the sutures. The three subcommissural sutures were tied first, creating a small graft plication under each commissure to narrow the valvular commissural angle. The remaining sutures were then tied firmly but not snugly all the way around, keeping the Hegar dilator in place to prevent narrowing of the left ventricular outflow tract. Following suture tying, a small amount of resistance was felt when removing the Hegar dilator.

By this time, the bladder temperature reached 20C. The patient was placed in Trendelenburg position, the head was packed in ice, and 15 mg/kg IV of sodium pentobarbital and 1 g IV methylprednisolone were administered. A woven Dacron graft sized 2 to 3 mm larger than the Hegar dilator used to size the graft for the valve-sparing root replacement was selected. A graft with a 10 mm sidebranch for later cannulation was chosen. The pump was discontinued and the aorta quickly resected. The trimmed graft was brought into the operative field and the distal anastomosis performed with a running 3-0 polypropylene suture such that the side limb of the graft pointed directly anterior. A small amount of biological glue was used to seal needle holes. Pump flow was commenced at 1 L/min and the side limb of the graft cannulated. Circulatory arrest time was **XX** minutes. The side limb, arch, and graft were carefully de-aired before the cross-clamp applied to the graft just proximal to the entrance of the side limb. The hemiarch anastomosis was inspected for leaks as cardiopulmonary bypass was brought back up to full flow. When surgical hemostasis was obtained, rewarming was begun and the residual graft folded under the innominate vein for later graft-to-graft anastomosis. Attention was turned back to the valve-sparing aortic root replacement.

3-0 Polypropylene sutures were placed in horizontal mattress fashion from inside to out anchoring the tops of the valve commissures to the graft at 120° intervals. To achieve the appropriate graft height, gentle traction was placed on the graft to slightly unravel its corrugations before placing the sutures. It was verified at this point that these commissural attachment sites would not obstruct the direct re-implantation of coronary arteries. The aortic root was irrigated with a small amount of cold saline and the valve leaflets inspected to ensure coaptation on the same plane with no prolapse into the left ventricular outflow tract. The commissural suspension sutures were then gently tied with three knots, each leaving two equal lengths of suture loaded with a needle.

One limb of one polypropylene suture was then brought from outside to in just over top of the aorta surrounding one commissure. The aortic cuff around the valve was sutured carefully to the graft in running fashion. Care was taken not to take excessive bites of the graft and that the bites were taken very close to the annulus of the aortic valve to prevent subsequent dilation of both the annulus and the intervening aortic segment. Following complete running of one of the commissures, the suture was brought outside and tied to one of the next Prolene commissure sutures. These were cut and the remaining suture on that side used to run to the next commissure and so on circumferentially. [To deal with a prolapsing leaflet, a 6-0 polytetrafluoroethylene (Gore-Tex) suture is doubly run in continuous fashion along the free margin of the leaflet reinforced with small pledgets placed on the outside of the graft. This suture is tied when traction on it pulls the free margin of the valve leaflet up to the same level as the other two leaflets.]

Ophthalmic cautery was used to create appropriately sized defects in the left and right neo-sinuses of the graft for re-implantation of the coronary arteries, performed with 5-0 polypropylene suture. Following completion of these two anastomoses, the reconstructed root was carefully inspected from the inside to make sure that the suture lines on the coronaries were uniform. Biological glue was applied to the anastomoses to seal needle holes.

Following completion of this portion of the operation, the graft was then trimmed to approximately 5 mm above the implanted aortic valve commissures. The previous graft used for the hemiarch anastomosis was unraveled, measured, and trimmed appropriately. The graft-to-graft anastomosis was then constructed with running 3-0 polypropylene suture.

Next, an ascending aortic vent with cardioplegia infusion line was inserted in the graft and 500 mL of warm cardioplegia given with the first 100 mL used to de-air the root. The ventricular vent was removed and oversewn with a running 2-0 polypropylene suture. The retrograde cardioplegic catheter was removed. Ventricular and atrial pacing wires as well as a 36 F mediastinal and 19 F left pleural Blake drain were placed. The cross-clamp was removed and sinus rhythm resumed. During myocardial recovery, careful interrogation of the valve was undertaken by TEE to assess for any residual insufficiency and to measure the coaptation distance of the valve leaflets. Following an appropriate period of rewarming (to at least 36.5°C) and de-airing, the ascending aortic vent was removed and reinforced with 4-0 polypropylene suture. The patient was then weaned from cardiopulmonary bypass. The venous cannula was removed. Protamine was administered directly down the side limb of the hemiarch graft. Following completion of protamine administration, the side graft was tied at its point of insertion into the larger graft with two #2 silk ties. The graft was then divided, resulting in arterial separation from bypass. Once adequate hemostasis was ensured, the chest was closed in the usual manner.

All instrument, sponge and needle counts were confirmed to be correct x 2 at the end of the operation. The patient was subsequently transferred to the postoperative cardiac surgical intensive care unit in critical condition.

Dr. **[BLANK]** was present and scrubbed for **[BLANK]** elements of this procedure.

III. Congenital Cardiac Surgery

III. Congenital Cardiac Surgery

III. Congenital Cardiac Surgery

1. Repair of Atrial Septal Defect- Secundum Atrial Septal Defect

Fahd Makhdom MD and Christo I. Tchervenkov MD.

McGill University, Montreal, Canada

Essential Operative Steps

1. Monitoring and central line.
2. General anesthesia with endotracheal intubation.
3. Intra-operative Transesophageal Echocardiogram (TEE)
4. Positioning; supine.
5. Median sternotomy (**Variation:** Right anterior thoracotomy, Ministernotomy, Submammary skin incision and sternotomy).
6. Opening the pericardium
7. Preserve portion of the pericardium to use as a patch for closure (**Optional**), Other alternates include: Bovine pericardium, or Gore-TEX patch.
8. Systemic heparinization (400 U/kg).
9. Ascending aortic cannulation.
10. Bicaval venous cannulation and caval snares.
11. Antegrade cardioplegia line.
12. Check ACT (greater than 400 seconds), initiate CBP.
13. Aortic cross clamp.
14. Antegrade cardioplegia with mild hypothermia.
15. Snare both cavae.
16. Right atriotomy; oblique incision from base of right atrial appendage towards the IVC.
17. Examination of the interatrial septum and identify the defect margins.
18. Structure to be identified upon examining the right atrium
19. Superior Vena Cava and Inferior Vena Cava to ensure that there is no anomalous pulmonary veins returning to the right atrium or the SVC
20. Eustachian valve is identified to prevent baffling blood from the IVC to the left atrium
21. The coronary sinus is identified and must be protected from the suture line to avoid heart block
22. Closure of the defect (**Variation:** direct closure if defect is small. If the defect is large, a patch is used for closure)
23. The suture should be taken through a good tissue paying attention not to injure the surrounding structure.
24. De-airing of left side chambers.
25. Ventilate the lungs (**Note:** Avoid excessive suctioning of the left atrium to prevent air trapping in the left heart).
26. Tightening the suture line and tie.
27. Place additional interrupted sutures at several strategic places to further secure the closure.
28. Remove aortic cross clamp.

29. Start rewarming.
30. Fill the right atrium to perform deairing.
31. Close the atrial incision.
32. Temporary Pacing wires, atrial/ ventricular.
33. Wean from cardiopulmonary bypass.
34. Transesophageal echocardiogram (TEE) to evaluate the repair and rule out residual shunt.
35. Heparin reversal; protamine (4 mg/kg).
36. Sequential decannulation.
37. Meticulous hemostasis.
38. Chest tube placement.
39. Sternotomy closure.

Potential Complications and Pitfalls

1. Bleeding from suture lines.
2. Improper de-airing can lead to systemic air embolism.
3. Pulmonary hypertension with right ventricular failure.
4. Injury to conduction system; heart block.
5. Residual shunting can occur in case of patch dehiscence, a suture line with pulmonary vein/veins draining into right atrium or missed additional ASD.
6. Misidentifying the Eustachian valve can lead to closing the IVC to left atrium causing the post-operative cyanosis.
7. Post-operative cyanosis can also be due to missed PAPVC to right atrium or a coronary sinus ASD or the left SVC draining into left atrium with an unroofing of the coronary sinus

Template Dictation

Preoperative diagnosis: Secundum Atrial septal defect

Postoperative diagnosis: Same.

Procedure(s) Performed: Repair of Secundum ASD with Gore-TEX patch

Attending Surgeon: [BLANK]

Secondary Surgeon: [BLANK]

Assistants: [BLANK]

Anesthesia: [BLANK]

Indication(s) for Procedure: [AGE] year old [GENDER] with [DURATION] history of recurrent pneumonia. During the workup she was diagnosed with atrial septal defect secundum type. On echocardiogram, the atrial septal defect was found to be very large and missing an inferior rim precluding percutaneous device closure. A cardiac catheterization revealed a large left to right shunt with a QP/QS ratio of 3:1. There are no other abnormalities diagnosed. The pulmonary artery pressures were only mildly elevated. The patient was brought to the operating room for closure of the atrial septal defect.

Perfusion Data: For the purpose of the surgery, the patient was put on cardiopulmonary bypass. Following systemic heparinization, we proceeded with cannulation the distal ascending aorta and of both venae cavae. The patient's weight was [BLANK] kilograms. The estimated flow optimal for this patient was at [BLANK] liters per minute. Following cross-clamping of the aorta and arresting the heart with antegrade cold blood cardioplegia, both cavae were snared and the right atrium was opened. The ASD secundum was closed with a Gore-Tex patch and the aortic crossclamp time was [BLANK] minutes.

Operative findings: The patient had normal thymic tissue. The pericardium was not adherent to the heart. The great vessels were normally situated. There was a large secundum atrial septal defect with no rim near the inferior vena cava. The systemic and pulmonary venous drainage was normal.

Description of the procedure: After informed consent and patient identification the patient was brought to the operating room and placed on the operating table in a supine position. After induction of general anesthesia with single lumen endotracheal tube intubation, arterial and central venous monitoring lines were placed. A transesophageal echocardiogram (TEE) was performed and the above findings were noted. The patient was positioned; chest, abdomen, groins and upper thigh were prepped and draped in a surgical sterile fashion.

We proceeded with a median sternotomy by achieving careful hemostasis. The pericardium was opened and suspended. A full dose of intravenous heparin was given to achieve the systemic anticoagulation. We proceeded with cannulation of the ascending aorta as well as cannulation of the superior vena cava and inferior vena cava. After achieving an activated clotting time above 450 seconds, cardiopulmonary bypass was initiated and the aortic crossclamp was applied. Antegrade blood cardioplegia was used to arrest the heart. The right atrium was opened and the secundum atrial septal defect was visualized. The coronary sinus and the ostia of both venae cavae were located. No anomalous pulmonary veins or additional defects were identified. A Gore-Tex patch (0.6 mm) was tailored to fit the size of the atrial septal defect. Using a 5-0 polypropylene, the patch was sutured around the rim of the atrial septal defect in a continuous fashion. Excessive suctioning of blood from the left atrium was avoided, in order to prevent trapping air on the left side of the heart. Just before completing the suture line, using Valsalva maneuver, the left atrium was allowed to fill and air was expelled towards the right atrium. Then the suture was tied. The suture line was reinforced in a few additional places with interrupted 5-0 mattress sutures. Next the patient was rewarmed and the aortic crossclamp was removed. The right atrium was allowed to fill partially. The atriotomy was closed using running 5-0 polyproplyene suture and was reinforced by another layer. Temporary ventricular and atrial pacing wires were placed. With the patient warm and normal sinus rhythm recovered, cardiopulmonary bypass was discontinued successfully.

Transesophageal echocardiogram confirmed a secure ASD closure, with no residual shunting, and no air on the left side of the heart. After protamine administration, the heart was decannulated. One mediastinal drain was placed. Once hemostasis was achieved the chest was closed in the usual fashion, sterile dressing was applied.

Dr. [BLANK] was present and scrubbed for [BLANK] elements of this procedure.

2. Ventricular Septal Defect: Perimembranous

Keerit Tauh, MD and Andrew I.M. Campbell, MD

Division of Cardiovascular and Thoracic Surgery, BC Children's Hospital

University of British Columbia

Vancouver, BC, Canada

Essential Operative Steps

1. Lines and Monitoring.
2. General anesthesia.
3. Intraoperative transesophageal echocardiogram.
4. Median sternotomy.
5. Open pericardium and inspect cardiac anatomy.
6. Right sided pericardial suspension.
7. Systemic heparinization.
8. Arterial cannulation.
9. Bi-caval cannulation.
10. Myocardial protection cannula placement (DLP Aortic Root Cannula)
11. Initiate cardiopulmonary bypass
12. Ensure ACT > 400
13. Systemic cooling to 34 degrees (**Variation:** For complicated cases requiring a longer cross clamp more significant hypothermia may be necessary).
14. Consider ligation of ductus arteriosis (routine in infants)
15. Right superior pulmonary vein (RSPV) vent is placed in absence of a patent foramen ovale (**Variation:** If a PFO is present, it may be used to directly vent the left side, once the right atrium is opened).
16. Encircle caval tourniquets around SVC and IVC.
17. Cross-clamp the aorta and administer cardioplegia.
18. Snare caval tourniquets and ensure aortic root is being vented.
19. Open and retract the right atrium to facilitate viewing of all borders of the VSD.
20. Cut an appropriately shaped patch.
21. Continous or interrupted closure of the VSD.
22. Place horizontal mattress pledgeted sutures starting at the inferior border of the VSD and moving in a counter-clockwise fashion towards the superior margin of the defect and the antero-septal commissure.
23. Continue placing interrupted pledgeted sutures through the septal leaflet with the pledgets on the atrial side of the tricuspid valve - starting at the anteroseptal commissure and running down to the posteroseptal commissure.
24. Close the inferior margin of the VSD with the other end of the running suture used to initially start the patch (**Variation:** place additional horizontal mattress pledgeted sutures in the ventricular septum in a

clockwise manner beginning from the original starting point up until the posteroseptal commissure is again reached).
25. Pass the interrupted sutures through the patch to ensure closure of the defect.
26. Parachute the patch into place and the pledgeted sutures are tied down.
27. Inspect the ASD, if the PFO has been used to vent the left side it is closed with a 5-0 suture.
28. Closure of right atrium.
29. Rewarm to normothermia.
30. Heart is de-aired and cross clamp is removed.
31. Ensure adequate hemostasis.
32. Place atrial and ventricular pacing wires.
33. Place chest tubes.
34. Wean from CPB.
35. Venous decannulation.
36. Administration of Protamine.
37. Aortic Decannulation.
38. Assess Hemostasis.
39. Close Sternotomy.

Note: - Similar Operative set up is utilized during repair of other types of VSD's including Muscular VSD's and conoventricular VSD's. Subpulmonic VSD's are approached with similar principles except a transverse incision in the pulmonary artery is utilized. Inlet VSD's will be covered in a separate chapter.

Potential Complications and Pitfalls

1. Remaining midline during sternotomy is crucial.
2. Avoid injury to innominate vein during pericardial dissection and suspension.
3. Cannulation complications include aortic dissection, SVC/IVC tears, hepatic vein cannulation, azygous vein cannulation, embolism with aortic manipulation.
4. Insufficient myocardial protection can occur due to the cross clamp not completely across the aorta, aortic insufficiency and cardiac distension due to inadequate venting and should be avoided.
5. Failure to address the patent ductus arteriosus may lead to air embolism and flooding of operative field.
6. Failure to securely snare the caval tourniquets can result into venous air lock and flooded operative field.
7. Transection of SA nodal artery by too far superior extension of the atriotomy should be avoided.
8. Overly aggressive tricuspid retraction can lead to tricuspid regurgitation and conduction anomalies.
9. Poor exposure of the VSD can potentially result into incomplete closure of VSD, technical difficulty and injury to conduction system or aortic valve.

III. Congenital Cardiac Surgery

10. Poor patch sizing can lead to a persistent VSD due to redundancy or insufficient patch material.
11. Careful attention must be paid to passing sutures near the posteroseptal commissure as damage to the bundle of His and potentially the AV node can occur as the suture is transitioned onto and through the septal leaflet.
12. The aortic valve leaflets are situated below the superior margins of the VSD and can be caught into the deep needle bites.
13. Sutures should be gently tied as excessive torque on the tissue can result into tearing of septum or septal leaflet when tying the sutures.
14. Adequate warming, de-airing and obtaining a meticulous hemostasis prior to sternotomy closure are of paramount importance.

Template Dictation

Preoperative Diagnosis: (**INDICATION** – e.g. Perimembranous VSD)

Postoperative Diagnosis: Same or other findings

Procedure(s) Performed: Repair of Perimembranous (**Variation:** type of VSD) VSD

Attending Surgeon: [BLANK]

Secondary Surgeon: [BLANK]

Assistants: [BLANK]

Anesthesia: [BLANK]

Indication(s) for Procedure: [AGE] year old [GENDER] with [DURATION] history of [COMPLAINT – Failure to thrive, Poor Feeding, Exercise intolerance, Shortness of Breath, Cyanosis etc]. Preoperative echocardiogram demonstrated a (FINDINGS – e.g. 1.4 cm perimembranous VSD with a Qp: Qs ratio of [VALUE] and pulmonary pressures of [VALUE] mm Hg.

Description of Procedure: After informed consent the patient was taken to the operating room on [DATE]. The patient's identity and planned procedure were verified, and the patient was placed on the operating table in a supine position. After appropriate IV access, arterial lines were established and general anesthetic was administered with endotracheal intubation. A central line was placed. Preoperative transesophageal echocardiogram was then performed to evaluate cardiac function and anatomy. We then proceeded to prep and drape the patient in the usual sterile fashion. Time out was performed. Median sternotomy was performed and the thymus [was/was not removed]. Following identification of the innominate vein, the pericardium was opened and right-sided pericardial stay sutures were placed. Once dissected, intravenous heparin was administered and an ACT was drawn. After the aorta was separated from the pulmonary artery and assessed, aortic cannulation sutures using [SIZE] polypropylene were placed. The aortic cannula was then inserted, secured and de-aired. SVC cannulation sutures were then placed and the right angle SVC cannula was inserted and connected to the bypass circuit. IVC cannulation sutures were then placed and the IVC cannula was inserted. The IVC and SVC cannulas were then connected using a Y connector to the common venous drainage line and tourniquets were encircled around each using umbilical tape. Once the ACT was greater than 480 seconds, the patient was placed on bypass and gradual systemic cooling to 34 degrees Celsius was begun. An aortic root cannula was then inserted into the ascending aorta for the cardioplegia administration and venting. The aortic cross clamp was applied and antegrade cold cardioplegia solution was administered for arrest and myocardial protection. Following cardioplegia administration, the caval tourniquets were snared and the aortic root vent was turned on.

An incision was then made in the right atrium starting at the right atrial appendage then moving obliquely towards the IVC. Drop-in cardiotomy suction was used to aid in visualization of the tricuspid valve and right atrial retraction sutures were placed. The inter-atrial septum was examined. The patent foramen ovale (PFO) was identified and used to vent the left side of the heart. The tricuspid valve was then gently retracted using an aortic root retractor such that the circumferential border of the perimembranous VSD could be clearly visualized and the repair could be planned. A double velour patch was then approximated and cut to the size of the defect to ensure that there would be a sufficient overlap. Starting from the inferior border of the VSD, pledgeted [SIZE] ethibond sutures were placed in a sequential interrupted manner using a mattress technique progressing in a counter-clockwise direction. Care was taken to avoid the conduction system deep to the ventricular septum. Once the antero-septal commissure was reached horizontal mattress sutures were then placed through the septal leaflet in a similar fashion. Care was taken to avoid entering the tricuspid annulus. Once the interrupted sutures were run down to the postero-septal commissure, sutures were then placed in a clockwise manner starting again from the inferior border of the defect. Once the septal leaflet was met, a double pledgeted transition stitch was applied with one pledget adjacent to the ventricular septum and one pledget on the atrial side of the septal leaflet. Cardioplegia was infused to help identify the aortic valve to ensure that it was not entrapped by a suture. Once the sutures encircled the defect, they were then passed through the pericardial patch. The patch was then parachuted down over the defect. In a sequential fashion, sutures were then gently tied ensuring appropriate pledget orientation. Prior to tying the last set of sutures, cardioplegia was again instilled and gross de-airing of the left ventricle was conducted. Once all sutures were secured, the patch and remainder of the interventricular septum was inspected to ensure no residual or additional VSD was present. The atrial retraction sutures were then removed and the tricuspid valve was interrogated using saline to assess for any signs of damage or new regurgitation. With the aortic vent on high, deairing of the left atrium and ventricle was performed. The atrium was then closed using a 2 layer running technique and [SIZE] polypropylene following gross de-airing. Once closed, the atrium was inspected for hemostasis and the caval tourniquets were then released and removed.

III. Congenital Cardiac Surgery

Once gross de-airing was complete, the CPB flow was reduced, the root vent was placed on high, and the cross clamp was removed. The patient was then rewarmed and further de-airing was conducted using transesophageal echocardiography and pulmonary recruitment. Chest tubes were placed into the mediastinum. [ATRIAL/VENTRICULAR] pacing wires were then inserted and tested for good capture. Once rewarmed to [NUMBER] degrees Celsius, the patient was slowly weaned from the CPB circuit. The SVC cannula was first clamped then removed. The SVC suture was then tied in place and checked for hemostasis. The IVC cannula was then removed. The IVC sutures was snared and left in place to allow reinstitution of cardiopulmonary bypass if necessary. A test dose of protamine was given, and the patient was monitored for a hemodynamic reaction. Protamine was then resumed and transfusion of pump blood via the aortic cannula was given as needed. Once the protamine was complete, the aortic cannula was then removed and the aortic sutures were tied. Once de-airing was complete the aortic root vent was then removed and the cannulation sutures were tied and assessed for hemostasis. The IVC purse string was also secured. Hemostasis of all intra pericardial sites was assessed. The chest wall was then examined for hemostasis. Sternum was then approximated using stainless steel wires. Hemostasis of wire sites was then assessed. The overlying fascia and soft tissue and skin were approximated using absorbable sutures in a running fashion. The wound was then dressed with a sterile dressing.

Instruments, sponges and needles counts were confirmed to be correct following conclusion of the operation. The patient was then transferred to the Cardiac Surgery Intensive Care Unit in a stable fashion.

Dr. [BLANK] was present and scrubbed for [BLANK] elements of this procedure.

3. Partial AV Canal Repair

Sandeep Sainathan, MD, and Paul Kirshbom MD

Yale University, New Haven, CT.

Essential Operative Steps

1. Informed consent
2. Peripheral IV insertion and general endotracheal anesthesia.
3. Arterial line, central venous line, and urinary catheter insertion
4. Intraoperative Transesophageal echocardiogram (Avoid in infants less than 3 kg as the probe can cause compression and distortion of the left atrium, interfering with the assessment and repair of the defect)
5. Median sternotomy with subtotal thymectomy
6. Asymmetric pericardiotomy to the left of the midline in order to harvest a pericardial patch.
7. Mobilization of aorta, ductus arteriosus and SVC.
8. Systemic heparinization.
9. Aortic and bicaval cannulation.
10. Initiate total cardiopulmonary bypass.
11. Ligation of PDA.
12. Snare the cavae.
13. Cool down to 34 degrees centigrade.
14. Apply aortic cross clamp with instillation of antegrade cardioplegia via the aortic root.
15. Right atriotomy parallel to the AV groove
16. Place left atrial vent via right upper pulmonary vein. (Rule out the presence of a small VSD under the septal leaflet of the tricuspid valve).
17. Assess the mitral valve for morphology and competence through the atrial septal defect.
18. Close the commissure between the superior and inferior bridging leaflets on the left side with either interrupted or running technique, typically with 5-0 or 6-0 monofilament suture. Commisuroplasties may be necessary in cases of annular dilation causing residual regurgitation.
19. Repair the atrial septal defect with the native pericardial patch +/- with preservation with glutaraldehye, bovine pericardium or PTFE patch.
20. Visualize the IVC orifice on right side of the patch.
21. Close of the atriotomy.
22. De-air the left heart via the aortic root and RSPV vent.
23. Remove the aortic cross-clamp.
24. Rewarm and remove the left atrial vent (**Optional:** Left atrial line, a LA line is generally not necessary).
25. Wean from CBP and decannulate.
26. Protamine administration.
27. Ventricular and atrial epicardial pacing wires
28. Place chest drains

29. Ensure adequate hemostasis.
30. Sternal closure.

Potential Complications and Pitfalls

1. The inferior vena caval cannula should be placed low enough to facilitate the adequate visualization of the inferior aspect of the defect.
2. Excessive suturing of the free edges of the mitral cleft may cause the worsening of the mitral insufficiency. Hence, just the opposing 'Kissing edges' should be approximated.
3. In order to carefully assess the mitral valve morphology and competence through the atrial septal defect, the defect may need to be enlarged towards or into the fossa ovalis. The defect may range from a partial cleft in the anterior leaflet to a complete cleft up to the base dividing the anterior leaflet into superior and inferior bridging segments. Cold saline with a red rubber catheter is often used to test the mitral valve. The regurgitant jet either is through the cleft or can be central after an adequate repair of the cleft due to annular dilation.
4. Central jet of mitral regurgitation from annular dilation after adequate repair of the cleft mitral leaflet can be treated with either commisuroplasty or posterior annuloplasty.
5. Large bites taken on the anterior leaflet of the mitral valve or bites skewed towards the mitral valve side of common annulus between the mitral and tricuspid valves may cause mitral insufficiency.
6. Repair of the atrial septal defect is done by placement of initial suture in the raphe between the mitral and tricuspid valve orifices. After this is completed, the rest of the patch is trimmed and sutured to close the remaining septal defect. The coronary sinus can be placed either on the right or left atrial side of the patch, but care must be taken to avoid the conduction system as it crosses inferior to the coronary sinus. The coronary orifice needs to be kept on the right side in presence of a left SVC.
7. Too much traction by the patch on the common annulus between tricuspid and mitral valve can potentially cause the mitral annulus to tent up, resulting into mitral insufficiency. The patch should be tailored after completing the suture line along the common annulus.
8. Friable tissue near the common annulus area can tear during suturing. Interrupted sutures reinforced with pericardial strip pledgets should be used.
9. Insufficient tissue near the common annulus to suture the patch can be problematic. In such cases, the bites are taken on the opposing leaflets of the tricuspid and mitral valve from the ventricular side near their insertion into the common annulus. Deep bites should be avoided in the ventricular crest near the region of the conduction system.
10. Deep bites near the tricuspid annulus into the ventricular crest and in the region of the coronary sinus can potentially cause AV block from injury

to the conduction system. This can be avoided by taking superficial endocardial bites in this region or suturing the right hand side of the patch over the coronary sinus.
11. Use of synthetic patch with residual mitral regurgitation may cause hemolysis, especially if the mitral regurgitation jet impacts the patch.
12. Incorporation of the IVC on the left side of the patch can happen when there is a prominent Eustachian valve. Similarly, when the defects extend high up superiorly or there is an associated secundum defect, the superior vena caval orifice can be accidentally incorporated into the left atrium.
13. Deep bites in the superior aspect of the septal defect can cause the damage to the aortic valve
14. Deep commisuroplasty or annuloplasty stitches during mitral valve repair can potentially injure the circumflex coronary artery.

Template Dictation

Preoperative Diagnosis: [INDICATION – Partial atrio-ventricular canal defect]

Postoperative Diagnosis: Same

Procedure(s) Performed: Repair of partial atrio-ventricular canal defect

Attending Surgeon: [BLANK]

Secondary Surgeon: [BLANK]

Assistants: [BLANK]

Anesthesia: [BLANK]

Indication(s) for Procedure: [AGE] year old [GENDER] with [DURATION] history of [COMPLAINT – e.g. - shortness of breath]. Preoperative echocardiography revealed an atrial septal defect with left to right shunting and an associated moderate to severe mitral regurgitation. The atrioventricular and arterioventricular concordance was normal with a normal pulmonary venous drainage.

Description of Procedure: After informed consent the patient was taken to the operating room on [DATE]. The patient's identity and planned procedure was verified, and the patient was placed on the operating room table in the supine position. General anesthesia was administered via an endotracheal tube. A right internal jugular central venous line, radial arterial line, and a urinary catheter were placed.

Preoperative transesophageal echocardiogram was then performed.

It confirmed the preoperative findings. We then proceeded to prep and drape the chest, abdomen, and groins in a sterile fashion. A time out was performed.

III. Congenital Cardiac Surgery

Median sternotomy was then performed. A subtotal thymectomy was carried out. After identification of the innominate vein, the pericardium was opened to the left of the midline. There were no pericardial adhesions. A pericardial patch of 3 by 4 cm was harvested from the right half and pericardial stay sutures were placed. The ascending aorta, SVC and PDA were mobilized. A total of [UNITS] of systemic heparin was administered. The aortic cannula was then inserted, secured and de-aired. Bicaval venous cannulation was performed and caval snares were placed. Cardiopulmonary bypass was initiated. The PDA was ligated with 6/0 polypropylene suture. Both the venae cavae were snared down. The patient was cooled to 34 degrees centigrade. The aorta was cross-clamped, antegrade cardioplegia was administered via the aortic root and a rapid diastolic arrest was achieved. A right atriotomy was made parallel to the AV groove. A left ventricular vent was placed through the right superior pulmonary vein with the help of a right angle clamp placed into it across the atrial septal defect. The atrial septal defect was inspected and an associated VSD was ruled out by thoroughly inspecting under the septal leaflet of the tricuspid valve. Through the atrial septal defect, the mitral valve was inspected. There was a cleft in the anterior leaflet of the mitral valve extending up to its base, dividing it into superior and inferior bridging segments. On testing the valve, a regurgitant jet through the defect was found. The defect was adequately repaired with simple interrupted 5/0 polypropylene with a complete resolution of the regurgitant jet. The raphe between the mitral and tricuspid valve orifices was of sufficient strength and amount to anchor the pericardial patch, in order to repair the atrial septal defect. The repair was started with a simple continuous 5/0 double armed polypropylene suture at the base of the mitral cleft repair. The suture was run in a clockwise fashion to the inferior aspect of the defect. In the region of the coronary sinus, the suture bites were kept superficial by taking subendocardial bites. The coronary sinus was positioned to the right side of the patch in the right atrial cavity. The second arm of the suture was run in an anticlockwise manner. After completion of the annular side of the repair, the pericardial patch was carefully tailored and sutured to rest of the defect avoiding any tenting of the annulus. Both caval and coronary sinus orifices were visualized in the right atrial cavity. The left atrium was purged of air before tying down the suture. The right atriotomy was closed with a 5/0 polypropylene suture in a simple continuous fashion and the right atrium was purged of air before tying the suture.

A hot shot cardioplegia was administered. The patient was rewarmed and caval snares were removed. The heart was de-aired through the aortic root and LV vent. The aortic cross-clamp was then removed. A total 2 mediastinal drains were placed in the mediastinum. Atrial and ventricular pacing wires were then inserted and tested for appropriate capture. The patient was weaned from the cardiopulmonary bypass. Postoperative TEE showed no residual atrial septal defect and complete resolution of the mitral regurgitation.

The venous cannulae were removed, and the cannulation sutures were secured. The LV vent was removed. A test dose of protamine was administered and the patient was monitored for adverse reaction before the protamine was resumed. The aortic cannula was then removed, and the cannulation sutures were tied.

An adequate hemostasis was then ensured within the mediastinum. All instruments, sponges and needles counts was confirmed to be correct x 2.The sternum was then approximated with stainless steel sternal wires. There was no change in the hemodynamics after sternal closure. The wound was irrigated with antibiotic solution. The presternal fascia was then closed with absorbable sutures in a running fashion. The skin and subcuticular layer was closed with 5-0 polyglactin suture in a running fashion. Sterile occlusive dressing was applied to the skin incision. The mediastinal drains were connected to bulb suction.The patient was subsequently transferred to the postoperative cardiac surgical intensive care unit in a satisfactory condition.

Dr. [BLANK] was present and scrubbed for [BLANK] elements of this operation.

4. Complete Atrioventricular Canal Repair

Julia C. Swanson, MD and James J. Gangemi, MD

University of Virginia, Charlottesville, VA

Essential Operative Steps

1. Lines and monitoring
2. General endotracheal anesthesia
3. Intraoperative transesophageal echo (measure defect size, assess valvular pathology)
4. Median sternotomy
5. Prepare patch material
6. Pericardial well, circumferential dissection of superior and inferior vena cava
7. Systemic heparinization (300u/kg)
8. Single arterial cannulation, bicaval venous cannulation.
9. Place umbilical tape with snare around the SVC and IVC and test snare to ensure inferior cannula not in hepatic vein. Leave tapes loose.
10. Confirm appropriate ACT.
11. Establish CPB and utilize moderate hypothermia (28-30C).
12. Place left ventricular vent (usually through right upper pulmonary vein).
13. DLP for antegrade cardioplegia.
14. Cross-clamp, give cardioplegia (single shot of Del Nido plegia 20ml/kg), ensure electromechanical arrest and then apply ice for topical cooling.
15. Snare caval tapes.
16. Long, medial right atriotomy is made parallel to the right coronary artery extending to a point medial to the IVC
17. Place silk stay sutures x3 to allow for visualization as well as use of Regnel or similar retractors
18. Position LV vent into left atrium
19. Gently fill the ventricular chambers with cold saline to float the AV valve leaflets to their closed position. This helps identify the line of apposition between the superior and inferior bridging components of the left AV valve which is then approximated with a 6-0 polyproplyene suture.
20. Measure the extent of ventricular defect inferiorly and cut a half-circle shaped Gore-Tex patch.
21. Measure the extent of atrial defect superiorly and cut an appropriate bovine pericardial patch.
22. Examine anterior mitral leaflet cleft and decide on approach for closure.
23. The septal leaflet of the right-sided AV-valve may need to be mobilized to visualize the ventricular defect, if so this will be closed at the completion of the repair.
24. Using a running 6-0 polypropylene close the VSD by placing the stitches on the right ventricular side of the crest of the septum to avoid the left bundle and the AV node.

25. Use interrupted horizontal mattress suture coming from right to left through the Gore-Tex patch, the left-sided AV-valve and the inferior aspect of the bovine pericardial patch and tie these down, thus recreating the AV valve separation.
26. Close the mitral valve cleft with interrupted 6-0 polypropylene.
27. Ensure mitral (and tricuspid) valve is not stenotic (**Note:** Gently pass a Hagar dilator through the orifice, know the z-score for the mitral and tricuspid valves in your patient)
28. Position the LV vent just across the valve into the LV.
29. Using the previous 6-0 polypropylene sutures complete the atrial defect closure.
30. De-air the left side of the heart as much as possible prior to completely closing the ASD.
31. Assess the right-sided AV valve; perform a valvuloplasty with 6-0 polypropylene.
32. Close the right atriotomy with 5-0 polypropylene while re-warming.
33. Institute inotropic support, suction lungs by anesthesia prior to instituting ventilation
34. Remove the cross-clamp and wean off bypass in concert with anesthesia
35. Ensure post-op echo shows acceptable valve function, cardiac function and no residual intra-cardiac shunts
36. Place atrial and ventricular pacing wires
37. Separate from bypass
38. Give protomine and ensure hemostasis and place a chest tube (consider 19 Fr round, fluted Blake drain circling the chest and draining both thoracic spaces)
39. Close chest in standard fashion

Potential Complications and Pitfalls

1. Persistent left superior vena cava may be encountered. If present, this may need to be snared during the repair to allow for visualization. Even in the absence of a bridging vein it may be safe to snare this, though some surgeons may choose to cannulate this as well.
2. The conduction system can be injured and either temporary or permanent heart block may occur. Knowledge of the location of the conduction system is imperative. Superficial bites need to be taken in this area.
3. Mitral stenosis needs to be avoided, thus it is important to ensure that appropriate orifice area is left after mitral cleft closure.
4. The presence of a patent ductus arteriosus should be noted on pre-op TTE or TEE and if present should be dissected carefully and then ligated prior to the induction of cardiopulmonary bypass.
5. The LVOT should also be assessed on pre-op TEE to ensure there is no narrowing.
6. These patients can have pulmonary hypertension that is reactive. This may result into right heart dysfunction and difficulty in weaning from

bypass. It should be diagnosed early and addressed. Nitric oxide (NO) should be in the room and available when initiating ventilation if pulmonary hypertension has been diagnosed or his likely. In the setting of pulmonary hypertension PO2 should be maximized and PCO2 kept low to optimize pulmonary blood flow. Infants brought for repair at an older age are at greater risk for this.

7. There are multiple variations to the surgical management of complete AV canal. This operation can be performed with deep hypothermic circulator arrest. A single patch technique can be used as compared to the double patch technique described herein. The left AV valve ("mitral") valve can be repaired to create a tri-leaflet valve as compared to the bi-leaflet valve, as described herein. If sufficient tissue AV valve tissue is not present, the valve may not be repaired, however this places the patient at risk for valve regurgitation and the need for reoperation and higher long-term mortality.

8. A comment should be made about the appearance of the AV valve leaflets, the repair and the satisfaction with the repair in the operative dictation.

Template Dictation

Preoperative Diagnosis: [INDICATION – Complete atrioventricular canal]

Postoperative Diagnosis: Same

Procedure(s) Performed: Repair of complete atrioventricular canal.

Attending Surgeon: [BLANK]

Secondary Surgeon: [BLANK]

Assistants: [BLANK]

Anesthesia: [BLANK]

Indication(s) for Procedure: [AGE] year old [GENDER] with [DURATION] history of [**COMPLAINT** – e.g. - shortness of breath, **COMORBIDITIES** –e.g.- Down Syndrome]. The patient was discussed at cath conference and it was decided to proceed with surgical intervention. After informed consent was obtained, the patient was set for surgery.

Description of the procedure: After informed consent the patient was brought to the operating room and placed in supine position. After general endotracheal intubation occurred without difficulty, a (**LOCATION**) central line and the (**LOCATION**) arterial line were placed. Systemic IV antibiotics were given. The chest was sterilely prepped and draped in the usual sterile fashion. Standard median sternotomy incision was made. The thymus was removed and the pericardium opened and standard pericardial well was made. At this point, the patient was systemically heparinized. A standard aortic and bicaval venous cannulation were carried out. The patient was placed on cardiopulmonary bypass. An LV vent was placed the right superior pulmonary vein and a cardioplegia needle was placed in midportion ascending aorta. The aorta was cross clamped and cold blood antegrade cardioplegia was given with an excellent diastolic arrest. The caval tapes were snared and the right atrium was opened and a right atriotomy was performed.

We then visualized the complete canal through the right atrium. We began by re-approximating the mid-point of the bridging leaflet that would become the anterior leaflet of mitral valve with a #6-0 polypropylene suture. We then measured out the ventricular septal defect and a half-moon patch of Gore-Tex was obtained. We then closed the ventricular septal defect portion using a running #6-0 polyproplyene suture. At this point, we then obtained a piece of bovine pericardium and trimmed this according to the size of the ASD. Next we placed multiple interrupted horizontal mattress sutures going through the tip of the Gore-Tex patch then through the left-sided AV valve and then through the bovine pericardium. These were then subsequently tied down thus creating the septum of the heart. We then addressed the cleft in the anterior mitral valve leaflet. This was then closed using multiple interrupted #6-0 polypropylene sutures. (**Note:** Make a comment on the appearance and nature of the cleft and the manner and satisfaction with which it was closed). The valve was then tested and did not appear to be stenotic. We were able to put a (SIZE) mm Hegar dilator through the orifice. The ASD was then closed using bovine pericardium and a running #6-0 polypropylene suture. Next we re-approximated the septal leaflet to the septal portion of the patch using a running #6-0 polypropylene suture in 2 layers (**Variation:** There was small PFO, which was closed using a running #6-0 polypropylene suture.) The patient was rewarmed.

The right atriotomy was closed using a running #5-0 polypropylene suture. De-airing maneuvers were performed. The aortic cross-clamp was removed and the patient was subsequently weaned off cardiopulmonary bypass on a (QUANTIFY) amount of inotropic support and excellent hemodynamics. The patient's LV function was (QUANTIFY). The patient (DID/DID NOT) have heart block (**Note:** report the rhythm and rate coming off bypass).

Atrial and ventricular pacing wires were placed (**Note:** "subsequently atrial/AV pacing was/was not utilized). [**Variation:** We did perform modified ultrafiltration for total of (DURATION) minutes with removal of (QUANTIFY) ml of volume taken off]. The protamine was given.

All cannulas were then removed and the purse strings tied and found to be hemostatic. A #19-French Blake drain was placed at the inferior portion incision and sewn in place with #2-0 silk suture then positioned in the chest and subsequently connected to Pleur-evac suction. Adequate hemostasis noted. We then re-approximated the sternum using several interrupted #1 stainless steel wires. The wounds were closed in multiple layers of vicryl followed by monocryl suture followed by benzoin, Steri-Strips and an occlusive dressing.

Instruments, sponges and needles counts were confirmed to be correct following conclusion of the operation. The patient was then transferred to the Cardiac Surgery Intensive Care Unit in a stable fashion.

Dr. **[BLANK]** was present and scrubbed **[BLANK]** elements of this procedure.

5. Repair of Partial Anomalous Pulmonary Venous Return

Thomas Caranasos MD, Mark Bleiweis MD

University of Florida, Gainesville, FL

Essential Operative Steps

1. Preoperative imaging to determine the type of PAPVR, directing repair.
2. Lines and monitoring.
3. General endotracheal anesthesia.
4. Intraoperative TEE to confirm diagnosis.
5. Median Sternotomy.
6. Pericardial well and harvesting of native pericardium (if elected to use pericardium).
7. Identify and dissect Right Sided Pulmonary Veins.
8. Systemic heparinization.
9. Arterial cannulation.
10. Bicaval venous cannulation (High SVC or Innominate vein and IVC cannulation).
11. Antegrade and/or retrograde cardioplegia (direct cannulation after atriotomy) for myocardial protection.
12. Opening the right atrium to allow for repair.
13. Evaluation of the location of the anomalous pulmonary veins and their draining location.
14. Enlarging the Atrial Septal Defect if needed.
15. Creation of a baffle from the ostia of the anomalous pulmonary veins to the left atrium through the Atrial Septal Defect or if needed disconnection of the SVC and drainage of the anomalous pulmonary vein through the ASD and attachment of the SVC to the Right atrium (Warden Procedure).
16. Closure of the right atriotomy.
17. Rewarming, Warm blood cardioplegia "hot shot".
18. Deairing of the left side of the heart.
19. Removal of the aortic cross-clamp.
20. Hemostasis of the atriotomy and/or SVC to Right Atrial connection.
21. Pacer wire placement.
22. Separate from CPB.
23. Venous decannulation.
24. Protamine administration.
25. Aortic decannulation.
26. Chest tube drainage.
27. Hemostasis and sternotomy closure.

Potential Complications and Pitfalls

1. Stay midline during sternotomy.
2. Cannulation catastrophe (aortic dissection/bleeding).

3. Insufficient myocardial protection (inappropriate aortic cross clamp, AI, insufficient venous drainage, persistent LSVC)
4. Coronary sinus injury with retrograde cardioplegia cannulation.
5. Improper visualization of the draining veins.
6. Small ASD limiting flow and creation of a pressure gradient.
7. Improper size of the baffle limiting flow.
8. Patency of the SVC to right atrial connection.
9. Improper deairing.
10. Bleeding from atriotomy.
11. Inadequate control of hemostasis prior to sternal closure.
12. Late obstruction of the pulmonary venous circulation, pulmonary hypertension.
13. Post Operative arrhythmia.

Template Dictation

Preoperative Diagnosis:

1. Partial anomalous pulmonary venous drainage of the right pulmonary veins to the right atrium.
2. Oval fossa atrial septal defect.

Postoperative Diagnosis: Same

Procedure(s) Performed:

1. Repair of partial anomalous pulmonary venous drainage by tunnel repair of the right pulmonary veins through the atrial septal defect using autologous pericardium.
2. Closure of atrial septal defect.

Attending Surgeon: [BLANK]

Secondary Surgeon: [BLANK]

Assistants: [BLANK]

Anesthesia: [BLANK]

Indication(s) for Procedure: [AGE] year old [GENDER] with [DURATION] history of [COMPLAINT – e.g. - newly discovered partial anomalous pulmonary venous drainage of the right pulmonary veins on imaging.] She has evidence of drainage of all the right pulmonary veins directly into the right atrium. There is also a small atrial septal defect. She has a history of polysplenia and developmental delay.

Description of Procedure: After informed consent and patient identification, the patient was brought to the operating room and placed in the supine position. After single lumen general endotracheal tube anesthesia appropriate monitoring lines were placed. Patient was then prepped and draped in the usual sterile fashion.

A median sternotomy incision was made, and dissection carried down to the level of the pericardium. The thymus was subtotally resected. The pericardium was then opened on the left side to preserve the pericardium for baffle repair if necessary. The aorta was separated from the pulmonary artery. The superior vena cava was dissected. A large azygous vein was identified which came in relatively close to the innominate vein. There were no pulmonary veins draining into the superior vena cava. We could identify the right pulmonary veins and they appeared to be in normal position, however they entered the right atrium proper. The patient had one episode of rapid supraventricular arrhythmia and synchronized cardioversion was necessary. The patient resumed a sinus rhythm at that point. Heparin was administered. After placing appropriate pursestring sutures, aortic and superior vena caval cannulation was performed. Cardiopulmonary bypass was instituted and an inferior vena caval cannula was added. An antegrade cardioplegia cannula was placed in the ascending aorta and this was also used as a root vent later in the case. The patient was allowed to drift to a low temperature of 34 degrees centigrade. The aorta was then cross clamped and a smooth diastolic cardiac arrest was achieved using antegrade cold potassium blood cardioplegia. Both caval snares were then applied.

An oblique right atriotomy was made. The retrograde cardioplegia cannula was placed directly into the coronary sinus os and held in place with polypropylene pursestring.

The retrograde cardioplegia was administered every 15-20 minutes during the cross clamp time. The pulmonary venous drainage from the right lung was noted to be to the right atrium. We also ensured that there were no other veins draining on the right side. The left veins drained normally into the left atrium. Since there was a small oval fossa defect, the remaining oval fossa tissue was excised. This produced a widely patent atrial septum. A patch of untreated pericardium was fashioned for baffling of the veins to the left atrium. This was then sutured in place using continuous fine polypropylene suture. The left side of the heart was de-aired prior to tying the knot.

[**Variation: For Warden Procedure**: A superior vena caval snare was placed above the level of the azygous. The azygous vein was controlled with a neurovascular clip. Clamps were placed at the SVC-RA junction. The patient remained in sinus rhythm. The superior vena cava was divided above the level of the pulmonary veins. The cardiac side was over sewn using a continuous polypropylene suture, in two layers, first a running horizontal mattress suture followed by simple continuous technique. The sutures were tied before releasing the clamp to prevent the pursestring effect. This was noted to be hemostatic. Next the aortic cross-clamp was applied, and a smooth diastolic cardiac arrest was achieved using a single dose of antegrade cold potassium blood cardioplegia. The inferior caval snare was applied. An oblique right atriotomy was made, avoiding the right atrial appendage. Superior sinus venosus defect was identified and defect was opened inferiorly and enlarged. We then ran a polypropylene suture to endothelialize the cut surface. Next a patch of autologous untreated pericardium

III. Congenital Cardiac Surgery

was fashioned for the patch closure of the sinus venosus atrial septal defect and baffling of the pulmonary veins to the left atrium. This was sutured in placed using continuous 5-0 polypropylene suture. The left side of the heart was deaired through this site before tying the suture. Then the aortic cross-clamp was removed and deairing was performed via the root vent. Patient resumed normal sinus rhythm spontaneously. Right atrial appendage was opened at its tip. The pectinate muscles were excised to ensure that the right atrial opening was widely patent. The anastomosis between the SVC and the right atrial appendage was constructed using continuous 5-0 polyproplyene suture. The anastomosis appeared to be widely patent and it was suture was tied this over a 10 mm dilator, which was the size of the vena cava. The right atriotomy was closed in two layers. Caval snares were removed and the patient was adequately rewarmed].

A hot shot was initiated in retrograde fashion. During this time, the left side of the heart was deaired. Next we completed the hot shot in an antegrade fashion and removed the retrograde catheter. The right atrial closure was initiated with continuous horizontal mattress polypropylene suture. Caval snares were then removed, the hot shot was completed, and the aortic cross clamp was removed. The right atrial closure was completed with a simple continuous technique. The patient resumed a normal rhythm spontaneously. He/She was rewarmed to normothermia.

An adequate deairing in the heart was ensured by the transesophageal echo. A double lumen right atrial catheter was tunneled from the upper abdomen. It was placed it in the right atrium and fixed in place using two pursestring polypropylene sutures. Patient was successfully weaned from the cardiopulmonary bypass. Post repair transesophageal echocardiogram revealed good biventricular function and no pulmonary venous obstruction.

Modified ultrafiltration was then performed **(Optional)**. The patient was decannulated while heparin was reversed with protamine sulfate. Atrial and ventricular pacing wires were placed. A right pleural drain was placed. A mediastinal chest drain was added. Excellent hemostasis was assured prior to closure. The sternum was reapproximated using interrupted #4 wires.

The presternal fascial, subcutaneous and cutaneous tissue layers were approximated with continuous absorbable sutures. Sterile dressings were applied. Sponges, needles and instruments counts were correct. The patient was taken to the intensive care in a stable condition. Cardiopulmonary bypass time was [BLANK] minutes and total clamp time was [BLANK] minutes.

Dr. [BLANK] was present and scrubbed [BLANK] elements of this procedure.

6. Supra-Cardiac Total Anomalous Pulmonary Venous Return (TAPVR)

Juan M. Lehoux, MD and Carlos M. Mery, MD, MPH

Texas Children's Hospital/Baylor College of Medicine, Houston, TX

Essential Operative Steps

1. Lines and Monitoring.
2. General endotracheal anesthesia.
3. Median sternotomy.
4. Perform partial thymectomy.
5. Open pericardium and set up pericardial well on stay sutures.
6. Dissect out the aorta, ligamentum arteriosum/PDA, SVC, and identify vertical vein.
7. Systemic heparinazation.
8. Bi-caval cannulation (may use single right atrial cannula).
9. Confirm ACT (>400).
10. Start cardiopulmonary bypass.
11. Ligate ligamentum arteriosum/PDA.
12. Cool to 18 degrees.
13. Dissect out the vertical vein.
14. Place apical stitch to aid in retraction of the heart.
15. Dissect out pulmonary venous confluence.
16. Cross clamp the aorta and instill cardioplegia once at desired temperature.
17. Start circulatory arrest.
18. Ligate the vertical vein.
19. Open the venous confluence widely with a longitudinal incision (may extend the incision into the vertical vein) without entering the pulmonary vein orifices.
20. Inspect the pulmonary venous orifices.
21. **Note:** The rest of the procedure may be performed with a combination of circulatory arrest, low-flow cardiopulmonary bypass, and full cardiopulmonary bypass if bicaval cannulation, or under circulatory arrest if single venous cannulation.
22. Snare IVC and SVC if bicaval cannulation; remove atrial cannula if single atrial cannulation.
23. Oblique right atriotomy.
24. Identify ASD.
25. May enlarge the ASD in order to inspect the left atrium and choose the best site for anastomosis.
26. Make incision on the posterior wall of left atrium corresponding to the incision on the pulmonary venous confluence (may include the left atrial appendage depending on the size and lie of the left atrium).
27. Perform anastomosis between pulmonary venous confluence and left atrium with 8-0 polypropylene in running fashion.

III. Congenital Cardiac Surgery

28. Close the ASD using either a patch or primary closure of the septum primum.
29. If single venous cannulation, close the right atriotomy, replace the cannula, and restart CPB.
30. Start rewarming.
31. De-air the left sided chambers.
32. Remove the aortic cross-clamp.
33. Vent the left heart via the left atrial appendage (if not included in the anastomosis) or the patch (prior to complete closure) until the left ventricle regains adequate function.
34. Close the right atriotomy (if bicaval cannulation).
35. May insert LA line through the left atrial appendage (if not included in the anastomosis). May insert PA line if patient had significant obstruction and there are concerns for pulmonary hypertension.
36. Resume ventilation.
37. Wean from cardiopulmonary bypass.
38. Sequential decannulation.
39. Place mediastinal tubes
40. May place peritoneal dialysis catheter to aid in postoperative fluid management
41. Sternal closure.

Potential Complications and Pitfalls

1. Avoid phrenic nerve injury during thymectomy.
2. Do not place too much tension on pericardial well in order to avoid worsening obstruction of the pulmonary veins.
3. Do not ligate vertical vein until in circulatory arrest or after the pulmonary venous confluence is open in order to avoid worsening pulmonary venous congestion.
4. Avoid right phrenic nerve injury when dissecting out the SVC.
5. Completely dissect SVC in order to avoid missing entry of a separate pulmonary vein
6. Make pericardiotomy towards the left side to allow for harvesting of patch material if autologous pericardium is to be used.
7. Limit incision to the venous confluence. Avoid manipulating pulmonary veins.
8. Avoid twisting/kinking of anastomosis.
9. Make anastomosis as wide as possible.
10. Do not allow the left ventricle to distend. Vent heart thru left atrial appendage if possible.
11. LA and/or PA lines may help for postoperative monitoring.
12. Peritoneal dialysis catheter may facilitate postoperative fluid management.

Template Dictation

Preoperative Diagnosis: Obstructed supra-cardiac total anomalous venous return (TAPVR)

Postoperative Diagnosis: Same

Procedure(s) Performed: Repair of obstructed supra-cardiac total anomalous venous pulmonary return via direct anastomosis.

Attending Surgeon: [BLANK]

Secondary Surgeon: [BLANK]

Assistants: [BLANK]

Anesthesia: [BLANK]

Indication(s) for Procedure: [AGE] year old [GENDER] with [DURATION] history of [COMPLAINT – e.g. - acute desaturations into the 70's soon after birth.] Patient was started on non-invasive respiratory support with no improvement. He was emergently intubated and transferred to the NICU. An Echocardiogram was performed which revealed supra-cardiac total anomalous pulmonary venous return with an obstructed vertical vein. Patient was taken urgently to the operating room for repair.

Description of Procedure [using bicaval cannulation]: The patient was brought to the operating room and placed on the operating table in the supine position. General anesthesia was induced. Monitoring lines were placed. The patient was prepped and draped in the usual fashion.

A median sternotomy was performed. A subtotal thymectomy was performed. The pericardium was opened and set on stays to create the pericardial well. A piece of autologous pericardium was harvested for future use. Dissection was performed around the aorta, superior vena cava and the ductus arteriosus. The aorta, superior and inferior vena cava were cannulated for cardiopulmonary bypass. After confirmation of adequate ACT, bypass was initiated. The ductus arteriosus was ligated. The patient was cooled to 18 degrees. During cooling, the vertical vein was identified entering the innominate vein. The vertical vein was dissected and followed inferiorly towards the pulmonary venous confluence. The confluence was dissected out by incising the posterior pericardium. Once the patient was at 18 degrees, the aorta was cross-clamped and antegrade cardioplegia was given. Smooth cardiac arrest was quickly achieved.

A pledgeted 6-0 polypropylene was placed on the apex of the heart to facilitate retraction upwards and rightwards. The dissection of the pulmonary venous confluence was then completed. Circulatory arrest was started and the vertical vein was ligated and divided at its entry point into the innominate vein. The venous confluence was incised longitudinally with care not to incise the individual pulmonary orifices. The veins were individually inspected.

Cardiopulmonary bypass was re-started. The SVC and IVC were snared, the right atrium was incised in the usual fashion. A large secundum ASD was identified. The left atrium was inspected through the ASD. The ideal area for the anastomosis was identified by lining up the left atrial wall to the previously made confluence incision. Special care was taken to avoid torsion at the site of the anastomosis by visualizing the area of the anastomosis from both inside and outside the heart.

The posterior wall of the left atrium was incised longitudinally up to the left atrial appendage mirroring the incision made in the pulmonary venous confluence. Using a combination of circulatory arrest and low-flow cardiopulmonary bypass, the anastomosis was performed between the pulmonary venous confluence and left atrium with 8-0 polypropylene suture in running fashion. After completion of the anastomosis, all 4 pulmonary veins were probed through the ASD and were found to be patent. Full cardiopulmonary bypass was restarted and the patient was rewarmed.

The ASD was closed (primarily/with a patch) using a running [Blank] polyproplyene (The left atrial appendage was incised to vent the left heart.). After de-airing, the cross-clamp was removed. The patient regained a spontaneous sinus rhythm. The right atriotomy was closed with running 6-0 polypropylene (**Optional:** A left atrial line was placed through the left atrial appendage in the usual fashion. A pulmonary arterial line was placed in the main pulmonary artery for pressure monitoring).

Once the patient was warm, ventilation was re-started. Cardiopulmonary bypass was weaned with (careful assessment of left atrial and pulmonary arterial pressures and) very judicious volume monitoring. The venous cannulas were removed. After confirmation of adequate hemodynamics, protamine was given. The aortic cannula was the removed.

A temporary peritoneal catheter and mediastinal tube were inserted. After confirmation of hemostasis, the patient's sternum was closed with steel wire in the usual fashion. The fascia, subcutaneous planes, and skin were closed in layers. The patient tolerated the procedure without complications and transported to the Pediatric Cardiac Intensive

Care Unit in a satisfactory condition. Sponge, needle and instrument counts were correct.

Cardiopulmonary bypass time was **[BLANK]** minutes. Hypothermic circulatory arrest time was **[BLANK]** minutes and cardiac ischemia time of **[BLANK]** minutes.

Dr. **[BLANK]** was present and scrubbed **[BLANK]** elements of this procedure.

7. Total Anomalous Pulmonary Venous Return (TAPVR) - Cardiac Type

Amit Pawale, MD, FRCS (CTh), Khanh Nguyen, MD

Mount Sinai Medical Center, New York, NY, 10029

Essential Operative Steps

1. General endotracheal anesthesia.
2. Median Sternotomy.
3. Partial thymectomy.
4. Opening pericardium, create pericardial well.
5. Systemic heparinization.
6. Aortic and bicaval cannulation.
7. Dissection of ductus arteriosus.
8. Initiation of cardiopulmonary bypass.
9. Ductus ateriosus ligation.
10. Perform right atriotomy.
11. Unroofing of coronary sinus.
12. Closure of atrial septal defect.
13. Weaning from cardiopulmonary bypass.
14. Venous decannulation.
15. Protamine administration and aortic decannulation.
16. Ensure excellent hemostasis.
17. Sternotomy closure.

Potential Complications and Pitfalls

1. Perioperative pulmonary vasodilators are useful to reduce the risk of pulmonary hypertensive crises.
2. Care should be taken dissecting and ligating the ductus arteriosus, as it can rupture during these maneuvers. It should be ligated as soon as initiating the cardiopulmonary bypass to avoid overflowing the pulmonary circulation.
3. A wide communication between the coronary sinus and left atrium should be ensured to prevent future narrowing.
4. During the atrial septal defect closure, care is taken to avoid the area anterior to the coronary sinus because it contains the atrioventricular (AV) node.
5. Postoperative diuretics are given for several days to minimize the pulmonary edema

Template Dictation

Preoperative Diagnosis:

1. Total anomalous pulmonary venous return (TAPVR), cardiac type
2. Patent foramen ovale

3. Patent ductus arteriosus

Postoperative Diagnosis: Same

Procedure(s) Performed:
1. Repair of total anomalous pulmonary venous return (Cardiac Type) with unroofing of coronary sinus ostium.
2. Patch closure of the atrial septal defect.

Attending Surgeon: [BLANK]

Secondary Surgeon: [BLANK]

Assistant: [BLANK]

Anesthesia: [BLANK]

Indication(s) for Procedure: A five month old baby girl, who was born at full term with caesarian section, had an echocardiogram for lower oxygen saturation after the birth. She was diagnosed to have an unobstructed total anomalous pulmonary venous return, with all the pulmonary veins draining into the coronary sinus. She also had atrial septal defect and a patent ductus arteriosus. Since the total anomalous pulmonary venous return was unobstructed type the baby was allowed to grow with close observation over the last five months and an elective repair was performed today.

Operative Findings: The right heart was significantly dilated. The systemic venous drainage was normal. Within the heart there was a small patent foramen ovale. The coronary sinus was severely dilated. After opening the atrial septum and the coronary sinus all 4 pulmonary veins could be seen draining directly into the coronary sinus.

Description of Procedure: After informed consent and patient identification the patient was brought to the operating room and placed on the operating table in a supine position. After induction of general anesthesia with single lumen endotracheal tube intubation, arterial and central venous monitoring lines were placed. The patient was positioned, prepped and draped in surgical sterile fashion. TEE was not performed.

A median sternotomy was performed and the partial thymectomy was undertaken. The pericardium was opened and a segment was harvested for later use in cardiac repair. Intravenous heparin was administered. Ascending aorta and both vena cava were cannulated. Having ascertained adequate ACT, total cardiopulmonary bypass was initiated. A small ductus arteriosus was ligated with a silk ligature. The child's temperature is decreased to 22°C. The aorta was cross-clamped and cold blood cardioplegia was given through the aortic root. A rapid diastolic arrest followed. The cavae were snared and the right atrium was opened with an incision parallel to the atrio-ventricular groove and intracardiac anatomy was noted. The atrial septal defect was found. The septum primum was resected. A vent was placed into the left atrium through the atrial septal defect to decompress the left side of the heart. The coronary sinus ostium was incised and the coronary sinus was completely unroofed to the left atrial chamber. Much of the superior margin of the coronary sinus was resected and the endocardium was reapproximated over the exposed muscle with running fine polypropylele. A piece of autologous pericardial patch was used to close this atrial septal defect with fine polypropelene running suture, such that the coronary sinus drains in to the left atirum. The suture line in the area anterior to coronary sinus was moved away from the edge of the septum into the floor of the coronary sinus to avoid injury to the atrioventricular (AV) node. The left atrial vent was removed and de-airing was performed before tightening the last few sutures. Once the atrial septal defect was closed, the cross-clamp was removed. A normal sinus rhythm returned rapidly. The right atriotomy was closed using running polypropelene suture.

The patient was weaned from cardiopulmonary bypass in sinus rhythm. Excellent hemodynamics were achieved. A left atrial pressure monitoring line was placed via the appendage and a peritoneal dialysis catheter was placed **(Optional)**. Modified hemofiltration was carried out. Single Blake drain was placed in the pericardium. Atrial and Ventricular pacing wires were placed. Sternotomy was closed in layers.

All instrument, sponge and needle counts were confirmed to be correct twice at the end of the operation. The patient was subsequently transferred to the postoperative pediatric cardiac surgical intensive care unit in stable but critical condition.

Dr. **[BLANK]** was present and scrubbed **[BLANK]** elements of this procedure.

8. Infra-Cardiac Total Anomalous Pulmonary Venous Return (TAPVR)

Muhammad Aftab, MD, Jeffrey S. Heinle*, MD

Baylor College of Medicine/Texas Heart Institute, Houston, TX

*Texas Children's Hospital/Baylor College of Medicine, Houston, TX

Essential Operative Steps

1. Lines and Monitoring.
2. General endotracheal anesthesia.
3. Bilateral cerebral near-infrared spectroscopy sensors (NIRS)
4. Transesophageal Echocardiogram (TEE) not performed (concern of compressing pulmonary veins confluence especially in small infants).
5. Median sternotomy.
6. Sub-total thymectomy.
7. Open pericardium, pericardial well.
8. Minimal initial dissection.
9. Systemic heparinization (3-4 mg/Kg).
10. Direct aortic cannulation (**Note:** small aorta-cannulation needs to be precise).
11. Single right atrial venous cannula- for emergent cases; (**Note:** Bicaval cannulation with caval snares – for elective cases)
12. Establish Cardiopulmonary bypass (CPB) circuit.
13. Check ACT >450
14. Initiate Cardiopulmonary bypass.
15. Immediately after initiation of CBP, dissect free and ligate the ductus arteriosus.
16. Slow cooling to 18°C (over 20-30 minutes) in anticipation of deep hypothermic circulatory arrest (DHCA).
17. Divide posterior pericardial attachments and mobilize pulmonary venous confluence while cooling.
18. Identify all four pulmonary veins and encircle the descending vein.
19. Once nasopharyngeal temperature 18°C, pack the head with ice.
20. Cross clamp ascending aorta.
21. Antegrade cold crystalloid cardioplegia with topical cooling.
22. Initiate deep hypothermic circulatory arrest (DHCA).
23. Remove right atrial cannula (If bicaval cannulation, snare both caval tapes.)
24. Rotate the apex of the heart towards patient's right shoulder.
25. Enter the posterior pericardium.
26. Mobilize vertically oriented pulmonary vein confluence.
27. Identify all four veins (with limited dissection on the veins).
28. Suture ligation of the descending vertical vein (**Optional**).
29. Perform right atriotomy and inspect the intracardiac anatomy.

III. Congenital Cardiac Surgery

30. Identify the atrial septal defect (ASD).
31. Longitudinally open the pulmonary venous confluence (steps 32-34 working from outside the heart).
32. Make a corresponding vertically oriented incision on posterior wall of left atrium.
33. Create a left atrium-to-pulmonary venous confluence anastomosis with fine suture and small bites.
34. Ensure a wide open anastomosis and probe the pulmonary veins (looking through right atrium).
35. Resume cardiopulmonary bypass followed by another period of brief circulatory arrest.
36. Harvest the autologous pericardium
37. Clean the redundant tissue [**Variation:** treat the pericardium with 0.6% glutaraldehyde solution for 20-30 min **(optional).**
38. Close the ASD with fresh autologous pericardium.
39. Resume bypass and de-air the left heart as ASD closure is completed.
40. Close the right atriotomy (either on pump sucker bypass or a brief period of DHCA).
41. Place the venous cannula (If single right atrial venous cannulation).
42. Resume full cold cardiopulmonary bypass.
43. Start re-warming after 5 minutes of reperfusion (remove the ice from head).
44. Perform de-airing of heart via aortic root.
45. Place patient in trendelenburg position and remove the aortic cross clamp.
46. Secure atrial/ventricular pacing wires (**Optional:** left atrial and PA lines, if needed).
47. Once re-warmed, resume the ventilation, fill the heart with blood and allow to eject.
48. Wean from CPB, inotropes and vasopressers as needed.
49. Ensure good gas exchange on 100% Oxygen, avoid hypercapnia (Optional: use of nitric oxide).
50. Goal of Pulmonary artery pressure < 2/3 to ½ of systemic pressures, within 15-30 minutes of weaning.
51. Administer protamine and sequential decannulation.
52. Assure excellent hemostasis.
53. Careful volume administration.
54. Place drain. Peritoneal dialysis catheter (**Optional**).
55. Sternal closure (temporary closure, if warranted).

Potential Complications and Pitfalls

1. Patient with obstructed TAPVR are critically ill, and sometimes in extremis, so an expeditious transfer to the operating room is of paramount importance.

2. Special attention should be paid to avoid any inadvertent injury to the phrenic nerves during partial thymectomy and dissecting the SVC.
3. Avoid rapid surface cooling in critically ill patients, as they may fibrillate at higher core body temperatures.
4. Special care should be exercised to avoid any disturbance to the myocardium after opening the pericardium, as any minimal retraction of ventricle can result in ventricular fibrillation.
5. Injury of the pulmonary artery during the cross clamp application should be avoided.
6. Gentle handling of myocardium, while tilting the apex of the heart up and to the right, is essential to avoid any crushing of myocardium (done after cross clamping).
7. Carefully matching incisions should be made on the pulmonary venous confluence and the posterior left atrial wall, such that the atriotomy should fall directly on the common venous confluence opening once heart resumes its normal position in the pericardium.
8. It is of paramount importance to insure a wide open left atrium-to-pulmonary venous confluence anastomosis.
9. To allow a widely patent anastomosis, the vertical incision on pulmonary venous confluence can be extended onto pulmonary vein or alternatively vertical vein can be divided to better conform the anastomosis. Similarly, the corresponding left atriotomy can be extended superiorly into the left atrial appendage. Left atriotomy should not be extended too close to mitral annulus, as this can result in injury to the circumflex coronary artery.
10. In the presence of a wide patent anastomosis, initially elevated pulmonary artery pressure should drop to < 2/3 of systemic pressures within 30 minutes of weaning from the CPB. Persistently elevated near systemic pulmonary artery pressure should be concerning for an obstructed anastomosis.
11. A secure and well hemostatic anastomosis is critical. Any anastomotic reinforcements in this area are technically very challenging and can also potentially distort the anastomosis.
12. Patients with TAPVR usually have small left heart chambers, so volume administration should be used judiciously and large volume administration should be avoided post-operatively.

Template Dictation

Preoperative Diagnosis:

1. Infra-cardiac total anomalous venous return (TAPVR), [**Variation:** Obstructed]
2. Secundum ASD (**Variation:** Patent foramen Ovale)
3. Patent ductus arteriosus
4. Cardiogenic shock

III. Congenital Cardiac Surgery

Postoperative Diagnosis: Same.

Drainage: Mediastinal chest tube(s).

Attending Surgeon: [BLANK]

Secondary Surgeon: [BLANK]

Assistant: [BLANK]

Anesthesia: [BLANK]

Procedure(s) Performed:
1. Emergent repair of obstructed infra-cardiac total anomalous pulmonary venous connection.
2. Autologous Pericardial patch closure of secundum atrial septal defect.
3. Ligation of patent ductus arteriosus.
4. Placement of temporary non-tunneled peritoneal dialysis catheter **(Optional)**
5. Placement of temporary pulmonary artery pressure monitoring line **(Optional)**
6. Placement of temporary left atrial pressure monitoring line **(Optional)**

Indication(s) for Procedure: This is an eight hours-old infant who was transferred from [BLANK] hospital to the neonatal intensive care unit at [BLANK] hospital [approximately one hour] prior to the initiation of this procedure. He/she was noted to be in extremis with oxygen saturations in the 50s, profound hypotension, and severe metabolic acidosis. Chest x-ray demonstrated severe bilateral pulmonary edema and echocardiogram showed obstructed infracardiac total anomalous pulmonary venous return. The patient was emergently/urgently taken to the cardiac operating room for repair.

Operative Findings: A thymus was present and there was atrial situs solitus with normal systemic venous return. There was severe pulmonary edema and hemorrhage. The pulmonary venous return was abnormal in that there was no direct pulmonary venous connection to the left atrium. All 4 pulmonary veins were identified draining to a vertically oriented confluence in the midline posterior to the pericardium. The confluence then drained inferiorly with a large descending vein traversing the diaphragm. The confluence was dilated and severely thickened. The ascending aorta was relatively hypoplastic and there was a patent ductus arteriosus. The right atrium was dilated. On intracardiac examination there was a large secundum atrial septal defect [**Variation:** sometimes there is just a PFO).

Repair consisted of a direct anastomosis between the vertically oriented confluences to an incision in the posterior left atrium. The atrial septal defect was augmented with an autologous pericardial patch. Post-repair pulmonary artery pressures were approximately one-half systemic.

Description of the Procedure: After informed consent and patient identification the patient was emergently brought to the operating room and placed on the operating table in a supine position. After induction of general anesthesia, the patient was intubated. Additional arterial and venous access was obtained. Transesophageal echo study not performed. The patient was then positioned supine, prepped, and draped in a standard sterile fashion. A complete median sternotomy was performed. A subtotal thymectomy was carried out. The pericardium was opened and a pericardial well was created. [**Variation:** Patient was in extremis, so monitoring lines were not obtained prior to sternotomy. An expeditious median sternotomy was performed and the thymus was removed. The pericardium was opened and a 2.5F arterial pressure monitoring line was placed in the aortic arch].

After preliminary dissection, pursestring sutures were placed in the ascending aorta and right atrial appendage. Heparin was administered and the ascending aorta and right atrium were directly cannulated utilizing single right atrial cannula [**Variation:** Bicaval cannulation was performed and both cavae were encircled with umbilical tapes]. These cannulae were secured, de-aired and connected to the bypass circuit. Having ascertained an adequate anticoagulation bypass was initiated. The ductus arteriosus was circumferentially dissected and ligated with a heavy silk ligature. A piece of fresh autologous pericardium was harvested for future use. The patient was slowly cooled to a nasopharyngeal temperature of 18°C over approximately 30 minutes. As we were cooling, posterior pericardial attachments were divided and the pulmonary venous confluence was mobilized. Then all four pulmonary veins were identified and the descending vein was encircled. After reaching a nasopharyngeal temperature of 18°C, the head was packed in ice. The ascending aorta was then cross-clamped and the myocardium was protected with cold crystalloid cardioplegia administered antegrade in the aortic root. A rapid diastolic arrest occurred. Additional cardioplegia was given at regular intervals during the crossclamp period.

The child was exsanguinated into the venous reservoir initiating a period of deep hypothermic circulatory arrest (DHCA). The right atrial cannula was removed, a right atriotomy was created and the intracardiac anatomy was inspected. [**Variation:** If bicaval cannulation: The caval tapes were snare. An oblique right atriotomy incision was performed and the intracardiac anatomy was inspected]. There was a large secundum atrial septal defect, which was further enlarged by incising the septum primum. The left atrium was inspected and was relatively small. The apex of the heart was rotated to the right shoulder and the vertically oriented pulmonary venous confluence was further mobilized. The descending vertical vein was suture ligated with 5/0 polypropylene, at the point where it pierces the diaphragm (**optional**).The vertically oriented pulmonary venous confluence was opened longitudinally with the incision carried on to the descending vertical vein. A corresponding vertically oriented incision was created on the posterior wall of the left atrium. Working from outside of the heart, a direct left atrium to pulmonary venous confluence anastomosis was accomplished with running 7-0 Prolene. A large connection was created. Looking back through the left atrium, the anastomosis was noted to be widely patent and the pulmonary veins were easily probed.

The harvested autologous pericardial patch was used to close the atrial septal defect with a running fine polypropylene suture. Cardiopulmonary bypass was resumed, on pump sucker bypass, and left-sided cardiac chambers were deaired as the atrial septal closure was completed. [**Variation:** Another brief period of circulatory arrest was utilized to close the right atrium]. The right atriotomy incision was closed using running Prolene suture and the right atrial cannula was replaced [**Variation** for Bicaval cannulation: Cardiopulmonary bypass was resumed. The harvested autologous pericardial patch was used to close the atrial septal defect with a running fine polypropylene suture. Prior to completing the suture line, the left-sided cardiac chambers were de-aired. Additional de-airing was carried out through the cardioplegia site in the ascending aorta. The right atriotomy incision was closed using running 6/0 Prolene suture].

The patient was then reperfused on full cold cardiopulmonary bypass for five minutes, removed the ice from the head, and then commenced rewarming. The heart was de-aired, patient was placed in trendelenburg position and the the aortic cross clamp was removed. A normal sinus rhythm returned rapidly. Temporary atrial epicardial pacing wires were placed. Additional de-airing was carried out through the cardioplegia site in the ascending aorta. [**Variation:** During rewarming, a left atrial monitoring catheter was placed via the left atrial appendage. A temporary pulmonary artery monitoring catheter was placed].

After complete rewarming, the lungs were ventilated and the heart was allowed to fill and eject. Patient was weaned from cardiopulmonary bypass without difficulty and with good hemodynamics. There was excellent gas exchange, and pulmonary artery pressures were approximately one-half systemic with/without the use of inhaled nitric oxide]. Protamine was given and the heart was sequentially decannulated. [**Variation:** A pressure monitoring line had been placed in the right atrial appendage immediately after weaning from bypass. **Note:** If arterial monitoring lines were not obtained prior to sternotomy; A 2.5F left femoral arterial catheter was replaced and the line in the aortic arch was removed.] A temporary non-tunneled peritoneal dialysis catheter (**Optional**) and mediastinal chest drains were placed. Hemostasis was assured. The sternal edges were reapproximated using stainless steel wires. The soft tissues were closed in multiple layers using running absorbable suture. The skin edges were reapproximated using a running absorbable subcuticular stitch. [**Variation:** If temporary sternal closure was performed: The sternum was supported in an open position with a strut fashioned from a 20 French chest tube and the skin was closed with a Gore-Tex membrane and then a sterile occlusive dressing applied]. The patient tolerated the procedure without complications. He was left intubated and was transported to the Pediatric Cardiac Intensive Care Unit in satisfactory condition. Sponge, needle and instrument counts were correct.

Cardiopulmonary bypass time was **[BLANK]** minutes, with a cross-clamp period of **[BLANK]** minutes. There were two/three periods of circulatory arrest of **[BLANK]** minutes each. The total circulatory arrest time was **[BLANK]** minutes.

Dr. **[BLANK]** was present and scrubbed **[BLANK]** elements of this procedure.

9. Patent Ductus Arteriosus Ligation

John R Spratt, MA, MD and Robroy MacIver, MD, MPH

University of Minnesota, Minneapolis, MN

Essential Operative Steps

1. Ensure adequate anesthesia/ nursing/ OR staff support if performing procedure in NICU
2. General endotracheal anesthesia with single-lumen tube
3. Right-lateral decubitus postioning.
4. Posterolateral thoracotomy incision, sparing latissimus and serratus if possible.
5. Enter left chest via third or fourth intercostal space.
6. Retract left upper and left lower lobes laterally.
7. Identify takeoff of head vessels and descending aorta as landmarks for incision of parietal pleura.
8. Divide crossing vein if necessary.
9. Expose duct with pleural retraction sutures.
10. Apply clip across duct.
11. Alternatively, encircle and tie off ductus.
12. Ensure hemostasis.
13. Place left chest tube or JP drain.
14. Re-approximate ribs with single suture.
15. Closure of muscle, fascia scarpa and skin incision in layers.

Potential Complications and Pitfalls

1. Consider performing in the NICU if patient requires oscillatory ventilation.
2. Failure to completely dissect can lead to incomplete ligation of duct by hemoclip, causing persistent flow.
3. Large ductus may be confused for aortic arch, leading to inappropriate ligation.
4. Each element of the arch should be identified prior to ligation. A large ductus may cause the aortic isthmus to be identified as the left subclavian and the left pulmonary artery as the ductus.
5. Division of periductal lymphatics may lead to chylothorax
    a. Higher risk in patients with upper respiratory infections.
    b. May benefit from the reapproximation of pleura.
6. Use of cautery around the ductus carries the risk of recurrent laryngeal nerve injury.

Template Dictation

Preoperative diagnosis: Patent ductus arteriosus

Postoperative diagnosis: Same

Procedure(s) Performed: Ligation of patent ductus arteriosus

Attending Surgeon: [BLANK]

Secondary Surgeon: [BLANK]

Assistants: [BLANK]

Specimens: [BLANK]

Fluids: [BLANK]

EBL: [BLANK]

Complications: [BLANK]

Drains: [BLANK]

Disposition: [BLANK]

Indication(s) for Procedure: Baby [NAME] is a [AGE/ GENDER] born at [GESTATIONAL AGE] with [HISTORY]. This child has been in the Newborn Intensive Care Unit with a persistent ductus arteriosus and pulmonary overcirculation, and was referred for surgical therapy. A lengthy preoperative consultation was carried with the patient's parents detailing the anatomy, planned surgery, and attendant perioperative risks. All of their questions were answered, and they were in favor of proceeding with the operation.

Operative Findings: There was significant chest wall and soft tissue edema. The lungs were morphologically normal but stiff, noncompliant and edematous. There was a moderate to large size patent ductus arteriosus with a normal-appearing aortic arch.

Description of Procedure: The patient was in the Newborn Intensive Care Unit intubated and sedated. After informed consent and patient identification, the patient was then moved into a right lateral decubitus position and the left chest was prepped and draped in the usual sterile fashion. A time out was performed, confirming the patient and procedure to be performed; all team members were in agreement.

A posterolateral thoracotomy incision was made and carried down to the chest wall. The latissimus muscle was divided in the line of the incision; care was taken to spare the serratus. The fourth intercostal space was identified and entered, taking care not to injure the underlying lung. A small Finochietto retractor was placed and narrow malleable retractors were used to retract the lung anteriorly and inferiorly, exposing the mediastinal pleura and aorta. The parietal pleura overlying the ductus was carefully opened, taking care not to damage the recurrent laryngeal nerve. The ductus was then identified between the aortic arch and the left main pulmonary artery and freed from surrounding structures. A single large hemoclip was applied across the ductus, completing the ligation [Note: Mention any hemodynamic changes]. A Jackson-Pratt drain was placed in the pleural cavity, brought out through the chest wall, and secured to the skin with nylon suture. The retractors were removed and the left lung was noted to re-inflate appropriately. The ribs were re-approximated with a single 2-0 pericostal suture, which was followed by reapproximation of the latissimus with running 4-0 vicryl. The skin was then closed using running subcuticular stitch and Dermabond was placed on the wound. The sponge and needle counts were correct at the end of the case. The patient will remain in the neonatal intensive care unit.

Dr. [BLANK] was present and scrubbed [BLANK] elements of this procedure.

10. Aortic Coarctation Repair with Extended End-to-End Anastomosis

Muhammad Aftab, MD, Ismael Alejandro Salas De Armas, MD, Carlos M. Mery*, MD, MPH

Baylor College of Medicine/Texas Heart Institute, Houston, TX

*Texas Children's Hospital/Baylor College of Medicine, Houston, TX

Essential Operative Steps

1. Lines and Monitoring.
2. General endotracheal anesthesia.
3. Right arterial radial line.
4. Blood pressure cuffs and pulse oxymeter in all extremities.
5. Right lateral decubitus position (for left-sided aortic arch).
6. Serratus-sparing left posterolateral thoracotomy.
7. Enter left pleural space through the 3rd or 4th intercostal space.
8. Retract the lung anteriorly to expose posterior mediastinum.
9. Longitudinal incision on the posterior parietal pleura, posterior to the vagus nerve, to expose the descending aorta and left subclavian artery. Ligate and divide the vein and lymphatic vessel that usually cross the base of the left subclavian artery.
10. Ligate and divide or cauterize any lympathic channels encountered.
11. Dissect the ductus arteriosus.
12. Identify and protect the recurrent laryngeal nerve.
13. If non-patent, ligate and divide the ligamentum arteriosum. If there is a patent ductus arteriosus, preserve at this time.
14. Widely mobilize the aorta from the level of the innominate artery onto the mid descending thoracic aorta.
15. Identify and preserve the intercostals vessels (may need to be looped with atraumatic snares). Some intercostal vessels in the area of the anastomosis may need to be ligated and divided.
16. Systemic heparinization (1 mg/Kg).
17. Allow the temperature of the child to drift down to ~35°C for additional spinal cord protection.
18. Ligate the ductus arteriosus (if left intact).
19. Place a C-clamp around the proximal aortic arch (just distal to the innominate artery), the left carotid artery, and the left subclavian artery. The left subclavian artery may also be controlled separately with an atraumatic snare.
20. Clamp the descending thoracic aorta below the level of coarctation.
21. Excise the coarctation segment and all ductal tissue.
22. Extend the proximal aortotomy onto the undersurface of the arch - to a point opposite to the origin of left common carotid artery.

23. Incise the distal aortotomy on its lateral aspect of to accommodate to proximal aortotomy.
24. Construct an extended end-to-end anastomosis.
25. De-air the aorta prior to completing the suture line with either heparinized saline solution or by unsnaring one of the intercostal vessels on the field.
26. Remove clamps and check for hemostasis.
27. Check pressure gradient between upper and lower extremities.
28. Approximate the parietal pleura.
29. Place a pleural drain.
30. Chest closure

Potential Complications and Pitfalls

1. Neonates with critical aortic coarctation are usually critically ill. If possible, an appropriate resuscitation in the Intensive Care Unit including prostaglandin to reopen the closing ductus arteriosus should be performed prior to the surgery. If the child is older or the ductus arteriosus is not responding to prostaglandin, urgent surgical intervention may be required.
2. Special attention should be paid to avoid any inadvertent injury to the vagus and recurrent laryngeal nerves during the dissection of the aortic isthmus and ductus arteriosus.
3. Gentle handling of the tissue is necessary to avoid inadvertent injury to the pulmonary artery, the ductus, or the aorta during ductus ligation.
4. The proximal aorta should be adequately mobilized. The proximal clamp onto the ascending aorta should be applied just distal to the innominate artery, so that the incision on the lesser curvature of the aorta can be extended proximally as far as the origin of the left common carotid.
5. Careful dissection should be performed during aortic mobilization, as intercostals arteries are usually enlarged and bronchial arteries sometimes arise from the posterior surface of aorta. An inadvertent injury to these thin walled vessels can result into the troublesome bleeding.
6. To prevent any tension on the aortic anastomosis suture line, the descending aorta should be mobilized as far distally as possible and atraumatic snares should be used to control collateral vessels that will be in the field of the anastomosis.
7. It is important to ensure that all coarctation and ductal tissue has been removed to prevent recurrent coarctation.
8. The descending aortotomy is enlarged laterally so that it will match to the size of proximal aortotomy.
9. Using absorbable suture or interrupted suture technique rather than a running monofilament non-absorbable suture anastomosis has not been shown to decrease the incidence of recurrent coarctation.
10. To minimize the risk of paraplegia the core body temperature should be allowed to drift to or below 35°C by keeping the room cold, utilizing cooling blankets and irrigation of the surgical field with cold saline. The

blood pressure proximal to the clamp should be allowed to be slightly higher than normal during the clamping period to allow distal collateral flow. Distal circulatory support (left heart bypass) should be used in older children if clamp time is anticipated to be more than 30 minutes.
11. If the proximal aortic arch (between the innominate artery and the left carotid artery) is hypoplastic as defined by a Z-score < -2 or an absolute size in mm less than the weight of the child in kilograms plus 1, consideration should be made to doing the repair through a median sternotomy and under cardiopulmonary bypass.

Template Dictation

Preoperative Diagnosis: Coarctation of the aorta.

Postoperative Diagnosis: Same

Procedure(s) Performed: Aortic coarctation repair with an extended end-to-end anastomosis.

Drainage: Left pleural chest tube.

Attending Surgeon: [BLANK]

Secondary Surgeon: [BLANK]

Assistants: [BLANK]

Anesthesia: [BLANK]

Indication(s): This is a [BLANK]-year/month/day old child who presented with [BLANK]. The workup revealed a moderate-severe coarctation of the aorta **[Variation: and patent ductus arteriosus/intracardiac anomalies]**. He/She was referred for surgical evaluation. The preoperative evaluation demonstrated an area of severe coarctation just distal to the isthmus with a peak velocity of **[BLANK]**. In addition, the pulses on his/her lower extremities were significantly diminished and there was a gradient on cuff pressures of **[BLANK]**. He/she was recommended surgical intervention.

Operative Findings: There was a left aortic arch with normal branching pattern. There was a severe juxta-ductal aortic coarctation. The coarctation was repaired with resection and extended end-to-end anastomosis, taking the proximal extent of the anastomosis into the distal aortic arch. Distal pulses were palpable and there was no blood pressure gradient between upper and lower extremities at the end of the procedure.

Description of Procedure: After obtaining appropriate consent, the patient was brought to the operating room and placed in supine position. Single lumen general endotracheal tube anesthesia was induced and necessary monitoring lines including a right radial arterial line were placed. The patient was placed on right lateral decubitus position and the left chest was prepped and draped. A serratus-sparing left posterolateral thoracotomy incision was performed and the left pleural space was entered through the third/fourth intercostal space. The lung was retracted anteriorly to expose the posterior mediastinum. The posterior mediastinal pleura was incised to expose the aorta. The aorta was then widely mobilized from the level of the innominate artery onto the mid descending thoracic aorta. The ligamentum arteriosum/ductus arteriosus was dissected, with care to avoid injuring the recurrent laryngeal nerve. **[The ligamentum arteriosum was suture-ligated and divided to facilitate mobilization.]** The above findings were noted. During dissection, the patient's nasopharyngeal temperature was allowed to fall to 35 degrees centigrade. Intravenous steroids were administered. The ligamentum arteriosum was suture ligated. Systemic heparin was administered at 100 IU/kg (1mg/kg). **[Variation: The first set of intercostal vessels below the coarctation were suture ligated and divided.]** All intercostal vessels expected to be within the clamped area were controlled with atraumatic snares **[Variation: The ductus arteriosus was suture-ligated]**. The proximal aortic arch, left carotid artery, and left subclavian artery were clamped with a Castaneda-type vascular clamp. The descending thoracic aorta was clamped below the level of the coarctation. The coarctation segment was excised. All ductal tissue was removed. The proximal aortotomy was extended onto the undersurface of the distal aortic arch to a point just opposite the distal left common carotid artery. The descending aorta was spatulated appropriately and then a long, sliding, extended end-to-end anastomosis was carried out with a fine running polypropylene suture. Prior to completing the suture line, the aorta was de-aired with heparinized saline solution. The suture line was completed. The vascular clamps were sequentially removed and the snares on the intercostal vessels were removed. There were excellent pulsations in the descending thoracic aorta. After the completion of the anastomosis the blood pressure gradient between upper and lower extremities was assessed and there was no significant gradient. Hemostasis was assured. The posterior mediastinum was irrigated with warm antibiotic saline irrigation. The pleural edges were reapproximated using running polypropylene suture. A **[BLANK]** French chest tube was placed through a separate incision and secured to the skin. The lung was re-expanded. The rib edges were reapproximated using interrupted absorbable pericostal sutures. Serratus anterior fascia, latissimus dorsi muscle, and subcutaneous tissue were reapproximated using running absorbable suture. The skin edges were approximated using a running absorbable subcuticular stitch. Dermabond skin adhesive was applied. The patient tolerated the procedure without complications. He/She was transported to the Pediatric Cardiac Intensive Care Unit in a satisfactory condition.

The aortic cross-clamp time was **[BLANK]** minutes. All instruments, sponges and needles counts were confirmed to be correct x 2 at the end of the case.

Dr. **[BLANK]** was present and scrubbed for **[BLANK]** elements of this operation.

Suggested Readings:

1. Khonsari S, Sintek CF. **Cardiac Surgery: Safeguards and Pitfalls in Operative Technique. 4th ed**. Philadelphia, PA: Lippincott Williams & Wilkins; 2008, p 209-217.

2. E. L. Bove and J. C. Hirsch. **Surgery for Congenital Heart Defects by** J. Stark and M. de Leval, VT Tsang. John Wiley & sons, Ltd; 2006, p 285-298.

3. Kaiser, Larry R.; Kron, Irving L.; Spray, Thomas L. **Mastery of Cardiothoracic Surgery**, 2nd Edition. Lippincott Williams & Wilkins; 2007. P 769-778

4. Backer CL, Kaushal S, Mavroudis S. Coarctation of the Aorta. In: Mavroudis C, Backer CL (eds). Pediatric Cardiac Surgery, 4th edition. Wiley-Blackwell; 2013, p 256-282.

III. Congenital Cardiac Surgery

11. Division of Vascular Ring

Wissam Raad, MD, MRCS[1,2] and Samuel Weinstein MD, MBA[1,2]

1. Montefiore-Einstein Center for Heart and Vascular Care, New York, NY
2. Albert Einstein College of Medicine, New York, NY

Essential Operative Steps

1. Lines and Monitoring
2. General endotracheal anesthesia
3. Appropriate positioning
4. Posterolateral thoracotomy
5. Identify aortic arch and descending aorta
6. Identify subclavian and carotid vessels, confirm presence of the ring
7. Confirm ligamentum arteriousm or patent ductus, if present
8. Divide the ring
9. Free the esophagus from adhesions
10. Chest tube
11. Close ribs, approximate the chest wall in layers

Potential Complications and Pitfalls

1. Avoid injury to the neurovascular bundle upon entering the chest
2. Identify and avoid injury to the vagus nerve
3. Identify and avoid injury to the recurrent laryngeal nerve
4. Avoid injury to the esophagus

Template Dictation

Preoperative Diagnosis: Vascular ring [**INDICATION** – e.g. stridor, dysphagia]

Postoperative Diagnosis: Same

Procedure(s) Performed: Division of vascular ring (**DETAILS** – e.g. PDA ligation)

Attending Surgeon: [BLANK]

Secondary Surgeon: [BLANK]

Assistants: [BLANK]

Anesthesia: [BLANK]

Indication(s) for Procedure: [AGE] year old [GENDER] with [DURATION] history of [**COMPLAINT** – e.g. increasingly worse stridor and shortness of breath]. Preoperative CT scan or echocardiogram reveals [**FINDINGS** - e.g. a descending right aorta with a rightward ductus] or barium swallow reveals

[FINDINGS - e.g. posterior indentation of the esophagus].

Description of Procedure: After informed consent the patient was taken to the operating room on [DATE]. The patient's identity and planned procedure were verified, and the patient was placed on the operating room table in a supine position. General anesthesia was induced. A right/left internal jugular central venous line and a right/left radial arterial line were inserted. The patient was then turned to the right/left, an axillary roll was placed underneath to protect the axilla and to prevent brachial plexus injury. We then proceeded to prep and drape the chest in the usual sterile fashion. A time out was performed. The right [**Variation:** in case of left arch and right ductus] or the left [**Variation:** in case of double arch with left-sided ligamentum, or in case of a right arch with retroesophageal component] chest was opened through a posterolateral thoracotomy. The latissimus dorsi was divided partially. Electrocautery was used for hemostasis. The serratus anterior muscle was spared, and the fourth intercostal space was entered. The lung was held anteriorly with stay sutures.

Variation: Right aortic arch with retroesophageal component. The descending aorta, ligamentum and vessels were all identified after opening of the chest. The ligamentum was mobilized from around the esophagus and divided. Clamping of this vessel does not result at all in blood pressure change in the arterial line in the left subclavien artery, and there is no change in the blood pressure cuff in the left arm. The vessel was then divided and ligated. Upon division it was obvious that there was ductal tissue within the structure. After division of the vessel the esophagus is relieved of the tethering. The incidental adhesions were taken down further to allow mobilization and freedom of the ring.

Variation: Left aortic arch and right sided ligamentum arteriosum. The descending aorta on the right was easily encountered. The vessels branching from the aortic arch were mobilized and identified. There was an additional vessel that leaves the aorta medially opposite the right subclavian branch and enters the pericardium towards the pulmonary artery. This vessel encircles the esophagus and there is obvious tension upon it. This vessel was mobilized and was temporarily clamped. Clamping of this vessel did not result in blood pressure change in the arterial line in the left subclavien artery, and there was no change in the blood pressure cuff in the right subclavian artery. Temporary clamping of the right subclavian artery does result in a blood pressure change in the blood pressure cuff in the right arm. The vessel was then divided and ligated taking care to avoid injury to the recurrent laryngeal nerve. Upon division it was obvious that there was ductal tissue within the structure [**Note:** This is the usual case for a vascular ring]. After division of the vessel the esophagus was relieved of the tethering. The incidental adhesions are further taken down to allow mobilization and freedom of the ring.

Variation: Double arch with left-sided ligamentum arteriosum. The atretic arch was easily identified after the thoracotomy. The arch vessels were identified from each limb of the aorta, and the posterior limb of the aorta was seen descending behind the esophagus. The arch was then divided between clamps close to its junction with the descending aorta to maintain patency of the arch vessels. Both ends were oversewn with two rows of 4-0 polypropylene sutures. Tissue bands were then divided away from the trachea and esophagus. The ligamentum arteriosum is divided, taking care to avoid injury to the recurrent laryngeal nerve.

A Marcaine block was given to the intercostal region. A 16-French straight chest tube was placed, and the ribs were approximated with #1 Vicryl. The remainder of the chest wall was closed in layers in the usual fashion. The fascia was then closed with #1 Vicryl suture in a running fashion. The deep dermal layer was then closed with #2-0 Vicryl suture in running fashion. The skin and subcuticular layer was closed with #3-0 Monocryl in running fashion. The skin of the wound was cleansed with sterile saline and dressed with antibiotic ointment and a sterile dressing. All instrument, sponge and needle counts were confirmed to be correct x 2 at the end of the operation. The patient was subsequently transferred to the postoperative pediatric cardiac surgical intensive care unit in critical condition.

Dr. [BLANK] was present and scrubbed for [BLANK] elements of this procedure.

12. Pulmonary Artery Banding

Raghav Murthy MD., Vinod Sebastian MD.

Children's Medical Center of Dallas, Texas.

Essential Operative Steps

1. Lines and monitoring.
2. General endotracheal anesthesia.
3. Median sternotomy.
4. Total/subtotal thymectomy.
5. Ligation of patent ductus arteriosus, if present.
6. Dissection of the pulmonary artery from the aorta.
7. Placement of band at the proximal pulmonary artery.
8. Depending on the specific lesion being palliated, adjustment of the band until the pressure distal to the band is 1/3 to ½ systemic pressure with an arterial oxygen saturation no less than 75% on 40% FiO2.
9. The constriction site of the band is secured with a hemoclip or permanent sutures.
10. The band is secured to the adventitia of the main pulmonary artery.
11. Assess hemostasis.
12. Mediastinal blake drain placement and closure of the pericardium.
13. Sternotomy closure.

Potential Complications and Pitfalls

1. Excessive banding may result in unacceptable cyanosis and hemodynamic collapse.
2. Inadequate banding may lead to persistent pulmonary overcirculation, possible pulmonary vascular disease and failure to thrive.
3. Placing the band too proximally can result into an incompetent pulmonary valve. This can also pose a problem during the debanding procedure. The sinus portion of the pulmonary artery often needs to be patched during the de-banding operation.
4. To avoid the band migration, the band should be sewn to the adventitia of the pulmonary artery. Band migration causes narrowing of the bifurcation and/or kinking/obstruction of the right pulmonary artery.
5. Damage from the band: Band material can potentially cut through the pulmonary artery and produce hemorrhage.
6. In case of difficulty in passing the band around the pulmonary artery, the 'subtraction technique' can be used to facilitate placement of the band around the pulmonary artery. The band is first passed around both the pulmonary artery and the aorta through the transverse sinus and then passed between the pulmonary artery and the aorta. This maneuver avoids passing a right angle solely around the friable pulmonary artery.

III. Congenital Cardiac Surgery

Template Dictation

Preoperative diagnosis: [Blank]

(**Possible Indications** –Swiss cheese ventricular septal defect, tricuspid atresia with normally related great vessels with pulmonary overcirculation, multiple ventricular septal defects with coarctation)

Postoperative diagnosis: Same

Procedure(s) Performed: Pulmonary artery banding

Attending Surgeon: [BLANK]

Secondary Surgeon: [BLANK]

Assistants: [BLANK]

Anesthesia: [BLANK]

Indication(s) for Procedure: [Age] week old [Gender] with history of [Complaint/Diagnosis].

Description of the Procedure: The patient was brought to the operation room on [Date]. The patient's identity and planned procedure were verified and the patient was placed supine on the operating table. General anesthesia was administered. Monitoring lines and foley catheter were placed. The chest and abdomen were prepped and draped in the usual sterile manner. A time out was performed. A median sternotomy was then performed. A total/subtotal thymectomy was performed. The pericardium was opened in the midline and a pericardial cradle created.

The patent ductus arteriosus was dissected out, ligated and divided (if present). The aorta and the pulmonary artery were then separated with cautery. The main pulmonary artery was then encircled circumferentially by blunt dissection [**Variation:** If difficulty is encountered while dissecting the main pulmonary artery the 'subtraction technique' can be used]. The banding material [**Options:** Teflon impregnated Dacron, Silastic or 3mm ePTFE] is passed around both the aorta and the pulmonary artery in the transverse sinus. The aorta is then dissected and the band was brought in between the pulmonary artery and the aorta. The band is sequentially tightened using hemoclips or 5-0 prolene sutures [**Note:** The approximate circumference of the band is determined using the Trusler's formula: 20mm+child's weight in kilograms]. Once the distal pulmonary artery pressure was reduced to 1/3 to ½ systemic pressure and the systemic arterial saturation was greater than 75% on 40% inspired oxygen the constriction site of the band was secured with a hemoclip or 5-0 prolene suture. With this a 10-15 mm of Hg rise in systemic arterial pressure was seen. The band was then secured to the adventitia of the main pulmonary artery using 6-0 prolene suture.

Hemostasis was confirmed. A mediastinal blake drain was placed. The median sternotomy was closed with stainless steel wires. The fascia was closed using 2-0 vicryl, the subcutaneous tissue using 3-0 vicryl and the skin was approximated using 4-0 vicryl in a subcuticular manner. Sterile dressing was applied to the incision.

All the needles, sponges and instruments counts were found to be correct at the end of the procedure. The patient was transferred to the intensive care unit in a stable condition.

Dr. [BLANK] was present and scrubbed for [BLANK] elements of this procedure.

III. Congenital Cardiac Surgery

13. Modified Blalock-Taussig Shunt (Using Interposition Gore-Tex Tube Graft)

Muhammad Aftab, MD, Ismael Alejandro Salas De Armas, MD, Carlos M. Mery*, MD, MPH

Baylor College of Medicine/Texas Heart Institute, Houston, TX

*Texas Children's Hospital/Baylor College of Medicine, Houston, TX

Essential Operative Steps
1. Lines and Monitoring.
2. General endotracheal anesthesia.
3. Left radial/femoral/pre-existing umbilical arterial line.

OPTION A: RIGHT THORACOTOMY
- A4. Left lateral decubitus position.
- A5. Serratus-sparing right posterolateral thoracotomy.
- A6. Enter left pleural space through 4th intercostal space.
- A7. Retract the lung inferiorly and posteriorly for an optimal exposure.
- A8. Doubly-ligate and divide the azygos vein.
- A9. Open the mediastinal pleura posterior to the SVC and right phrenic nerve.
- A10. Dissect behind the SVC until the right pulmonary artery and its branches are identified. Circumferentially dissect the right pulmonary artery and its branches (perform the proximal dissection under the ascending aorta).
- A11. Identify the right subclavian artery on the apex of the pleural cavity and circumferentially dissect the artery with care not to injure the right recurrent laryngeal nerve.

OPTION B: MEDIAN STERNOTOMY (NO CPB)
- B4. Supine position.
- B5. Median sternotomy and thymectomy.
- B6. Open the superior portion of the pericardium and distract with stay sutures.
- B7. Dissect the innominate artery, right carotid artery, and right subclavian artery with care not to injure the recurrent laryngeal nerve.
- B8. Dissect the right pulmonary artery under the ascending aorta and SVC. Continue the dissection to include the first branches of the right pulmonary artery.

THORACOTOMY/STERNOTOMY
1. Select 3/3.5/4 mm Gore-Tex shunt and trim appropriately.
2. Systemic heparinization 100 IU/Kg (1 mg/Kg).

3. Control the right subclavian artery with atraumatic snares or a side-biting clamp. **[If through a sternotomy, control the innominate artery, the right carotid artery, and the distal right subclavian artery].**
4. A longitudinal incision on the inferior surface of the right subclavian artery to correspond to the size of the shunt.
5. An end-to-side shunt to subclavian artery anastomosis with fine poplypropelene suture.
6. Deair the shunt with heparinized saline solution.
7. Control the shunt with a clamp.
8. Unclamp the subclavian artery **[innominate artery/right carotid artery]**.
9. Assure hemostasis at the anastomotic site.
10. Snare the proximal right pulmonary artery with an atraumatic snugger and control the branches with Silastic vessel loops or atraumatic snuggers.
11. Make a longitudinal incision on the superior surface of the right pulmonary artery with care not to enter the right upper lobe branch of the artery.
12. Create an end-to-side shunt to pulmonary artery anastomosis with fine polypropelene suture.
13. Remove the pulmonary artery snare and vessel loops.
14. Remove the clamp from the shunt.
15. Ensure hemostasis and check for a thrill.
16. **[If through a median sternotomy, may ligate the patent ductus arteriosus].**
17. Irrigate with warm antibiotic saline irrigation.
18. Place an appropriate drain.
19. Chest closure

Potential Complications and Pitfalls

1. Modified Blalock-Taussig shunts can be performed through right or left posterolateral thoracotomies or through a median sternotomy. The approach depends on the anatomy of subclavian and pulmonary artery, the presence and location of the ductus arteriosus, the relationship of the great vessels, and surgeon/institutional preference. Advantages of a thoracotomy approach include the ability to place the shunt more distally in the subclavian artery potentially allowing for better control of pulmonary blood flow and the lack of mediastinal adhesions for future operations. Advantages of a sternotomy approach include less technical challenge and the ability to control the ductus arteriosus at the same time. If the patient is marginally stable, a median sternotomy approach with cardiopulmonary bypass may be necessary.
2. Special attention should be paid to avoid any inadvertent injury to the phrenic and recurrent laryngeal nerves during the dissection.

III. Congenital Cardiac Surgery

3. The right pulmonary artery should be clearly identified and circumferentially dissected. The right pulmonary artery should be dissected medially up to the location of the main pulmonary artery and laterally onto the first branches. The branches of the right pulmonary artery should be adequately identified in order to avoid placing the shunt into the right upper lobe branch.
4. The size of Gore-Tex graft is determined based on the size of the patient, the length of the shunt, and its location. Generally, when creating a shunt through a median sternotomy, a 3.5 mm shunt is used for most patients except for those <2.5 kg (3 mm shunt) or >4 kg (4 mm shunt). When creating a shunt through a thoracotomy, a 4 mm shunt is usually appropriate as the size of the subclavian artery will control the amount of flow into the shunt.
5. The graft should be trimmed to an accurate length. Too short of a graft will cause tension on the anastomosis leading to bleeding along the suture line, distortion of the pulmonary artery with resultant stenosis and possible thrombosis. Similarly, too long of a graft may cause kinking and distortion of the pulmonary artery and possibly compromise shunt flow.
6. At the completion of anastomosis, oxygen saturation should increase and diastolic blood pressure should decrease. A palpable thrill should be present in the shunt and the distal pulmonary artery. In patients with a very large ductus arteriosus that are undergoing a shunt through a contralateral thoracotomy, there may not be marked changes in oxygen saturation or diastolic blood pressure upon unclamping of the shunt.
7. Bleeding from the suture line is controlled by packing the anastomotic site lightly with Gelfoam soaked with topical thrombin or Surgicel for a few minutes. Protamine administration to reverse the heparin is usually avoided, unless there is excessive bleeding.
8. It is imperative to maintain an adequate systemic arterial pressure prior, during, and after the procedure to avoid early shunt thrombosis.
9. Aspirin or low-dose intravenous heparin are routinely administered and continued postoperatively to prevent shunt thrombosis.

Template Dictation

Preoperative Diagnosis: [BLANK]

Postoperative Diagnosis: [BLANK]

Procedure(s) Performed: Creation of right modified Blalock-Taussig shunt with [BLANK] mm Gore-Tex graft via right thoracotomy/median sternotomy.

Drainage: Right pleural/mediastinal chest tube.

Attending Surgeon: [BLANK]

Secondary Surgeon: [BLANK]

Assistants: [BLANK]

Anesthesia: [BLANK]

Indication(s) for Procedure: This is a [BLANK]-day-old, [BLANK] kilogram, full-term neonate with a pre-natal/post-natal diagnosis of [BLANK]. He was started on intravenous prostaglandins and transferred to the Neonatal Intensive Care Unit. An echocardiogram confirmed the diagnosis of [BLANK]. The branch pulmonary arteries were of good caliber and were confluent. He was felt to be an appropriate candidate for staged single ventricle palliation and is put forward now for placement of a systemic-to-pulmonary artery shunt.

Operative Findings: The right pulmonary artery and its branches were of adequate size. The right subclavian artery was of adequate size. The oxygen saturation and blood pressure responded as expected after placement of the shunt. There was a palpable thrill on the shunt and right pulmonary artery at the end of the procedure.

Description of the procedure: After obtaining appropriate consent, the patient was brought to the operating room and placed in a supine position. Single lumen general endotracheal tube anesthesia was induced and necessary monitoring lines, including a left radial arterial line, were placed (**Variation:** The patient was brought from the Intensive Care Unit with umbilical arterial and venous catheters in place).

RIGHT THORACOTOMY:

The patient was turned into the left lateral decubitus position and the right chest was prepped and draped. A serratus-sparing right posterolateral thoracotomy incision was performed and the pleural space was entered through the fourth intercostal space. The lung was retracted inferiorly and posteriorly. The azygos vein was doubly ligated and divided. The right pulmonary artery was identified and was circumferentially dissected distally onto the first branches. The right subclavian artery was identified medial/lateral to the recurrent laryngeal nerve, and was circumferentially dissected.

MEDIAN STERNOTOMY:

The patient was prepped and draped. A median sternotomy was performed. A thymectomy was undertaken. The upper pericardium was opened longitudinally and a series of pericardial stay stitches were placed in order to facilitate exposure. The innominate artery, right carotid artery, and right subclavian artery were dissected with care not to injure the recurrent laryngeal nerve. The right pulmonary artery was dissected up to its first branches.

THORACOTOMY/STERNOTOMY:

A [BLANK] mm Gore-Tex shunt was selected and tailored appropriately. Systemic heparin was administered at 100 IU/kg (1mg/kg). The right subclavian artery [**, right carotid artery and innominate artery**] was/were controlled with a vascular clamp/atraumatic snuggers. A longitudinal incision was made on the inferior surface of the right subclavian artery. An end-to-side graft to subclavian artery anastomosis was performed using running fine polypropylene suture. The shunt was deaired and controlled with a clamp. The clamp/snuggers was/were removed from the subclavian artery [, **carotid artery and innominate artery**]. Hemostasis was assured at the anastomotic site. The proximal right pulmonary artery was snared with an atraumatic snugger. The branches were controlled with silastic vessel loops. A longitudinal incision was made on the superior surface of the right pulmonary artery and an end-to-side shunt to pulmonary artery anastomosis was performed using running fine polypropylene suture. The pulmonary artery snare and the vessel loops were removed and the shunt was de-aired through the suture line. The clamp was then removed from the shunt, and there was an appropriate fall in mean and diastolic arterial pressure. There was a thrill in the shunt. Excellent hemostasis was assured. The incision was irrigated with warm antibiotic saline irrigation. A single right pleural/mediastinal chest tube was placed. **[The rib edges were re-approximated using interrupted absorbable pericostal sutures. Serratus anterior fascia, latissimus dorsi muscle, and subcutaneous tissue were re-approximated using running absorbable suture.] [The pericardium was loosely reapproximated. The sternum was reapproximated with interrupted stainless steel wire. The fascia and subcutaneous tissues were re-approximated with running absorbable suture]** The skin edges were approximated using a running absorbable subcuticular stitch. Dermabond skin adhesive was applied. The patient tolerated the procedure without complications. He/She was left intubated and was transported to the Pediatric Cardiac Intensive Care Unit in satisfactory condition.

Needles, sponges and instruments counts were correct at the end of the procedure.

Dr. **[BLANK]** was present and scrubbed for **[BLANK]** elements of this procedure.

Suggested Readings:

1. Khonsari S, Sintek CF. **Cardiac Surgery: Safeguards and Pitfalls in Operative Technique. 4th ed**. Philadelphia, PA: Lippincott Williams & Wilkins; 2008, p 221-235.
2. C. van Doorn, and M. de Leval. **Surgery for Congenital Heart Defects** by J. Stark and, VT Tsang. John Wiley & sons, Ltd; 2006, p 251-260.
3. Kaiser, Larry R.; Kron, Irving L.; Spray, Thomas L. **Mastery of Cardiothoracic Surgery**, 2nd Edition. Lippincott Williams & Wilkins; 2007. p 694-707.
4. Backer CL, Mavroudis C. Palliative Operations. In: Mavroudis C, Backer CL (eds). Pediatric Cardiac Surgery. 4th edition. Wiley-Blackwell; 2013, p160-163.

14. Norwood Procedure

Peter Sassalos, MD and Ming Si, MD

University of Michigan Health System, Ann Arbor, MI

Essential Operative Steps

1. General endotracheal anesthesia
2. Lines and monitoring
3. Median sternotomy
4. Subtotal thymectomy
5. Pericardial well
6. Systemic heparinization
7. Arterial cannulation of patent ductus arteriosus
8. Venous cannulation of right atrium
9. Full cardiopulmonary bypass
10. Cool to 18°C for deep hypothermic circulatory arrest
11. During cooling, dissection of ascending aorta, aortic arch, proximal descending aorta, head vessels, and pulmonary artery branches with placement of unengaged snares
12. Snare arterial cannula to direct flow into systemic circulation
13. Division of main pulmonary artery proximal to bifurcation
14. Closure of distal main pulmonary artery with Gore-Tex patch
15. If right ventricle to pulmonary artery shunt performed, proximal anastomosis using 5 mm or 6 mm ringed Gore-Tex graft with distal anastomosis performed following neoaorta construction
16. After cooling at least 20 minutes to 18°C, snare the head vessels
17. Cross clamp the descending aorta
18. Antegrade cold blood cardioplegia – 30- 40 cc per kg through arterial cannula.
19. Topical cooling of heart
20. Deep hypothermic circulatory arrest initiated and cannulae removed
21. Limited right atriotomy and atrial septectomy
22. PDA ligation and division
23. Aortotomy along lesser curvature on leftward side of aorta from level of divided proximal main pulmonary artery to normal descending aorta distal to PDA with resection of ductal tissue
24. Approximation of proximal most extent of aortotomy and adjacent divided proximal main pulmonary artery
25. Neoaorta augmentation with pulmonary homograft patch
26. De-air the neoaorta
27. Remove the Aortic cross clamp
28. Recannulation with partial cardiopulmonary bypass
29. Right atriotomy closure with full cardiopulmonary bypass and removal of head vessel snares
30. Rewarm to 37°C

III. Congenital Cardiac Surgery

31. If systemic (innominate artery or aorta) to pulmonary artery shunt performed, proximal and distal anastomoses using 3.5 mm or 4.0 mm heparin bonded Gore-Tex graft
32. Resume ventilation
33. Wean from cardiopulmonary bypass
34. Modified ultrafiltration if <15 kg
35. Sequential decannulation
36. Right atrial transthoracic intracardiac line placement
37. Protamine administration
38. Hemostasis
39. Atrial and ventricular pacing wire placement
40. Mediastinal chest tube placement
41. Sternum left open (or can be closed)
42. Skin closure with Silastic patch

Potential Complications and Pitfalls

1. PDA injury during arterial cannulation and dissection
2. Injury to pulmonary valve during placement of right ventricle to pulmonary artery shunt
3. Cooling less than 20 minutes prior to deep hypothermic circulatory arrest
4. Restricted atrial level shunting due to insufficient atrial septectomy
5. Insufficient length and/or spiraling of aortotomy
6. Distortion of native ascending aorta during creation of neoaorta
7. Bleeding from distal aortotomy suture line
8. Failure to de-air neoaorta prior to disengagement of head vessel snares
9. Overwarming with neurologic sequelae
10. Using innominate artery of unsuitable size for shunt rather than central aorta shunt

Template Dictation

Preoperative Diagnosis: Hypoplastic left heart syndrome (HLHS)

Postoperative Diagnosis: Same

Procedure(s) Performed: Norwood procedure with **[Variation: Right ventricle to pulmonary artery shunt or Modified Blalock-Taussig Shunt OR Central shunt]**

Attending Surgeon: [BLANK]

Secondary Surgeon: [BLANK]

Assistants: [BLANK]

Anesthesia: [BLANK]

Indication(s) for Procedure: **[AGE]** day old **[GENDER]** diagnosed with the Hypoplastic Left Heart Syndrome (HLHS). The procedure as well as its potential benefits, risks, and other treatment options were discussed with the patient's parents. They consented to the above procedure.

Description of Procedure: After informed consent and patient identification, the patient was brought to the operating room and placed in the supine position. After induction of general anesthesia, a single lumen endotracheal tube was placed. A central venous catheter and arterial line were placed for the hemodynamic monitoring. An oropharyngeal tube, foley catheter and rectal temperature probe were placed. Preoperative antibiotics were administered. The chest was prepped and draped in the usual sterile fashion. A second time out was performed to identify correct patient, procedure and site.

A standard median sternotomy was performed. A subtotal thymectomy was carried out. The pericardium was opened and marsupialized. The patient was systemically heparinized with 400 units per kg of heparin. Arterial cannulation was performed in the patent ductus arteriosus. Venous cannulation was performed in the right atrium. After a satisfactory activated clotting time, full cardiopulmonary bypass was initiated. Cooling to 18°C was begun for deep hypothermic circulatory arrest.

During cooling, dissection of the ascending aorta, aortic arch, descending aorta, head vessels and pulmonary artery branches was performed with unengaged snares placed. The arterial cannula was then snared to direct flow into the systemic circulation. The main pulmonary artery was then divided just proximal to the bifurcation. The distal main pulmonary artery was closed with a Gore-Tex patch using running 6-0 Gore-Tex suture.

[If right ventricle to pulmonary artery shunt performed: A stab incision was made to create a right ventricular infundibulotomy. A right angle clamp was carefully passed into the proximal main pulmonary artery through the pulmonic valve to exit the infundibulotomy. A [5 MM OR 6 MM] ringed Gore-Tex graft was selected and passed with the right angle clamp through the wall of the right ventricle. It was cut flush to a ring and pulled back such that one ring was inside the ventricular wall and the other at the level of endocardium. The graft was then secured to the epicardium using two pursestring polypropylene sutures. The distal end was left for anastomosis following neoaorta construction.]

At this point, the patient was cooled for greater than 20 minutes to a temperature of less than 18°C. A cross clamp was placed on the descending aorta and the head vessels were snared. Antegrade cold blood cardioplegia was administered at a dose of [30-40 cc] per kg through the arterial cannula. Topical cooling of the heart was achieved with ice slush. The pump was stopped and deep hypothermic circulatory arrest was initiated. The cannulae were removed.

A limited right atriotomy was made and an atrial septectomy performed to allow unrestricted atrial level shunting. The patent ductus arteriosus was then ligated and divided. An aortotomy was created along the lesser curvature on the leftward side of the aorta from the level of the divided proximal main pulmonary artery to normal descending aorta distal to the patent ductus arteriosus with resection of all ductal tissue. The most proximal extent of the aortotomy and the adjacent divided proximal main pulmonary artery were approximated using three interrupted [6-0 or 7-0] polypropylene sutures. A pulmonary homograft patch was then sewn with running [6-0 or 7-0] polypropylene suture to augment the arch from the proximal descending aorta through the arch and down the ascending aorta with incorporation of the main pulmonary artery to form the neoaorta.

A pursestring suture was then placed in the neoaorta homograft to de-air the reconstruction. The aortic cross clamp was removed. Recannulation with partial cardiopulmonary bypass was initiated. The right atriotomy was closed and full cardiopulmonary bypass was achieved. The head vessel snares were removed. Rewarming to 37°C was begun.

[If right ventricle to pulmonary artery shunt performed: The distal main pulmonary artery was transposed to the rightward side of the aorta. The right ventricle to pulmonary artery shunt was cut to an appropriate length and beveled to reach the main pulmonary artery. The distal anastomosis was then performed in an end-to-side fashion between the graft and the anterior aspect of the main pulmonary artery using running [6-0 OR 7-0] polypropylen suture.]

[If modified Blalock-Taussig shunt or central shunt performed: A Castaneda clamp was used for vascular control of the [INNOMINATE ARTERY OR NEOAORTA]. A [3.5 MM OR 4.0 MM] heparin bonded Gore-Tex graft was selected, cut to length and beveled appropriately. An [ARTERIOTOMY OR AORTOTOMY] was made and the proximal anastomosis was then performed in an end-to-side fashion between the graft and the [INNOMINATE ARTERY OR NEOAORTA] using a running [6-0 OR 7-0] polypropylene suture. [SNARES OR CLAMPS] on the branch pulmonary arteries were then used for vascular control of the main pulmonary artery. An arteriotomy was made and remaining ductal tissue resected. The distal anastomosis between graft and main pulmonary artery was then performed in a similar fashion. The graft was de-aired in the usual fashion.]

After rewarming, ventilation was resumed. The patient was weaned from cardiopulmonary bypass on [INOTROPES/VASOPRESSORS]. Modified ultrafiltration for 10 minutes was then performed. The cannulae were removed. The right atrial cannulation site was replaced with a transthoracic intracardiac line. Protamine sulfate was administered at a dose of 1 mg per 100 units of heparin given. Hemostasis was obtained. Atrial and ventricular pacing wires were placed. A mediastinal chest tube was placed through a separate stab incision and secured in the usual fashion. The sternum was left open. The skin was closed with a Silastic patch. A sterile dressing was applied. The patient tolerated the procedure well with no apparent complications and was transferred to the Pediatric Cardiothoracic Intensive Care Unit for further evaluation and management.

Cardiopulmonary bypass data included a height [CM], weight [KG], body surface area [M^2] and blood type [BLANK]. Total cardiopulmonary bypass time was

[MIN], aortic cross clamp time [MIN] and deep hypothermic circulatory arrest time [MIN].

All instruments, sponges and needles counts were correct twice at the conclusion of the procedure.

Dr. [BLANK] was present and scrubbed for [BLANK] elements of this procedure.

III. Congenital Cardiac Surgery

15. Bidirectional Glenn Procedure

Muhammad Aftab, MD, Ismael Alejandro Salas De Armas, MD, E. Dean McKenzie*, MD

Baylor College of Medicine/Texas Heart Institute, Houston, TX

*Texas Children's Hospital/Baylor College of Medicine, Houston, TX

Essential Operative Steps

1. Lines and Monitoring (Note: IJ line in SVC for PAP monitoring postop and NTG delivery).
2. General endotracheal anesthesia.
3. Bilateral cerebral near-infrared spectroscopy sensors (NIRS).
4. Transesophageal Echocardiogram (Not useful unless AV valve regurgitation).
5. Redo median sternotomy with oscillatory saw.
6. Lysis of adhesions under direct vision between the heart, the sternum and the diaphragm.
7. Dissect around the SVC, right atrium and Neoaorta (extreme care with phrenic nerve).
8. **Dissect the pulmonary artery (PA) from the hilum on the right onto the left PA. (Note: mostly done prior to heparinization).**
9. Identify the BT shunt and perform circumferential dissection.
10. Systemic heparinization (3-4 mg/Kg).
11. Direct aortic cannulation (Neoaorta).
12. Direct distal SVC cannulation.
13. Right atrial (IVC) cannulation (Note: IVC cannulation is necessary only if intracardiac procedure required).
14. Establish Cardiopulmonary bypass (CPB) circuit.
15. Check ACT >350.
16. Initiate Cardiopulmonary bypass.
17. Immediately after initiation of CBP, ligate the BT Shunt or clip the Sano shunt (Ultimately the shunt needs to be divided).
18. Normothermic beating heart.
19. Snare the SVC proximal to the cannula, divide azygous vein to prevent retrograde flow.
20. Apply a vascular clamp to the SVC-right atrial junction.
21. Divide the SVC and suture closure the cardiac end.
22. Ligated the azygos vein to further mobilize the SVC.
23. **Excise the shunt from the PA and extend the arteriotomy medially and laterally on the superior aspect of the branch pulmonary arteries. with Hegar dilators)**
24. Construct the end to side cavopulmonary anastomosis.
25. Resume mechanical ventilation.

26. Wean from CPB.
27. Place common atrial, **if no femoral venous catheter.**
28. TEE evaluation, hemodynamic and oxygen saturation assessment
29. Protamine and sequential decannulation.
30. Assure hemostasis.
31. Place mediastinal drains.
32. Sternal closure.

Potential Complications and Pitfalls

1. A safe sternal reentry is one of the major steps to the successful outcomes of redo operations.
2. Careful evaluation of preoperative imaging to assess the proximity of vital structures to the sternum, use of an oscillating saw for the anterior table, lifting the sternal edges and incising the posterior table under direct vision, removing the sternal wires sequentially after incising the posterior table are some of the considerations for a safe sternal reentry.
3. Special attention should be paid to avoid any inadvertent injury to the right phrenic nerve during the lysis of adhesions between the right side of the heart and pericardium and dissecting the SVC. A combination of sharp and blunt dissection should be carried out and use of electrocautery should be avoided.
4. Sinoatrial (SA) node is located on the lateral aspect of the SVC-right atrial junction. The inferior vascular clamp should be applied across the SVC just above the atrio-caval junction and SVC should be divided above the clamp and the stump is oversewn.
5. The azygous vein should be doubly ligated and divided to avoid the postoperative decompression of superior cavopulmonary shunt (Glenn) flow into the IVC.
6. Entire procedure can be performed on full flow bypass with beating heart and normothermia.
7. To avoid pulmonary over circulation during the procedure, the systemic-pulmonary shunt (BTS) should be ligated and proximally divided immediately after instituting the cardiopulmonary bypass.
8. The correct orientation of the proximal SVC should be maintained and any twisting should be avoided to create an optimal cavopulmonary anastomosis. This can be facilitated by placing the marking sutures on the SVC and dividing the azygous vein.
9. The SVC should be completely mobilized and opening on the right pulmonary artery (RPA) should be made as close to the SVC as possible to perform a tension free cavopulmonary anastomosis. In case of previous systemic-pulmonary shunt, all the shunt material should be completely removed and incision should be extended few millimeters medially before creating the SVC to RPA anastomosis.
10. To avoid purse-stringing of the cavopulmonary anastomosis, two separate sutures can be used for anterior and posterior rows. Alternatively, the

interrupted suture technique may be prudent to construct the anterior aspect of the anastomosis.
11. If it is decided to eliminate the source of additional pulmonary blood flow at the time of second stage procedure, the main pulmonary artery should be divided just above the valve and pulmonary valve should be either excised or over-sewn (Note: this will require myocardial arrest). Proximal and distal pulmonary stumps should be closed with running polypropylene. Simple suture ligation of main pulmonary artery should be avoided as it creates a space between the valve and ligature where thrombosis occurs which can result into systemic emboli and stokes.
12. A monitoring catheter should inserted in the common atrium and needle measurements of SVC and PA pressure should be done at the time of weaning from bypass to evaluate for any anastomotic problems. The common atrial pressure should be no more than 5-6 mm Hg. The pulmonary artery pressure, which should be equal to SVC pressure, should be no more than 12-15 mm Hg.

Template Dictation

Preoperative Diagnosis:

1. Hypoplastic left heart syndrome
2. Status post Norwood palliation with placement of systemic-to-pulmonary artery shunt.

Postoperative Diagnosis: Same

Procedure(s) Performed:

Repeat median sternotomy for:

1. Creation of bidirectional cavopulmonary shunt (bidirectional Glenn anastomosis).
2. Takedown of previous systemic to pulmonary artery shunt.
3. *Pulmonary patch arterioplasty with pulmonary homograft* ***[Variation]***

Drainage: Mediastinal chest tube(s).

Attending Surgeon: [BLANK]

Secondary Surgeon: [BLANK]

Assistants: [BLANK]

Anesthesia: [BLANK]

Indication(s) for Procedure: Patient is a [BLANK] -month-old infant with single ventricle congenital heart disease consisting of [BLANK] who underwent Norwood palliation with placement of a systemic-to-pulmonary artery shunt as a neonate. Clinically, *he/she* has done well and is being put forward now for the next stage of his/her single ventricle palliation.

Operative Findings: The systemic and pulmonary venous drainage were normal. There were significant adhesions between the heart and the chest wall and pericardium. The neo-aorta was of adequate caliber. The superior vena cava was of low normal size. *[Variation: There was an area of stenosis on the pulmonary artery at the level of the insertion of the ligamentum arteriosum].* The coronary arteries were normal. There was trace tricuspid regurgitation and good ventricular function at the end of the case.

Description of Procedure: After informed consent and patient identification the patient was brought to the operating room and placed on the operating table in a supine position. After induction of general endotracheal anesthesia and placement of monitoring lines the patient was positioned, prepped and draped in routine sterile manner. A transesophageal echocardiogram (TEE) was not performed.

A reoperative median sternotomy was performed and preliminary dissection was carried out. There were expected adhesions in the mediastinum, which were taken down sharply. A sternal retractor was placed. The phrenic nerves were identified bilaterally, and care was taken to avoid injuring these structures. The innominate vein and superior vena cava (SVC) were dissected. The SVC was circumferentially dissected on its entirety from the innominate vein down to the right atrium. The dissection was performed around the inferior vena cava (IVC) and right atrium. The neoaortic reconstruction was mobilized. The previous systemic-pulmonary shunt /**Blalock-Taussig Shunt (BTS)** was identified and circumferentially dissected. A limited dissection was carried out on the right pulmonary artery.

Heparin was administered and aorto-bicaval cannulation was performed. These cannulae were secured, deaired and connected to the bypass circuit. Having ascertained an adequate anticoagulation, bypass was initiated. The temperature was allowed to drift to 34°C. The heart was allowed to maintain a normal sinus rhythm throughout the procedure. Immediately after instituting bypass the shunt was doubly suture-ligated and divided. The proximal end was oversewn using running polypropylene suture.

The azygos vein was divided between silk ligatures. The superior vena cava was snared just proximal to the level of the venous cannula. An angled vascular clamp was placed across the cardiac end of the SVC. The SVC was transected at the cavoatrial junction with the cardiac end being over-sewn with running polypropylene. The pulmonary artery was then circumferentially dissected from the hilum on the right onto the left pulmonary artery. Upon inspection of the pulmonary artery there was no stenosis and we were able to pass a normal-sized Hegar dilator upto the branch pulmonary arteries *[Variation for pulmonary artery stenosis: There was an area of stenosis of the pulmonary artery to the right/left of the shunt. The decision was made to do a pulmonary artery patch augmentation. A longitudinal pulmonary arteriotomy was performed and extended with Pott's scissors. A patch was tailored as appropriate and sutured to the pulmonary artery with fine 7-0 polypropylene suture in a running fashion].*

All of the systemic-pulmonary shunt material was removed from the main pulmonary artery. The resulting arteriotomy was extended both medially and laterally on the anterior superior surface. An end-to-side cavopulmonary anastomosis was then created using running 7-0 polypropylene suture. The patient was rewarmed. Temporary atrial epicardial pacing wires were placed. Patient was weaned from cardiopulmonary bypass without difficulty and with good hemodynamics. Pressures in the Glenn circuit were 9-11 mmHg. Systemic arterial saturations were 90% on an FIO2 of 1.0 [**Optional:** A *right atrial line was inserted through the right atrial appendage and secured].* Protamine was administered and the patient was sequentially decannulated. Hemostasis was assured. The mediastinum was irrigated with copious amounts of warm antibiotic saline irrigation. A single mediastinal chest tube was placed. The sternal edges were re-approximated using stainless steel wires. The soft tissues were closed in multiple layers using running absorbable suture. The skin edges were re-approximated using a running absorbable subcuticular stitch and steristrips. Sterile dressings were placed.

The patient tolerated the procedure without complications. The patient was extubated in the operating room and transported to the Pediatric Cardiac Intensive Care Unit in a satisfactory condition.

Sponge, needle and instrument counts were correct at the end of the procedure.

Cardiopulmonary bypass time was **[BLANK]** minutes.

Dr. **[BLANK]** was present and scrubbed for **[BLANK]** elements of this procedure.

Suggested Readings:

1. Khonsari S, Sintek CF. **Cardiac Surgery: Safeguards and Pitfalls in Operative Technique. 4th ed**. Philadelphia, PA: Lippincott Williams & Wilkins; 2008, p 354-366.

2. Jonas R. (editor) **Comprehensive Surgical Management of Congenital Heart** Disease, Hodder Arnold Publication; 2004, p 357-385.

3. Kouchoukos NT, Blackstone EH, Hanley FL, Kirklin JK. Kirklin/Barratt-Boyes **Cardiac Surgery: 4th ed**. Elsevier Saunders, Philadelphia, PA; 2013, p 1533-1540.

16. Completion Lateral Tunnel Fontan

Jonathan C. Hong, MD and Andrew I.M. Campbell, MD

Division of Cardiovascular Surgery, BC Children's Hospital

University of British Columbia, Vancouver, BC

Essential Operative Steps

1. Lines and monitoring
2. General anesthesia
3. Intraoperative transesophageal echocardiogram (TEE)
4. Redo median sternotomy
5. Systemic heparinization
6. Arterial cannulation of ascending aorta
7. Venous cannulation (right angle cannula in the superior vena cava and flexible straight/right angle cannula in the inferior vena cava encircled with tourniquet)
8. Insert cardioplegia cannula in the ascending aorta
9. Establish cardiopulmonary bypass (CPB)
10. Ensure ACT>480 seconds
11. Systemic hypothermia (24° C).
12. Ensure all systemic-to-pulmonary artery shunts are controlled (if present).
13. Cross clamp the aorta
14. Antegrade cardioplegia
15. Snare IVC and SVC tourniquet
16. Left atrial vent through right superior pulmonary vein
17. Make oblique incision along the free wall of the right atrium parallel to sulcus terminalis
18. Confirm intracardiac anatomy
19. Excise previously constructed patched orifice between the pulmonary artery and right atrium
20. Cut appropriately shaped baffle out of polytetrafluoroethylene (PTFE)/Gore-Tex graft
21. Suture in a baffle in right atrium directing blood flow from the IVC to the right pulmonary artery
22. Create fenestration in baffle
23. Rewarm to normothermia
24. De-air the heart
25. Remove the cross clamps
26. Atrial and ventricular pacing wires
27. Ensure hemostasis
28. Wean from CPB
29. Measure PA pressure, consider leaving catheter if pressures elevated (>15)
30. Venous decannulation

III. Congenital Cardiac Surgery

31. Administer the Protamine
32. Aortic decannulation
33. Ensure hemostasis
34. Placement of chest tubes
35. Sternotomy closure

Potential Complications and Pitfalls

1. Catastrophic hemorrhage during redo sternotomy.
2. Cannulation complications.
3. Inadequate myocardial protection.
4. Obstruction of pulmonary venous return by the lateral tunnel prosthesis.
5. Failure to securely snare the tourniquets may result in venous air lock and flooding of the operative field.
6. The superior extension of the right atrial incision must not injure the sinus nodal artery.
7. Manipulation of the crista terminalis, atriocaval junction and area around the sinoatrial node may increase the risk of atrial arrhythmias, so a gentle tissue handing is prudent.
8. The fenestration of the baffle must be created in a location amenable to device closure
9. Acute thrombosis of the baffle fenestration.
10. Collateral blood flow to the pulmonary circulation is often significant, so the left atrium and ventricle must be adequately vented to prevent any distension.
11. Incomplete de-airing.
12. Incomplete hemostasis prior to the sternotomy closure

Template Dictation

Preoperative Diagnosis:

1. Hypoplastic Left Heart Syndrome (HLHS)
2. Post hemi-Fontan

Postoperative Diagnosis: Same

Procedure(s) Performed: Lateral Tunnel Fontan

Attending Surgeon: [BLANK]

Secondary Surgeon: [BLANK]

Assistants: [BLANK]

Anesthesia: [BLANK]

Indication(s) for Procedure: [AGE] year old [GENDER] with [DIAGNOSIS – e.g. hypoplastic left heart syndrome, post hemi-Fontan]. Cardiac catheterization demonstrated [suitability of anatomy and hemodynamics – e.g. pulmonary vascular resistance, unobstructed flow between systemic veins and pulmonary arteries]. An echocardiogram revealed [e.g. assessment of chamber size and function, valvular function]. It was felt that the patient was suitable for completion lateral tunnel Fontan.

Description of Procedure: The patient was taken to the operating room on [Date]. The patient's identity, consent, and planned procedure were verified. The patient was placed on the operating table in the supine position. The procedure was performed under general anesthesia with left radial arterial line and right internal jugular central venous line access. A preoperative transesophageal echocardiogram (TEE) was performed to evaluate anatomy and function. The patient was prepped and draped in the standard fashion including both groins for emergency access. A redo median sternotmy was performed. Cannulation sites and the right atrium were exposed. Limited dissection of the superior vena cava was performed taking care not to injure the phrenic nerve. The pericardium was retracted to create a well using [#2-0] silk sutures. The patient was systemically heparinized with [IU] of heparin.

A right angle venous cannula was placed in the SVC and an arterial cannula was inserted into the ascending aorta. After ensuring that the ACT was > 480 seconds, cardiopulmonary bypass was initiated. A right angle venous cannula was placed in the inferior vena cava (IVC). IVC was encircled with a tourniquet. The patient was cooled to moderate hypothermia [e.g. 28° C]. The ascending aorta was clamped and antegrade cardioplegia was delivered into the aortic root. A left atrial vent was placed through the right superior pulmonary vein. There was rapid arrest of the heart. [Blank] mL of cardoiplegia was administered. The tourniquets around the IVC and left innominate vein were snared. The right atrial free wall was opened with an oblique incision parallel to the atrioventricular groove with the superior end veering anterior to the sinus node taking care not to injure the sinus nodal artery. The intra-cardiac anatomy and previous hemi-Fontan shunts were examined including the previously constructed patched orifice between the right pulmonary area and right right atrium. A 15-blade scapel was used to excise the right atrial patch and it was removed.

A PTFE baffle was shaped appropriately to divert blood from the IVC to the pulmonary circulation. A 10-mm PTFE tube graft was cut longitudinally to create a half-cylinder. The two ends were beveled with the medial side longer than the lateral side running along the free edge of the right atrium. The baffle was sewn in place using a #5-0 polypropylene running technique starting medial to the IVC orifice then posterior to the IVC then cephalad along the lateral wall of the atrium and then around the SVC orifice. After three quarters of the SVC circumference was sewn, the other end of the #5-0 polypropylene was used to complete the anastomosis. The two ends of the suture were tied together to secure the baffle. A 4 mm punch was used to create a fenestration in the medial aspect of the baffle opposite to the ASD to allow for device closure at a later date. The right atrial free wall was sutured obliquely over the anterior surface of the PTFE baffle using a running #5-0 polypropylene.

III. Congenital Cardiac Surgery

The patient was rewarmed to normothermia. The heart was de-aired in the usual fashion. The cross clamp to the aorta was removed. Atrial and ventricular pacing wires were placed epicardially. Hemostasis was confirmed. The patient was weaned from cardiopulmonary bypass. A transesophageal echo was performed to confirm appropriate deairing of the systemic atrium and ventricle and good systemic ventricular function. The patient was decannulated and protamine was administered. A fine pressure line was inserted through the previous SVC cannulation site and secured with the pursestring suture. Three [Size] chest tubes were placed in the left pleural, right pleural and mediastinum. The sternum was closed with stainless steel wires. The fascia was closed with #2-0 Vicryl in continuous fashion. The deep dermal layer was closed with #2-0 Vicryl. The subcuticular layer was closed with running #3-0 Monocryl.

All instruments, sponges and needles counts were confirmed to be correct x 2 at the end of the operation. The patient was subsequently transferred to the postoperative cardiac surgical intensive care unit in stable condition.

Dr. [BLANK] was present and scrubbed for [BLANK] elements of this procedure.

17. Extra-Cardiac (Non-Fenestrated) Completion Fontan Procedure

Muhammad Aftab, MD, Ramanan Umakanthan*, Jeffrey S. Heinle*, MD

Baylor College of Medicine/Texas Heart Institute, Houston, TX

*Texas Children's Hospital/Baylor College of Medicine, Houston, TX

Essential Operative Steps

1. Lines (central venous line, arterial line, volume line) and Monitoring.
2. General endotracheal anesthesia.
3. Intra-operative Transesophageal Echocardiogram (TEE)
4. Redo-median sternotomy.
5. Lysis of adhesions.
6. Dissection of superior cavopulmonary shunt (Glenn)
7. Dissection of branch pulmonary arteries to the hilum.
8. Systemic heparinization (3-4 mg/Kg).
9. Direct aortic cannulation.
10. Bicaval cannulation, both Cavae encircled with the tourniquets.
11. Establish Cardiopulmonary bypass (CPB) circuit
12. Check ACT >450
13. Initiate Cardiopulmonary bypass.
14. Systemic hypothermia (cooling to 34°C).
15. Ensure that all the systemic to pulmonary shunts are controlled or ligated.
16. Prepare the GORE-TEX (or PTFE) conduit beveled.
17. Snare the branch Pulmonary Arteries (PAs) and SVC tourniquets.
18. Longitudinal pulmonary arteriotomy – along inferior aspect of the right PA and carried centrally.
19. End-to-side conduit-to-PA anastomosis (running 6-0 GORE-TEX suture).
20. Clamp across the right atrium at the right atrial-IVC junction.
21. Snare the Inferior vena cava (IVC) tourniquet
22. Transect the IVC.
23. Oversew the cardiac end (double running layer of 4-0 Polypropylene).
24. Trim the conduit - transected to an appropriate length.
25. End-to-end conduit-to-IVC anastomosis (using running 5-0 GORE-TEX suture).
26. Start rewarming.
27. Atrial epicardial pacing wires.
28. Start ventilation and suction the lungs.
29. Remove the caval snares.
30. Allow the heart to fill and eject.
31. Wean from cardiopulmonary bypass.
32. Check pressure in the Glenn circuit and systemic arterial saturations.
33. Venous decannulation.
34. Administer protamine to reverse heparin.

35. Aortic decannulation.
36. Ensure excellent hemostasis.
37. Placement of mediastinal drain and bilateral pleural Blake drains.
38. Sternotomy closure.
39. Attempt extubation in the operating room.

Potential Complications and Pitfalls

1. A safe sternal reentry is one of the major steps to the successful outcomes of redo operations.
2. Special attention should be paid to avoid any inadvertent injury to the phrenic nerves during the lysis of adhesions between the right side of the heart and pericardium and dissecting the SVC/superior cavopulmonary shunt.
3. Injury to sinoatrial (SA) node during dissection should be avoided.
4. Purse string for the IVC cannulation should be placed as low a possible on the IVC.
5. Occasionally, a relatively short intrathoracic segment of IVC may require taking down the diaphragmatic reflection onto the IVC for an optimal exposure. Alternatively, the femoral vein can be cannulated in larger patients.
6. Placing the clamp on the right atrium can result into an inadvertent injury to the coronary sinus or right coronary artery. This can be avoided by careful inspection prior and after the clamp placement.
7. An adequate rim (1-2 cm) of right atrial tissue should be left beyond the clamp for the suture line on the cardiac stump. An accidental slipping of right atrial tissue can result into catastrophic air embolism.
8. Any areas of branch pulmonary artery stenosis should be addressed by either the direct patch augmentation (GORE-TEX/pericardial patch) or the long beveled proximal anastomosis should be fashioned to patch augment the pulmonary artery narrowing, if possible.
9. To maintain the laminar flow in the main pulmonary artery the anastomosis of the GORE-TEX conduit to Pulmonary artery should be as central as possible, thus offsetting the flows from IVC and SVC to the pulmonary artery and avoiding direct collision of two blood streams.
10. There is no growth potential growth for the extra cardiac conduits. Simultaneous placing a larger conduit will result into IVC-conduit diameter mismatch, with an increased risk of stasis and thrombosis. Typically an 18-22mm GORE-TEX conduit will be used.
11. Keep the conduit short.
12. Avoid obstruction of right sided pulmonary veins due to compression by the conduit. Confirm an unobstructed ASD and unobstructed pulmonary venous return after conduit placement.
13. Significant atrioventricular valve regurgitation should be addressed at the time of Fontan.

Template Dictation

Preoperative Diagnosis:

1. Hypoplastic left heart syndrome (**Variation:** Aortic Atresia/Mitral Stenosis)
2. Post Norwood procedure
3. Post bidirectional Glenn (cavopulmonary shunt).

Postoperative Diagnosis: Same

Procedure Performed:

1. Third redo-sternotomy.
2. Completion Fontan: Total cavopulmonary connection with non-fenestrated extra-cardiac conduit (20-mm GORE-TEX conduit).

Drainage: Mediastinal chest tube and bilateral pleural Blake drains were placed.

Attending Surgeon: [BLANK]

Secondary Surgeon: [BLANK]

Assistants: [BLANK]

Anesthesia: [BLANK]

Indication(s) for Procedure: This is a 4 year old with hypoplastic left heart syndrome (aortic atresia/mitral stenosis) who is status-post the first 2 stages of his single-ventricle palliation and is now being put forward for completion Fontan. Preoperative echocardiogram and cardiac catheterization show favorable anatomy and hemodynamics for Fontan operation. There is a normal right ventricular function with mild tricuspid regurgitation. There is good development of the branch pulmonary arteries, pulmonary arterial resistance was 2.0 Wood units and pulmonary artery pressure 14 mm Hg with an end diastolic pressure 9 mmHg.

Operative Findings: The branch pulmonary arteries were of good caliber. Transesophageal echocardiogram showed good right ventricular function with mild tricuspid regurgitation and an unobstructed intra-atrial communication. Completion Fontan was performed using total cavopulmonary connection with 20-mm GORE-TEX non-fenestrated extra-cardiac conduit. Pressures in the Fontan circuit were 12-14 mmHg with systemic arterial saturations in the high 90s. [*Variation: There was small venous collateral in the form of a persistent left vein of Marshall, which was ligated at the level of the innominate vein.*]

Description of the Procedure: After informed consent and patient identification the patient was brought to the operating room and placed on the operating table in a supine position. After induction of general anesthesia with single lumen endotracheal tube intubation, arterial and central venous monitoring lines were placed. A transesophageal echocardiogram (TEE) was performed and the above findings were noted. The patient was positioned, prepped and draped in a surgical sterile fashion.

A repeat median sternotomy was performed. For this purpose, the previous scar was excised and the incision was carried down to the sternum. The sternal wires were removed and the anterior table of the sternum was divided with the use of an oscillating sternal saw. The posterior table of the sternum was divided with scissors and electrocautery after dissecting the structures attached to posterior sternum under direct visualization. Chest wall adhesions were taken down bilaterally. There were dense adhesions in the mediastinum, which were divided using electrocautery. The phrenic nerves were identified bilaterally, and care was taken to avoid injuring these structures. The superior vena cava and cavopulmonary anastomosis were dissected. A limited dissection was carried out on the branch pulmonary arteries. Pursestrings were placed on the ascending aorta, superior vena cava and the inferior vena cava for cannulation. The patient was then systemically heparinized and cannulated for cardiopulmonary bypass using direct aorto-bicaval cannulation. After reaching appropriate ACT, bypass was established and the patient was cooled to 34 °C. The procedure was performed with the beating heart.

The branch pulmonary arteries were further dissected. [*Variation:* *The innominate vein was dissected, and the venous collateral in the form of left vein of Marshall was identified and ligated.*] A [20-mm] GORE-TEX (or PTFE) conduit was then brought onto the field and beveled on its distal end. The branch Pulmonary arteries were controlled with atraumatic snares and the SVC tourniquet was snared. A longitudinal arteriotomy was created on the inferior aspect of the right pulmonary artery and carried centrally. An end-to-side conduit-to-pulmonary-artery anastomosis was performed using running 6-0 GORE-TEX suture. A large vascular clamp was placed across the right atrium at the right atrial-inferior vena caval junction and the inferior vena cava (IVC) tourniquet was snared. The IVC was transected and the cardiac end was over-sewn using double running layer of 4-0 polypropylene suture. The conduit was transected to an appropriate length, and an end-to-end conduit-to-IVC anastomosis was performed using running 5-0 GORE-TEX suture.

During the final anastomosis, the patient was rewarmed. Temporary atrial and ventricular epicardial pacing wires were placed. The lungs were suctioned and ventilated. The patient was weaned from cardiopulmonary bypass without difficulty and with good hemodynamics. Pressure in the Fontan circuit was 12-14 mmHg with systemic arterial saturations in the high 90s. The TEE showed an unobstructed atrial septal defect and unobstructed right-sided pulmonary veins. Protamine was administered, and the patient was sequentially decannulated. Hemostasis was assured. The mediastinum was irrigated with copious amounts of warm antibiotic saline irrigation. A mediastinal chest tube and bilateral pleural Blake drains were placed. The sternum was re-approximated using stainless steel wires. The soft tissues were closed in multiple layers using running absorbable suture. Skin edges were re-approximated using a running absorbable subcuticular stitch.

The patient tolerated the procedure without complications. The patient was extubated in the operating room and transported to the Pediatric Cardiac Intensive Care Unit in a satisfactory condition. Sponge, needle and instrument counts were correct.

Cardiopulmonary bypass time was **[BLANK]** minutes.

Dr. **[BLANK]** was present and scrubbed for **[BLANK]** elements of this procedure.

Suggested Readings:

1. Khonsari S, Sintek CF. Cardiac Surgery: Safeguards and Pitfalls in Operative Technique. 4th ed. Philadelphia, PA: Lippincott Williams & Wilkins; 2008, p 354-366.

2. Jonas R. (editor) Comprehensive Surgical Management of Congenital Heart Disease, Hodder Arnold Publication; 2004, p 376-382.

3. Kouchoukos NT, Blackstone EH, Hanley FL, Kirklin JK. Kirklin/Barratt-Boyes Cardiac Surgery: 4th ed. Elsevier Saunders, Philadelphia, PA; 2013, p 1540-1563.

4. de Leval MR, Dubini G, Migliavacca F, Jalali H, Camporini G, Redington A, Pietrabissa R. Use of computational fluid dynamics in the design of surgical procedures: application to the study of competitive flows in cavo-pulmonary connections. J Thorac Cardiovasc Surg. 1996 Mar; 111(3):502-13.

18. Repair of Supravalvular Aortic Stenosis

Raghav Murthy MD, David Graham MD, Vinod Sebastian MD

Children's Medical Center of Dallas, Texas

Essential Operative Steps

1. Lines and monitoring.
2. General endotracheal anesthesia.
3. Intraoperative transesophageal echocardiogram (generally if > 2.5kg).
4. Median sternotomy.
5. Total/subtotal thymectomy.
6. Open pericardium, create pericardial well.
7. Ligation of patent ductus arteriosus, if present.
8. Dissection of the pulmonary artery from the aorta.
9. Assess location of supravalvular stenosis and size of ascending aorta and arch.
10. Systemic heparinization.
11. Arterial cannulation in the distal ascending aorta or proximal arch.
12. Single venous dual-stage cannula.
13. Placement of antegrade cardioplegia cannula.
14. Initiate cardiopulmonary bypass when ACT in acceptable range.
15. Placement aortic cross clamp.
16. Antegrade cardioplegia (40ml/kg).
17. Reverse Trendelenburg position to better view aortic pathology.
18. Aortotomy (longitudinal for Option A, transverse for Option B).
19. Reconstruction Options:

    a. Inverted 'Y' Incision, vertical over the ascending aorta and the thickened sinotubular ridge and bifurcate into the non-coronary sinus and the right coronary sinus, staying to the left of the RCA; assess the valve and the coronary ostia; pantaloon shaped patch is sutured using 6-0 polypropylene; aortic anastomosis created.

    b. 3-patch technique (Brom) with incisions into each coronary sinus; assess the valve and coronary ostia; shield shaped patch is sutured using 6-0 polypropylene in each sinus; aortic anastomosis created.

20. Patch options include: Dacron/Gore-Tex, pulmonary homograft, bovine pericardium and autologous pericardium.
21. Deep Tredelenburg position, de-airing at the cardioplegia cannula site, removal of aortic cross clamp.
22. Assess hemostasis.
23. Atrial and ventricular wire placement.
24. Wean from cardiopulmonary bypass.
25. Venous decannulation.
26. Assess gradient with TEE.
27. Protamine administration.

28. Aortic decannulation.
29. Assess hemostasis.
30. Mediastinal Blake drain and intracardiac line placement.
31. Sternotomy closure.

Potential Complications and Pitfalls

1. While making the incision into the right coronary sinus it is important to visualize the right coronary ostium so that the incision has adequate clearance from the ostium to allow subsequent suturing.
2. The pantaloon shaped patch should be rather generous to create bulging sinuses of Valsalva similar to the normal aorta.
3. Special attention should be focused on cardioplegia protection of the myocardium in view of the severe left ventricular hypertrophy associated with supravalvular aortic stenosis.
4. If extensive narrowing of the sinotubular junction is seen, a more extensive augmentation of all the three sinuses as advocated by Brom may be required.
5. Inspection of the aortic valve leaflets and coronary ostia are important. Careful separation of the adhered leaflets from the ridge may be required.
6. Careful and extensive de-airing must be performed to prevent air embolism and stroke.
7. Injury to the aortic leaflets: the aortic valve leaflets must be protected while making the incision into the sinuses.
8. Incisions into the coronary sinuses should never extend beyond the maximal width of the proximal aortic segment nor near the aortic commissures. If they do, the patch will distort the base of the valve or alter the commissural geometry resulting into postoperative aortic incompetence.

Template Dictation

Preoperative diagnosis: (Indication –Supravalvular aortic stenosis, Williams syndrome)

Postoperative diagnosis: Same

Procedure(s) performed: Inverted 'Y' patch aortoplasty

Attending Surgeon: [Blank]

Secondary Surgeon: [Blank]

Assistants: [Blank]

Anesthesia: [BLANK]

Indication(s) for Procedure: (Age) month old **(Gender)** with history of **(Complaint/Diagnosis).**

III. Congenital Cardiac Surgery

Description of the Procedure: The patient was brought to the operation room on **(Date)**. The patient's identity and planned procedure were verified and the patient was placed supine on the operating table. Single lumen general endotracheal tube anesthesia was administered. Monitoring lines and foley catheter were placed. The chest and abdomen were prepped and draped in the usual sterile manner. A time out was performed. A median sternotomy was then performed. A total/subtotal thymectomy was performed. The pericardium was opened in the midline and a pericardial cradle created.

The patent ductus arteriosus was dissected out, ligated and divided (if present). Aortic cannulation sutures were placed as distal on the ascending aorta as possible. The patient was then systemically heparinized. The aortic cannula was then inserted, secured and de-aired. A single right atrial venous cannula was placed. An antegrade cardioplegia cannula was then placed in the ascending aorta. CPB was initiated after appropriate ACT levels were obtained. The aorta was cross-clamped and antegrade cardiopledia delivered. Rapid arrest of the heart was achieved. Ice was applied to the heart.

A longitudinal aortotomy was made over the narrow segment of the ascending aorta. The coronary ostia and the valve leaflets were then visualized. The aortotomy was then extended in a bifurcated manner, inverted 'Y' configuration, onto the non- coronary sinus and onto the right coronary sinus staying to the left of the right coronary artery ostium. A generous pantaloon shaped autologous pericardial/homograft/ Dacron/Gore-Tex patch was then fashioned. This was sutured to the aorta in a continuous manner using 6-0 polypropylene suture. The patient was then placed in a steep Trendelenburg position and de-airing was performed through the antegrade cardioplegia site. The aortic cross clamp was removed. Hemostasis was confirmed at the suture line.

Atrial and ventricular pacing wires were placed. The patient was weaned from cardiopulmonary bypass. Calcium was administered. The venous cannula was removed from the right atrium. TEE was used to check the repair and any residual gradient. Protamine was administered. The aortic cannula was removed. Intracardiac lines were placed and secured in place. All the cannulation sites were checked for hemostasis. A mediastinal Blake drain was placed. The median sternotomy was closed with stainless steel wires. The fascia was closed using 2-0 Vicryl, the subcutaneous tissue using 3-0 Vicryl and the skin was approximated using 4-0 Vicryl in a subcuticular manner. Sterile dressing was applied to the incision.

All needles, sponges and instruments counts were found to be correct at the end of the procedure. The patient was transferred to the intensive care unit in a stable condition.

Cardiopulmonary bypass time was **[BLANK]** minutes, with a cross-clamp period of **[BLANK]** minutes.

Dr. **[BLANK]** was present and scrubbed for **[BLANK]** elements of this procedure.

19. Ross Procedure for the Correction of Congenital Aortic Stenosis

Ala Al-Lawati, MD and Andrew I.M Campbell, MD

Division of Cardiovascular and Thoracic Surgery, BC Children's Hospital

University of British Columbia Vancouver, BC, Canada

Essential Operative Steps

1. Lines and monitoring
2. General anesthesia
3. Intraoperative Trans-esophageal echocardiography (TEE)
4. Median sternotomy
5. Open pericardium
6. Create pericardial well and inspect cardiac and coronary anatomy
7. Systemic heparinization
8. Aortic and bicaval cannulation
9. Establishing cardiopulmonary bypass (CPB) with ACT > 400 seconds
10. Systemic hypothermia to 28° C
11. Mobilizing aorta and pulmonary artery
12. Insertion of LV vent via right superior pulmonary vein
13. Cross clamp and administration of cardioplegia
14. Aortotomy & inspection of aortic valve, root and left ventricular outflow tract (LVOT)
15. Transect the PA and inspect pulmonary valve for suitability
16. Harvest pulmonary autograft and prepare it for implantation
17. Transect the aorta and excision of aortic valve; root and annular decalcification
18. Prepare the aortic root and harvesting coronary buttons
19. Implant pulmonary autograft in the aortic position [performing proximal anastomosis]
20. Re-implant coronary buttons
21. Perform distal neoaortic anastomosis
22. Start rewarming
23. Right ventricular outflow tract (RVOT) reconstruction with pulmonary homograft
24. De-airing and removal of cross clamp
25. Atrial and ventricular pacing wires
26. Weaning from CPB
27. Hemostasis
28. Postoperative TEE
29. Venous decannulation
30. Protamine administration and aortic decannulation
31. Ensure excellent hemostasis
32. Chest tube placement

33. Sternotomy and soft tissue closure

Potential Complications and Pitfalls

1. Correct patient selection – no distal obstruction
2. Inadequate myocardial protection
3. Preoperative AI
4. Preoperative aortic dilatation
5. Aortic root autograft size mismatch
6. Damage to left main coronary during posterior PA root mobilization
7. Bicuspid pulmonary valve or valve leaflet perforation
8. Damage to pulmonary valve during autograft harvest
9. Inadequate muscular rim below the harvested pulmonary valve autograft
10. Damage to first septal perforator during autograft harvest
11. Inadequate aortic valve/annulus decalcification
12. Injure the coronary arteries with button mobilization
13. Improper anatomic alignment of autograft
14. Excessive tension, kinking, or twisting of coronary arteries with button re-implantation
15. Injuring the coronary artery with deep suture placement while performing the posterior suture line of the RVOT reconstruction

Template Dictation

Preoperative Diagnosis: Congenital, severe aortic stenosis

Postoperative Diagnosis: Same

Procedure(s) Performed: Ross Procedure

Attending Surgeon: [BLANK]

Secondary Surgeon: [BLANK]

Assistants: [BLANK]

Anesthesia: [BLANK]

Indication(s) for Procedure: [AGE] year old [GENDER] with symptomatic severe aortic stenosis and anatomy suitable for Ross procedure.

Description of Procedure: After patient identification, surgical site confirmation and informed consent, the patient was taken to the operating room and placed in a supine position. Single lumen general endotracheal tube anesthesia was induced and all the necessary monitoring lines including a left radial arterial line and right internal jugular central venous line were placed. A preoperative transesophageal echocardiogram was performed to confirm the diagnosis, rule out other associated congenital anomalies and establish the presence of a structurally normal pulmonary valve and a baseline cardiac function assessment. The patient was prepped and draped in standard fashion, including both groins for emergency access.

A median sternotomy was performed. The thymus was excised and innominate vein identified. The pericardium was opened and retracted to create a well using 2-0 silk sutures. Cardiac anatomy was inspected to rule out any obvious anomalies. The patient was then systemically heparinized with [UNTIS] of heparin.

Aortic and bicaval cannulation sutures were placed in standard fashion. The aorta was cannulated using a [SIZE] cannula. The cannula was secured, de-aired and connected to the pump circuit. The superior vena cava (SVC) was then cannulated using a [SIZE] cannula and the inferior vena cava (IVC) was also cannulated using a [SIZE] cannula. Both cannulae were secured and connected to the pump circuit. SVC and IVC snares were then placed and laid loose. A purse string for the antegrade cardioplegia cannula was placed in the ascending aorta and the cannula was inserted. Another purse-string suture was placed in the right atrium for placement of a retrograde catheter. The left ventricle was vented by inserting a catheter through the right superior pulmonary vein.

The aortic root size and pulmonary valve size were measured externally to ensure size match. These measurements were correlated with the echocardiographic measures. Extensive aortic and pulmonary trunk dissection was performed including both pulmonary artery (PA) branches. Once ACT exceeded 480 seconds, cardiopulmonary bypass was established. The ductal tissue remnants were ligated and transected to provide further mobility. The Patient was cooled to 28° C. An aortic cross-clamp was applied and [VOLUME] of antegrade cardioplegia solution infused. A dose of cardioplegia was repeated every 20 minutes in a retrograde fashion to ensure an adequate myocardial protection.

An aortotomy was made at a level 1-2 cm above the sinotubular junction to inspect the aortic valve, root and LVOT for procedure suitability. Both cavae were snared and the main PA was incised below the bifurcation to assess the pulmonary valve (PV). The Pulmonary valve was assessed for its tri-leaflet structure, intact leaflets and other structural or functional abnormalities. We judged it appropriate to proceed with the Ross procedure, and the pulmonary trunk was transected below its bifurcation. We then harvested the pulmonary autograft by inserting a right-angled forceps through the pulmonary valve to identify our first incision site on the right ventricle's anterior wall, 1-1.5cm below the valve. The ventriculotomy was extended circumferentially with sharp dissection in both directions, staying below the valve and leaving a rim of at least 5mm of myocardial tissue. Extra caution was taken in the leftward posterior dissection, to avoid injuring the first septal coronary perforator as well as noting any other coronary anomalies. This part was done under direct visualization of the left main coronary artery and its branches. After harvesting the pulmonary autograft, a dose of cardioplegia was administered to identify and control bleeding points from the dissection area. The autograft size was measured, scalloped in preparation for its insertion, and kept in a clearly marked bowl. The pulmonary homograft was then thawed and rinsed.

The aorta was transected above the sinotubular junction. Three commissural stiches were placed above the aortic commissures as guides for re-implanting the coronary arteries. The aortic valve was excised. The annulus was decalcified and debrided. The aortic annulus was measured and no further modification of the aortic root annulus was required. The aortic root was further prepared by excising the aortic sinuses. The right and left coronary buttons were dissected with excess tissue. Both coronary arteries were mobilized extensively to facilitate reimplantation.

The pulmonary autograft was implanted in the aortic position at a sub-annular level maintaining its anatomic alignment, using interrupted pledgeted 3-0 ethibond sutures sewn in a horizontal mattress fashion. This suture line was reinforced with a second running suture line with 4-0 polypropylene.

A #11 blade scalpel was used to create two arteriotomies in the pulmonary autograft at the positions of the left and right coronary buttons, respectively. The left coronary button was re-implanted using a running 6-0 polypropylene suture. Similarly, the right coronary button was re-implanted using a running 6-0 polypropylene suture. Care was taken to anastomose the right coronary button high onto the new right cusp to avoid kinking. Reconstruction was then completed by performing the distal anastomosis with running 4-0 polypropylene suture.

The cardioplegia cannula was then reinserted into the neo-aorta. Antegrade cardioplegia was administered and the coronary button suture lines were inspected for hemostasis.

The patient was rewarmed, and we proceeded with reconstruction of an appropriately sized pulmonary homograft. The homograft was sutured first to the RVOT with running 4-0 polypropylene suture. While completing the posterior suture line, special care was taken to avoid injury to the coronary arteries. This was followed by completion of the proximal pulmonary anastomosis.

The left side of the heart was then de-aired and the cross-clamp was removed. The heart started beating in a normal sinus rhythm. Both atrial and ventricular pacing wires were placed. At normothermia, after 15 minutes of reperfusion, mechanical ventilation was resumed and patient was weaned from the cardiopulmonary byass uneventfully. The post operative TEE showed no gradient or regurgitation across the neoaortic valve, and a satisfactory pulmonary homograft with preserved left ventricular function. Venous cannulae, left sided vent and cardioplegia lines were sequentially removed. Protamine was administered. The aorta was subsequently decannulated.

Hemostasis was secured, and two [SIZE] chest drains were inserted. The sternum was approximated using [SIZE] wires. The subcutaneous layer was closed using [SIZE] vicryl in two layers, followed by subcuticular skin closure using [SIZE] monocryl. The patient tolerated the procedure well. He/she was then transferred to the cardiac surgery intensive care unit in stable condition.

Needles, sponges and instruments counts were correct at the end of the procedure. Cardiopulmonary bypass time was **[BLANK]** minutes, with a cross-clamp period of **[BLANK]** minutes.

Dr. **[BLANK]** was present and scrubbed for **[BLANK]** elements of this procedure.

20. Repair Of Obstructive Hypertrophic Cardiomyopathy: (Septal Myomectomy)

Justin R. Van Meeteren, D.O., Joseph A. Dearani, MD

Mayo Clinic, Rochester, MN

Essential Operative Steps

1. Lines and Monitoring
2. General endotracheal anesthesia
3. Intraoperative transesophageal echocardiogram (TEE)
4. Median sternotomy
5. Open pericardium
6. Create pericardial wall, survey ascending aorta for plaque burden and cannulation sites
7. Systemic Heparinization (400 u/kg)
8. Arterial Cannulation
9. Venous Cannulation
10. Myocardial protection cannula placement (aortic tack vent in the aortic root)
11. Check ACT (>400 sec)
12. Initiate CPB
13. Systemic hypothermia to 28° C
14. Aortic cross clamp (reduce CPB flow rate, apply cross clamp, increase CPB flow to 2.0-2.5L/min/m2)
15. Antegrade cardioplegia (+/-1000 ml for satisfactory asystolic arrest)
16. Create an oblique aortotomy (Note: Aortotomy is carried down toward the noncoronary sinus)
17. Suspend the aortotomy with pledgeted polypropylene sutures
18. Perform septal myectomy
19. Inspect Mitral valve
20. Inspect Aortic valve
21. Close the aortotomy closed
22. Removal aortic cross clamp
23. Post-Operative transesophageal echocardiogram (TEE)
24. Check for hemostasis
25. Wean from CPB
26. Venous decannulation
27. Protamine administration
28. Aortic decannulation
29. Asses hemostasis
30. Sternotomy closure

Potential Complications and Pitfalls

1. Incomplete (inadequate) septal myectomy towards mid-ventricle resulting in residual obstruction and systolic anterior motion (SAM) of mitral valve

2. Injury to the mitral valve or aortic valve
3. Complete heart block
4. Ventricular septal defect or free wall perforation

Template Dictation

Preoperative Diagnosis: [Indication: - e.g. hypertrophic obstructive cardiomyopathy, left ventricular outflow tract obstruction]

Postoperative Diagnosis: Same

Procedure(s) Performed: Extended left ventricular septal myectomy

Attending Surgeon: [Blank]

Secondary Surgeon: [Blank]

Assistants: [Blank]

Anesthesia: [BLANK]

Indication(s) for Procedure: [Age] year old [Gender] with [Duration] history of [Complaint – e.g. shortness of breath, diastolic heart failure, syncope, chest pain]. Preoperative echocardiogram reveals [Findings – e.g. hypertrophic cardiomyopathy with obstruction, basal septal thickness, left ventricular outflow gradient].

Description of Procedure: The patient was taken to the operating room on [DATE]. The patient's identity and planned procedure verified, and the patient was placed on the operating room table in the supine position. Single lumen General endotracheal tube anesthesia was obtained. A right internal jugular central venous line and pulmonary artery catheter and radial arterial line were inserted. Preoperative transesophageal echocardiogram was performed to evaluate ventricular outflow tract anatomy, septal thickness, ventricular function and valve function. We then proceeded to prep and drape the chest, abdomen, groins, and lower extremities in sterile fashion. A time out was performed. Median sternotomy was then performed. After identification of the innominate vein, the pericardium was opened and a pericardial well was created. The aortic cannulation sutures were then placed in the distal ascending aorta below the level of the innominate artery. The right atrial cannulation sutures were placed within the right atrium. A total of [UNITS] of systemic heparin was administered. The aortic cannula was inserted, secured and de-aired. The venous cannula was placed and secured in the right atrium. Total cardiopulmonary bypass was instituted and cooling for moderate hypothermia was begun (28° C). An aortic tack vent was then inserted into the ascending aorta on aspiration for administration of antegrade cardioplegia and venting of the left heart. The aortic cross-clamp was placed. Cold blood antegrade cardioplegia was administered obtaining asystolic arrest of the heart. Additional cold blood cardioplegia was administered via the coronary ostia at 20-minute intervals during the cross clamp period.

III. Congenital Cardiac Surgery

After administrating [Blank] ml of cardioplegia, an oblique aortotomy was made and carried down toward the noncoronary sinus. The aortotomy was suspended with pledgeted polypropylene sutures. The septal myectomy was performed by making an incision at the nadir of the right coronary cusp and extending this in a counterclockwise manner, around toward the mitral valve. Further resection was done on the apical third of the resection to the right of the right coronary cusp incision. The base of the resection was deepened with a rongeur. The mitral and aortic valves were inspected and noted to be intact. The aortotomy was closed with running polypropylene suture in two layers. Air was evacuated from the suture line before securing it. The cross-clamp was released with suction on the aortic root vent was turned on. Cardiopulmonary bypass was gradually discontinued with satisfactory hemodynamics. Postcardiopulmonary bypass transesophageal echocardiogram showed [Findings]. Decannulation was accomplished and surgical sites were over-sewn. Protamine was administered and hemostasis was achieved. A total of [Number] of chest tubes were placed in the mediastinum. The sternum was closed with interrupted wires in the usual manner and the soft tissue was approximated in layers using absorbable sutures.

All instruments, sponges and needles counts were confirmed to be correct x 2 at the end of the operation. The patient was subsequently transferred to the postoperative cardiac surgical intensive care unit in critical condition.

Cardiopulmonary bypass time was [BLANK] minutes, with a cross-clamp period of [BLANK] minutes.

Dr. [BLANK] was present and scrubbed for [BLANK] elements of this procedure.

21. Arterial Switch Procedure

Muhammad Aftab, MD, Charles D. Fraser, Jr.*, MD

Baylor College of Medicine/Texas Heart Institute, Houston, TX

*Texas Children's Hospital/Baylor College of Medicine, Houston, TX

Essential Operative Steps

1. Lines and Monitoring.
2. General endotracheal anesthesia.
3. Intraoperative TEE.
4. Median sternotomy.
5. Partial thymectomy.
6. Open the Pericardium.
7. Harvested pericardium (for reconstruction of the defects created by excision of coronary buttons from the native aortic root).
8. Create a pericardial well.
9. Ascending aortic cannulation.
10. Bicaval cannulation.
11. Establish total Cardiopulmonary bypass circuit.
12. Systemic hypothermia - cooling to 28-30°C (deep hypothermic circulatory arrest 18°C with antegrade cerebral perfusion is employed only if an arch repair is needed).
13. Dissect out, doubly ligate and divide the PDA.
14. Extensive mobilization of pulmonary arterial branches (past their first-order divisions).
15. Cross clamp the Aorta.
16. Administer anetgrade cardioplegia.
17. Vent the left atrium utilizing transseptal approach / ASD after right atriotomy.
18. Repair the VSD, if present, through the right atriotomy with trans-triscupid approach using autologous pericardium (**Variation:** in case of TGA/VSD).
19. Interval doses of cardioplegia every 15-20 minutes – antegrade cardioplegia directly into the coronary ostia.
20. Divide both aorta and the main PA above the semilunar valves.
21. Reposition the aortic cross clamp.
22. Excise the coronary ostia from the native aortic root.
23. Reimplant the coronary buttons into the native pulmonary root (neoaortic root).
24. Perform Lecompte maneuver (translocation of the pulmonary artery confluence in front of the aorta).
25. Establish the aortic continuity by anastomosing the native pulmonary root (neoaortic root) to the ascending aorta.

26. Patch the defects of coronary buttons in the native aortic root (neopulmonary root) using the autologous pericardium.
27. Re-establish the Pulmonary arterial continuity by anastomosing the neopulmonary root to the pulmonary artery bifurcation.
28. Close the ASD primarily or by patch the closure.
29. Start rewarming and de-airing- trendelenburg position.
30. Remove the aortic cross clamp.
31. Start de-airing; confirm complete de-airing under TEE guidance.
32. Wean from the cardiopulmonary bypass.
33. Venous decannulation
34. Protamine administration
35. Aortic decannulation
36. Ensure excellent hemostasis.
37. Place mediastinal drains and peritoneal dialysis catheter.
38. Standard sternotomy closure.

Potential Complications and Pitfalls

1. Special attention should be paid to avoid any inadvertent injury to the phrenic during partial thymectomy.
2. The preliminary dissection includes mobilization of aorta (**Variation:** mobilize beyond the origin of innominate artery if the arch repair is planned). Aorta should be dissected free from the main pulmonary artery to the level of coronary ostia. Similarly, the branch pulmonary arteries should mobilized well out past their first-order divisions to allow for anterior translocation.
3. Pulmonary valve should be carefully assessed by the preoperative TTE and intra-operative TEE (**Optional**). A competent and non-stenotic pulmonary valve (neo-aortic valve) must be ensured prior to excising the coronary ostia.
4. Injury to the sinoatrial (SA) node during SVC cannulation or placement of the SVC snare should be avoided.
5. To prevent the flooding of lungs from the run off of aortic cannula flow, the ductus arteriosus should be immediately ligated or occluded after the institution of cardiopulmonary bypass.
6. If a VSD is present, it can be repaired through the right atrium across the tricuspid valve with an adequate exposure. Alternative approaches include through the anterior great vessel or pulmonary artery.
7. Intracardiac repair (VSD and ASD repair), if needed, should be performed after the application of initial cross-clamp and administration of cardioplegia. This allows additional doses of cardioplegia to be administered prior to the aortic reconstruction.
8. Prospective sites of coronary reimplantation onto the proximal main pulmonary artery can be marked with marking fine polypropylene sutures.

9. While performing the Lecompte maneuver, to bring the ascending aorta behind the pulmonary artery bifurcation, extreme care should be exercised not to twist the aorta as this will result into the torsion of the suture line.
10. To prepare the coronary arteries, a D-shape cuff of coronary artery ostia with at least 2-3 mm rim of the surrounding aortic tissue is usually excised. The proximal coronary arteries should also be mobilized using a low-voltage electrocautery.
11. Any injury to neo-aortic leaflets should be avoided while making medially-based trap-door flap incisions in the neoaorta.
12. During coronary reimplantation special care should be taken to avoid rotation and distortion of the coronary arteries.

Template Dictation

Preoperative Diagnosis:

1. D-transposition of the great arteries with intact ventricular septum.
2. Yacoub type A coronary branching (**Variation:** Yacoub A, B, C, D).
3. Large secundum atrial septal defect after balloon atrial septostomy.
4. Small patent ductus arteriosus.
5. Small perimembranous ventricular septal defect (**Variation: in patient with TGA/VSD**).

Postoperative Diagnosis: Same

Procedure(s) Performed:

Via median sternotomy on cardiopulmonary bypass support:

1. Arterial switch operation.
2. Direct suture closure of secundum atrial septal defect.
3. Ligation and division of patent ductus arteriosus.
4. Direct suture closure of small perimembranous ventricular septal defect (**Variation: in TGA/VSD**).
5. Insertion of left atrial catheter.
6. Insertion of peritoneal dialysis catheter.

Drainage: Left pleural chest tube(s).

Attending Surgeon: [BLANK]

Secondary Surgeon: [BLANK]

Assistants: [BLANK]

Anesthesia: [BLANK]

Indication(s) for Procedure: This is a [BLANK]-day-old, [BLANK] kilogram, full-term neonate with a prenatal diagnosis of transposition with intact ventricular

III. Congenital Cardiac Surgery

septum. He was attended to immediately at birth. He had a restrictive atrial level of communication and was very hypoxic. He underwent urgent balloon atrial septostomy and improved rapidly. He was subsequently weaned off of prostaglandin and has been in the Cardiac Intensive Care Unit being prepared for surgery. A lengthy preoperative consultation was carried out with the patient's parents detailing the anatomy, planned surgery and attendant perioperative risks. All of their questions were answered, and they are in favor of proceeding with the operation.

Operative Findings: The patient had normal thymic tissue. The pericardium was not adhered to the heart. The great vessels were situated in an anterior-posterior relationship. There was Yacoub type A coronary branching. The semilunar valves both were tricuspid, but the pulmonary valve (neoaortic valve) had asymmetric sinuses. The leftward anterior sinus was somewhat rudimentary, although the leaflet tissue appeared adequate. There was a large secundum ASD after balloon atrial septostomy. There was a small patent ductus arteriosus. (**Variation:** There was a small perimembranous ventricular septal defect).

Description of Procedure: After informed consent and patient identification, the patient was taken to the operating room and placed on the operating table in a supine position. After induction of general anesthesia, the patient was intubated. Central venous and arterial lines were placed. The patient was then positioned, prepped, and draped in standard sterile fashion. A complete median sternotomy was performed. A partial thymectomy was carried out. The pericardium was opened, and patches were harvested and kept fresh for later use. After our preliminary dissection, pursestring sutures were placed in the ascending aorta and superior and inferior venae cavae. Heparin was administered. The heart was then cannulated for cardiopulmonary bypass utilizing bicaval venous drainage. Bypass was initiated. The patient was cooled to a nasopharyngeal temperature of 30 degrees centigrade (Variation: Lower temaprature 22-25°C if VSD repair is required). The ductus arteriosus was dissected out, doubly ligated, and divided. The branch pulmonary arteries were mobilized well out past their first-order divisions. The ascending aorta was cross-clamped, and the heart was arrested with potassium cardioplegic solution instilled in the aortic root. The heart became flaccid. An oblique right atriotomy was performed, and a pump sucker was placed into the left atrium to act as a vent. (**Variation for TGA/VSD:** Working through the tricuspid valve, the VSD was visualized. It was quite small and very difficult to see underneath the septal leaflet of the tricuspid valve. After careful deliberation, it appeared that the only safe way to address the VSD would be with a primary mattress suture buttressed with Teflon felt.Therefore, 6-0 polypropylene pledgeted horizontal mattress sutures were placed across the VSD and then tied and cut.). We then turned our attention to the arterial switch operation. The ascending aorta was transected just above the sinotubular junction. The coronary ostia were visualized. They were centrally located in their respective aortic sinuses of Valsalva. There was type A branching. The coronary ostia were then mobilized as buttons of aortic wall. The main pulmonary artery was then transected. As mentioned, the leftward anterior sinus was somewhat rudimentary but suitable for translocation of the left main ostium. Appropriate medially-based trap-door flap incisions were made in the neoaorta. The coronary ostia were translocated to these incisions and then sewn in with running fine polypropylene sutures. A LeCompte maneuver was performed. Aortic continuity was then reestablished with the primary anastomosis between the ascending aorta and neoaortic root with a running fine polypropylene. At this time, the patient was rewarmed. The ASD was closed primarily with a running fine polypropylene. Multiple additional de-airing maneuvers were then carried out with the heart venting through the anterior ascending aorta. The aortic cross-clamp was removed. Normal sinus rhythm resumed spontaneously, and the electrocardiogram normalized. The right atriotomy was closed with a running fine polypropylene. We then reconstructed the neopulmonary sinus of Valsalva with liberal patches of the previously harvested autologous pericardium, sewn in with running fine polypropylene. Pulmonary arterial continuity was then reestablished with an anastomosis between the neopulmonary trunk and the pulmonary artery bifurcation, also with a running fine polypropylene. As we finished warming the patient, a left atrial catheter was placed. Ventilation was commenced. The heart was then allowed to fill and eject, and the patient separated from cardiopulmonary bypass without difficulty. The heart was sequentially decannulated. Protamine was administered to counteract the heparin. The suture lines and cannulation sites were inspected and found to be hemostatic. The wound was irrigated with copious amounts of antibiotic irrigation. Chest drains were placed. A peritoneal dialysis catheter was placed, and then the wound was closed in layers. All needle, sponges and instruments counts were correct at the end of the case, as indicated by the circulating nurse. The patient tolerated the procedure well and returned to the Pediatric Cardiac Surgical Intensive Care Unit in a good hemodynamic state.

Cardiopulmonary bypass time was [BLANK] minutes. Cross-clamp time was [BLANK] minutes.

Dr. [BLANK] was present and scrubbed for [BLANK] elements of this procedure.

Suggested Reading:

1. Khonsari S, Sintek CF. **Cardiac Surgery: Safeguards and Pitfalls in Operative Technique. 4th ed**. Philadelphia, PA: Lippincott Williams & Wilkins; 2008, p 303-323.
2. R. B B. Mee **Surgery for Congenital Heart Defects by** J. Stark and M. de Leval, VT Tsang. John Wiley & sons, Ltd; 2006, p 471-487.
3. Spray, Thomas L **Mastery of Cardiothoracic Surgery** by Kaiser, Larry R.; Kron, Irving L.; Spray, Thomas L., 2nd Edition. Lippincott Williams & Wilkins; 2007. P 856-872.

22. Tetralogy of Fallot: Transventricular Repair

Juan M. Lehoux, MD and E. Dean Mckenzie, MD

Texas Children's Hospital/Baylor College of Medicine, Houston, TX

Essential Operative Steps

1. Lines and Monitoring
2. General endotracheal anesthesia
3. Intraoperative transesophageal echocardiography (TEE)
4. Median sternotomy
5. Partial Thymectomy
6. Open pericardium
7. Harvest pericardial patch (place in glutaraldeyde for 10 min)
8. Set up pericardial well
9. Preliminary dissection of aorta and main pulmonary artery
10. Systemic heparinization (3-4 mg/Kg).
11. Cannulation, direct aortic and single venous cannula.
12. Confirm ACT (>400)
13. Start cardiopulmonary bypass
14. Systemic hypothermia (cooling to 28°C).
15. Place vent in right superior pulmonary vein
16. Cross clamp the aorta
17. Antegrade cardioplegia.
18. Incise RVOT and pass hagar dialator antegrade through the pulmonary valve [Note: if it is too small, carry the incision thru the pulmonary valve annulus into the main pulmonary artery].
19. Identify location of VSD, tricuspid valve and subvalvar apparatus of the tricuspid valve.
20. Resect hypertrophied septoparietal muscle bundles avoiding the infundibular septum and subvalvar aparatus of the tricuspid valve.
21. Place interrupted 6-0 pledgeted polypropylene stitches circumferentially around VSD and secure to perforated sheet.
22. Pass circumferential stitches into appropriately sized and trimmed pericardial patch.
23. Parachute patch into position and tie down sutures.
24. De-air the left heart
25. Remove cross clamp
26. Remove vent from left upper pulmonary vein
27. Place pericardial patch over infundiblar incision.
28. Place left atrial line through the left atrial appendage.
29. Resume ventilation
30. Wean cardiopulmonary bypass
31. Remove venous cannula
32. Confirm adequate repair with TEE

33. Place needle into RV through the infundibular patch and measure pressure
34. Administer protamine
35. Decanulate the aorta
36. Obtain hemostasis
37. Mediastinal drain
38. Sternotomy closure

Potential Complications and Pitfalls

1. Avoid phrenic nerve injury during partial thymectomy
2. Identify coronary anatomy prior to infundibular incision. The anterior descending may come from the right, crossing the site of planned incision.
3. Avoid injury to subvalvar aparatus of the tricuspid valve when resecting septo-parietal muscle bands
4. Do not resect muscle over the infundibular septum, as it forms part of the margin of the VSD.
5. Sutures will not hold through cut endocardium.
6. In order to preserve the long term right ventricular function, the ventriculotomy incision should be just larger enough to adequately visualize and relieve the infundibular obstruction.
7. Identify aortic valve and its annulus.
8. The patch should be secured to aortic valve annulus to avoid a residual VSD.
9. The aortic valve leaflets are situated immediately below the superior margin of the ventricular septal defect. The injury to the aortic valve leaflets should be avoided when placing sutures.

Template Dictation

Preoperative diagnosis: Tetralogy of Fallot

Postoperative diagnosis: Same

Procedure(s) performed: Trans-ventricular Tetralogy of Fallot repair

Attending surgeon: [Blank]

Secondary surgeon: [Blank]

Assistants: [Blank]

Anesthesia: [BLANK]

Indication(s) for Procedure: [AGE] month old [GENDER] with prenatal diagnosis of tetralogy of fallot.

Description of procedure: The patient was taken to the operating room and placed in the supine position. General endotracheal anesthesia was induced.

Arterial and central venous access was obtained by the anesthesia team. Transesophageal echo probe was placed.

The patient was prepped and draped in the usual sterile fashion. A median sternotomy was performed. The thymus was excised. The pericardium was incised and a pericardial patch was harvested and placed in glutaraldehyde solution for 10 minutes. A pericardial well was set up. The aorta and pulmonary artery were dissected. After heparin administration, the patient was cannulated with single venous and arterial cannula. A vent was placed thru the right superior pulmonary vein. The patient was cooled to 28°C. The aorta was cross clamped and antegrade cardioplegia was administered with prompt cardiac arrest in diastole. Cardioplegia was given every 20 minutes while cross clamped.

The right ventricular outflow tract was incised. Hegar dialators were passed to size the pulmonary valve, which was found to be inadequate. The incision was thus carried through the pulmonary valve annulus into the main pulmonary artery.

The VSD margins, the aortic valve and the subvalvar apparatus of the tricuspid valve were identified. The aortic and tricuspid valves were in fibrous continuity. We then divided and resected hypertrophied septo-parietal muscle bands with special care taken not to injure the tricuspid valve subvalvar apparatus. The VSD was patched with pericardium of sufficient size to baffle the LVOT to the aortic valve using interrupted pledgeted polypropylene sutures.

After the VSD was closed, the left heart was de-aired and cross clamp was removed.

The heart restarted to contract spontaneously with a sinus rhythm. The infundibular incision was closed with a pericardial patch using running polypropylene suture.

A left atrial line was placed thru the left atrial appendage for post-operative monitoring of filling pressures.

Ventilation was resumed and the patient was weaned from cardiopulmonary bypass. The venous cannula was removed. The repair was confirmed by TEE. A needle was passed into the RV through the trans-annular patch to measure RV pressure. This was found to be less than 2/3 systemic. Protamine was administered and the arterial cannula was removed. After adequate hemostasis, a peritoneal dialysis catheter and mediastinal drains were placed. The sternum was approximated with the stainless steel sternal wires. The soft tissue and skin were closed in layers. A sterile dressing was applied. The child was transported to the cardiac intensive care unit stable having tolerated the procedure.

Sponges, needles and instruments counts were correct twice at the end of the procedure.

Cardiopulmonary bypass time was **[BLANK]** minutes, with a cross-clamp period of **[BLANK]** minutes.

Dr. **[BLANK]** was present and scrubbed for **[BLANK]** elements of this procedure.

III. Congenital Cardiac Surgery

23. Tetralogy of Fallot Repair - Infundibular Sparing (Transatrial Repair)

Muhammad Aftab, MD, Ismael Alejandro Salas De Armas, MD, E. Dean McKenzie*, MD

Baylor College of Medicine/Texas Heart Institute, Houston, TX

*Texas Children's Hospital/Baylor College of Medicine, Houston, TX

Essential Operative Steps

1. Lines and Monitoring.
2. General endotracheal anesthesia.
3. Intra-operative Transesophageal Echocardiogram (TEE).
4. Median sternotomy.
5. Partial thymectomy.
6. Open pericardium, Pericardial patch harvest (two segments)
7. Create pericardial well.
8. Dissection of SVC, aorta and main pulmonary artery.
9. Systemic heparinization (3-4 mg/Kg).
10. Direct aorto-bicaval cannulation.
11. Establish Cardiopulmonary bypass (CPB) circuit.
12. Both Cavae encircled with the tourniquets.
13. Check ACT > 350.
14. Initiate Cardiopulmonary bypass.
15. Systemic hypothermia (cooling to 28°C).
16. Cross clamp the aorta.
17. Antegrade cardioplegia-diastolic arrest.
18. Snare the SVC and IVC tourniquets.
19. Oblique right atriotomy.
20. Vent left heart chambers though the interatrial septum/PFO.
21. Evaluate right ventricular outflow tract and ventricular septal defect through the tricuspid valve.
22. Resection of obstructing muscle bundles (hypertrophied septoparietal trabeculations) at the right ventricular outflow tract (RVOT) obstruction. Preserve moderator band.
23. Baffle/closure of the ventricular septal defect (Avoiding conduction system). [**Note:** May require incision in anterior and septal leaflets of tricuspid valve parallel to the annulus].
24. Longitudinal Pulmonary arteriotomy.
25. Pulmonary valve assessment.
26. Incise the commissure to the level of annulus. May carry incision onto infundibulum for 2-5mm.
27. Reassessment of RVOT through the pulmonary valve.
28. Perform additional subvalvular infundibular resection.
29. Ensure adequate size of RVOT and branch PA's.

30. Start rewarming.
31. PFO/ASD closure and deairing.
32. Remove the aortic cross clamp.
33. Closure of right atriotomy.
34. Pulmonary artery/annulus pericardial patch plasty.
35. Left atrial catheter placement in LA appendage.
36. Temporary pacing wires.
37. Start ventilation and suction the lungs.
38. Remove the caval snares.
39. Allow the heart to fill and eject.
40. Wean from cardiopulmonary bypass (**Variation:** on Esmolol +/- Milrinone)
41. Confirm satisfactory post-operative TEE findings [Note: Anticipate mild residual dynamic RVOT obstruction].
42. Administer protamine.
43. Sequential decannulation.
44. Ensure excellent hemostasis.
45. Placement of mediastinal drains and peritoneal catheter (if indicated).
46. Standard Sternotomy closure.

Potential Complications and Pitfalls

1. To perform an optimal repair it is of paramount importance that surgeon should be thoroughly familiar with the patient's anatomy including the size and distribution of pulmonary arteries, extent of RVOT obstruction, size and nature of pulmonary annulus, coronary distribution, anatomy of VSD and any other anomalies.
2. Care should be exercised to perform as little manipulation of the heart as possible during the preliminary dissection, to avoid any precipitating severe hypoxemia from a "spell".
3. The patient should be outside the neonatal period and weigh >4 kg for considerations for the right ventricular infundibular sparing (RVIS) repair of Tetralogy of Fallot. The ideal weight for the RVIS repair of Tetralogy of Fallot is 5kg or greater. We wouldn't advocate for infundibular sparing repair in a child of weight less than 5 kg and would probably perform a BT shunt.
4. Avoid the injury of the phrenic nerve during partial thymectomy.
5. Injury to sinoatrial (SA) node during SVC cannulation or placement of the SVC snare should be avoided.
6. A high right atrial incision should be made close to the AV groove for a transatrial repair.
7. To achieve optimal exposure for evaluation intra-cardiac anatomy and repair, purse string for the IVC cannulation should be placed as low a possible. Occasionally, a relatively short intrathoracic segment of IVC may require taking down the diaphragmatic reflection onto the IVC for an optimal exposure.

8. Special care should be taken to avoid excessive resection of muscle from RVOT to avoid perforation of free anterior wall. Avoid unnecessary retraction to avoid junctional ectopic tachycardia (JET).
9. In younger children incision, rather than the excision, of the obstructing septal and parietal bands is all that is usually necessary [Note: Neonates are not considered good candidates for RVIS repair]. In older children fibrous and hypertrophied rim of septal and parietal bands must be resected.
10. Pulmonary valvotomy should be performed such that valve leaflets are mobilized and fused commissures are divided all the way to the pulmonary artery wall; up to but not through the annulus.
11. The pulmonary annulus and main pulmonary artery are evaluated with a Hegar dilator. Following completion of the infundibular resection and pulmonary valvotomy if the RVOT does not accept a Hegar dilator 1-2mm larger than the predicted Pulmonary Valve annulus based on BSA then a very limited transannular incision is created.
12. Conduction system is located close to inferior margin of the VSD. Aortic valve leaflets are situated immediately below the superior margins of the defect. Special care should be taken by avoiding deeper bites in above locations to prevent puncturing/tethering the aortic valve leaflets and damaging the conduction system.
13. Preserve the visible RV coronary artery branches. Also preserve the conal coronary branch during the limited infundibular incision.

Template Dictation

Preoperative Diagnosis: Tetralogy of Fallot

Postoperative Diagnosis: Same

Procedure(s) performed:

Infundibular sparing repair of tetralogy of Fallot including

1. Transatrial creation of intracardiac baffle from LV to the anteriorly displace aorta through the VSD (glutaraldehyde-prepared autologous pericardium).
2. Pulmonary valvotomy and Infundibular-sparing transannular patch augmentation of main pulmonary artery (autologous pericardium).
3. Transatrial/transpulmonary right ventricular outflow tract resection/Excision of right ventricular outflow tract muscle bundles.
4. Primary closure of patent foramen ovale
5. Insertion of peritoneal dialysis catheter [Optional].
6. Insertion of left atrial catheter [Optional].

Drainage: [BLANK] Fr. mediastinal chest tube.

Attending Surgeon: [BLANK]

Secondary Surgeon: [BLANK]

Assistants: [BLANK]

Anesthesia: [BLANK]

Indication(s) for Procedure: This is a 6 month old child with the prenatal diagnosis of tetralogy of Fallot with a large conoventricular malalignment ventricular septal defect, significant pulmonary valvar/subvalvar and supravalvar stenosis. He/she has been growing and developing well, with adequate oxygen saturations and has been followed with the diagnosis of tetralogy of Fallot. This child was recently referred to us for surgery and was felt to be a candidate for promotion to a complete repair. Lengthy consultation was carried out with the patient's family prior to surgery emphasizing the planned surgery, attendant perioperative risks, and the need for life-long medical follow-up and possible reintervention. All of their questions were answered and they were in favor of proceeding with the operation.

Operative Findings: A thymus was present. The pericardium was not adherent to the heart. The systemic and pulmonary venous drainage were normal. There was atrial solitus with atrioventricular concordance and ventriculoarterial concordance. The aorta was anterior, consistent with the lesion. There was a left aortic arch with normal branching. The coronary arteries were normal with just a small conal branch crossing the right ventricular outflow tract. There was a large conoventricular malalignment ventricular septal defect. There were a significant amount of muscle bundles in the right ventricular outflow tract. The pulmonary valve annulus was small, requiring creation of a transannular incision. There was a vertically oriented fishmouth-shaped bicuspid pulmonary valve with a functional orifice of 4mm. *[Variation: The Pulmonary Valve was unicuspid/trilaflet].* There was a mild to moderate supravalvar main pulmonary artery stenosis *[Variation: There was a mod/severe valvar/subvalvar and supravalvar main pulmonary artery stenosis].* The main pulmonary artery was small but both branch pulmonary arteries were of normal caliber. There was a small ligamentum arteriosum with no flow and a patent foramen ovale.

Description of Procedure: After obtaining appropriate consent, the patient was brought to the operating room and placed in supine position. General anesthesia was induced with the use of a single-lumen endotracheal tube. All monitoring lines were placed by the Anesthesia Service. A TEE probe was placed in the esophagus confirming the mitral/aortic continuity and preoperative diagnosis. The patient was prepped and draped in usual sterile fashion. A time out was performed confirming the patient's identity and procedure to be performed.

A primary median sternotomy was performed, sternal retractor was placed. A thymus was present and partial thymectomy was carried out. The phrenic nerves were identified and protected; the upper horns of the thymus were preserved. The pericardium was opened and two separate patches were harvested for later use and cardiac repair. One pericardial segment was treated with glutaraldehyde while the second one was left fresh in saline solution.

Pericardial stitches were placed in order to create a pericardial well. The superior vena cava and the aorta were circumferentially dissected. The pulmonary artery was dissected up to the level of the ligamentum arteriosum. Purse string sutures were placed in the ascending aorta, and superior and inferior venae cavae. Heparin (3-4 mg/kg) was administered and direct aorto-bicaval cannulation was achieved. These cannulae were secured, de-aired and connected to the bypass circuit. After confirmation of adequate ACT, cardiopulmonary bypass was initiated. There was excellent venous drainage. The patient was cooled down to 28°C. An antegrade cardioplegia catheter was placed on the proximal ascending aorta. An aortic cross-clamp was placed and antegrade cardioplegia was administered into the aortic root achieving a rapid diastolic cardiac arrest. Cardioplegia was administered every 20 minutes throughout the case. The superior and inferior vena caval tapes were snared. The patent foramen ovale was enlarged and a vent was placed into the left atrium, through which, the left side heart chambers were vented. Flow on CPB was decreased significantly until the left heart could be vented. We encountered significant collateral return to the left atrium.

The right ventricle was examined through the tricuspid valve. There was an anterior malalignment of the infundibular septum, with a ventricular septal defect and a significant hypertrophy of multiple septopareital trabeculations obstructing the right ventricular outflow tract. A trans-tricuspid right ventricular resection of hyperthrophied septoparietal trabeculations was performed. The muscle bundles were excised on the anterior, lateral, and posterior walls of the right ventricular outflow tract, just lateral to the infundibular septum.

Attention was then turned to the ventricular septal defect. The previously prepared glutaraldehyde-treated autologous pericardial patch was used to baffle the ventricular septal defect to the anteriorly displaced aortic valve. A series of interrupted pledgeted 6-0 polypropylene sutures were placed through the annulus of the tricuspid valve and into the medial edge of the ventricular septal defect. The previously harvested glutaraldehyde-prepared patch of autologous pericardium was brought to the field and was trimmed to the appropriated size and configuration. It was used to close the ventricular septal defect with a running 6-0 polypropylene and the previously placed tricuspid valve stitches. Care was taken to not damage the conduction system around the posterior inferior aspect of the defect. The patch was then inspected and found be seated nicely. The tricuspid valve was tested by inflating the right ventricle with cold saline and was found to be competent.

The main pulmonary artery was opened longitudinally and the incision carried to the bifurcation distally. The branch pulmonary arteries were assessed and both were of normal caliber. This incision on the main pulmonary artery was then carried proximally to the pulmonary annulus. The pulmonary annulus was *small/normal* and there was a very stenotic fishmouth shaped bicuspid pulmonary valve. The anterior commissure was incised down to the level but not through the pulmonary valve annulus and then working through the enlarged pulmonary valve an additional subvalvar infundibular resection was carried out. Having done this we could pass a Hegar dilator through the right ventricular outflow tract which is almost 2 mm larger than the mean expected pulmonary valve size for this child *[Variation, If Unicuspid valve: The unicuspid pulmonary valve had a posterior commissure. Anteriorly the valve leaflet was incised up to the level of the annulus. With a posterior commissurotomy and by extending the incision through the annulus for a distance of approximately 1 mm, a dilator 2 mm larger than the mean expected pulmonary valve size for this child could be passed into the relaxed right ventricle. Working through the enlarged pulmonary valve the infundibular resection was completed].*

We began to rewarm systemically and the atrial septal defect was closed primarily as the left heart was de-aired. Additional de-airing was accomplished via the ascending aorta and confirmed with TEE. The aortic cross-clamp was removed and a normal sinus rhythm returned rapidly. The right atriotomy was approximated with running polypropylene and the caval tourniquets were removed. A previously prepared pericardial patch was tailored and this was used to augment the main pulmonary artery incision. This was sewn and secured in place with running 7-0 polypropylene. A left atrial catheter was placed through the left atrial appendage. Temporary atrial/ventricular pacing wires were placed.

At this point the child was warmed systemically, the lungs were ventilated, and the heart was in sinus rhythm with good contractility. Having ascertained adequate de-airing utilizing the TEE the child was weaned from cardiopulmonary bypass and separated on a beta blocker infusion [**Variation:** on Esmolol +/- Milrinone]. The TEE demonstrated no residual ventricular septal defect, normal functioning tricuspid valve and acceptable velocity across the right ventricular outflow tract. Protamine was administered and the heart was sequentially decannulated. A peritoneal dialysis catheter and mediastinal chest drains were placed. *[Optional, If patient younger than a year: A non tunneled peritoneal dialysis catheter was placed by making an incision in the peritoneum under the diaphragm and placing the catheter through the abdominal wall and into the peritoneal cavity under direct visualization].*

The mediastinum was irrigated with antibiotic solution and aspirated. The sternum, fascia and skin were all approximated in a standard manner. The child was transported to the cardiac intensive care unit stable having tolerated the procedure.

Sponge, needle and instrument counts were correct.

Cardiopulmonary bypass time was **[BLANK]** minutes, with a cross-clamp period of **[BLANK]** minutes.

Dr. **[BLANK]** was present and scrubbed for **[BLANK]** elements of this procedure.

III. Congenital Cardiac Surgery

Suggested Readings:

1. Khonsari S, Sintek CF. **Cardiac Surgery: Safeguards and Pitfalls in Operative Technique. 4th ed.**
2. Philadelphia, PA: Lippincott Williams & Wilkins; 2008, p 276-287.
3. E. L. Bove and J. C. Hirsch. **Surgery for Congenital Heart Defects** by J. Stark and M. de Leval, VT Tsang. John Wiley & sons, Ltd; 2006, p 399-409.
4. Kouchoukos NT, Blackstone EH, Hanley FL, Kirklin JK. Kirklin/Barratt-Boyes **Cardiac Surgery: 4th ed.** Elsevier Saunders, Philadelphia, PA; 2013, p 1381-1392.

24. Pulmonary Valve Replacement and Reconstruction of Right Ventricle Outflow Tract

Muhammad Aftab, MD, Ramanan Umakanthan*, Jeffrey S. Heinle*, MD

Baylor College of Medicine/Texas Heart Institute, Houston, TX

*Texas Children's Hospital/Baylor College of Medicine, Houston, TX

Essential Operative Steps

1. Lines (central venous line, arterial line, volume line) and monitoring.
2. General endotracheal anesthesia.
3. Intra-operative Transesophageal Echocardiogram (TEE) to rule out residual intracardiac lesions (especially residual ventricular or atrial septal defects)
4. Redo-median sternotomy.
5. Lysis of adhesions.
6. Systemic heparinization (3-4 mg/Kg).
7. Direct aortic cannulation.
8. Bicaval cannulation, both cavae encircled with the tourniquets.
9. Establish Cardiopulmonary bypass (CPB) circuit.
10. Check ACT >450.
11. Initiate Cardiopulmonary bypass.
12. Systemic hypothermia (cooling to 34°C).
13. Dissect right ventricle outflow tract (RVOT) – dissection is facilitated once heart is decompressed on CPB.
14. Longitudinally open RVOT, main pulmonary artery (MPA) extending to the level of bifurcation. [**Variation:** RVOT was opened transversely at the level of the pulmonary valve annulus].
15. Excise the remnants of native pulmonary valve and inspect right ventricular outflow tract.
16. Measure the annulus and select the prosthesis (Bioprosthesis). NOTE: We do not use mechanical valves in the RVOT
17. Trim the redundant aneurysmal RVOT/main PA [**Variation:** completely excise the calcified outflow patch or previous RV-to-PA conduit].
18. Secure the prosthetic valve into orthotropic position using multiple horizontal mattress pledgeted sutures [**Variation:** Running 2-0 polypropylene].
19. Anteriorly, non-pledgeted sutures are placed through the valve sewing ring and tied exterior to the PA.
20. Re-approximate the edges of trimmed aneurysmal PA/RVOT [**Variation:** Augment the Pulmonary artery/RVOT using autologous pericardial/CorMatrix/Dacron patch etc.with an oval or diamond shape patch]. NOTE: we do not like nor do we use CorMatrix although others do.
21. Start rewarming.

22. Start ventilation and suction the lungs.
23. Allow the heart to fill and eject.
24. Wean from cardiopulmonary bypass
25. Administer protamine to reverse the heparin.
26. Aortic decannulation.
27. Ensure excellent hemostasis.
28. Placement of mediastinal drains and pleural chest tubes.
29. Sternotomy closure

Potential Complications and Pitfalls

1. A safe sternal reentry is one of the major steps to the successful outcome of redo operations. Typically the RV and RA will be dilated and immediately adjacent/adherent to the posterior aspect of the sternum. A previous RV-to_PA conduit may be densely adhered to the sternum.
2. Careful evaluation of preoperative imaging to assess the proximity of vital structures to the sternum, use of an oscillating saw for the anterior table, initially leaving the untwisted sternal wires in place, lifting the sternal edges and incising the posterior table under direct vision, removing the sternal wires after incising the posterior table and use of peripheral cannulation in high risk situations are some of the considerations for a safe sternal reentry.
3. Special attention should be paid to avoid any inadvertent injury to the phrenic nerves during the lysis of adhesions between the right side of the heart and pericardium and dissecting the SVC. The left phrenic nerve will be in close proximity to the lateral aspect of the dilated MPA and left PA.
4. Entire procedure can be performed on warm and beating heart, if no intracardiac defect (residual VSD or ASD) needs to be repaired. Residual intracardaic shunts allow for potential air entrainment into the left heart once the right heart is opened.
5. The incision along the anterior aspect of the main PA/RVOT can often be difficult due to severe calcification of the previous trans-annular patch.
6. A calcified transannular patch should be completely excised followed by anterior RVOT augmentation using autologous pericardial/Dacron/CorMatrix/bovine pericardial patch/Gore-Tex patch. If the RVOT patch is not clacified, it may be trimmed and closed primarily. **NOTE:** we do not use CorMatrix but others do.
7. The prosthetic valve is usually positioned in the annulus/RVOT at the orthotopic position with a slight posterior tilt.
8. The prosthesis is positioned such to avoid obstruction of the branch PA's.
9. The valve can be secured by either multiple horizontal mattress pledgeted sutures or running polypropylene suture.
10. For the reconstruction of RVOT, the oval or diamond shape patch should be secured starting from the apex of pulmonary arteriotomy with sutures lines running on both sides of the pulmonary atreriotomy upto to annulus. The patch is then folded on itself and running polypropylene suture will

incorporate the anterior annulus of prosthesis and the patch into the suture line. Alternatively, non-pledgeted sutures can be taken through the anterior aspect of valve sewing ring and then brought through the patch and tied exterior to the neo-pulmonary artery. The remaining portion of the patch is used to augment the RVOT.

Template Dictation

Preoperative Diagnosis:

1. Tetralogy of Fallot, status post repair with placement of a transannular right ventricular outflow tract patch
2. Severe pulmonary valve insufficiency.
3. Severe right ventricle dilatation.

Postoperative Diagnosis: Same

Procedure(s) Performed:

1. Repeat median sternotomy.
2. Total cardiopulmonary bypass
3. Pulmonary valve replacement with [BLANK] mm bioprosthetic valve
4. Right ventricular outflow tract reduction [**Variation**: Reconstruction of main pulmonary artery and right ventricular outflow tract with autologous pericardial/Dacron/CorMatrix/bovine pericardial patch/Gore-Tex patch].

Drainage: Mediastinal chest tube and right/left pleural drains were placed.

Attending Surgeon: [BLANK]

Secondary Surgeon: [BLANK]

Assistants: [BLANK]

Anesthesia: [BLANK]

Indication(s) for Procedure: This is a [AGE] -year-old [GENDER] who had undergone previous repair of the Tetralogy of Fallot with placement of a transannular RVOT patch when he was 9 months old. He has done well but has developed severe pulmonary insufficiency with severe right ventricular dilatation. He was, therefore, put forward for pulmonary valve replacement to preserve right ventricular function. A lengthy preoperative consultation was carried out with the patient and his family detailing the anatomy, planned surgery and attendant perioperative risks. All of his questions were answered.

Operative Findings: Intraoperative TEE confirmed no residual intracardiac lesions. The previously created sternotomy was well-healed. The patient had the expected pericardial adhesions consistent with his previous surgery. The right ventricle and right atrium were severely dilated. The main pulmonary artery and right ventricular outflow tract (RVOT) were severely dilated. The RVOT patch was densely adhered to the sternum. The ascending aorta was mildly dilated. The systemic venous drainage was normal. The branch pulmonary arteries were of excellent caliber bilaterally. No pulmonary valve tissue could be identified. A [BLANK] mm bioprosthesis was placed in an orthotopic position to restore pulmonary valve competency. [**Variation:** The RVOT reduction was performed by excising the redundant portion of the main pulmonary artery and the outflow tract patch].

Description of Procedure: After informed consent was obtained and the patient's identity and the surgical site were confirmed, the patient was brought to the operating room and positioned supine on the operating table. Adequate general anesthesia was induced and patient was intubated. Central venous and arterial lines were placed and a transesophageal echo (TEE) probe was passed. A preoperative TEE was carried out and contrast study was performed which demonstrated no residual intracardiac shunting. The patient was positioned supine and all the pressure sites were padded appropriately. The chest, abdomen and groins were prepped and draped in standard sterile fashion. A repeat median sternotomy incision was made over the sternum and carried down to the presternal fascia with electrocautery. The chest was entered through the previous median sternotomy with an oscillating sternal saw initially leaving the sternal wires in place, lifting the sternal edges and incising the posterior table under direct vision and removing the sternal wires after incising the posterior table. Hemostasis was achieved with electrocautery. Adhesions in the mediastinum were taken down with careful sharp dissection and electrocautery. The heart was dissected out from the surrounding mediastinal structures and ascending aorta was mobilized. The phrenic nerves were identified bilaterally, and care was taken to avoid injuring these structures.

Pursestrings were placed on the ascending aorta, superior vena cava and the inferior vena cava for cannulation. The patient was then systemically heparinized and cannulated for cardiopulmonary bypass using direct aorto-bicaval cannulation. After reaching appropriate ACT, bypass was established and the patient was cooled to 34 °C. The entire operation was carried out with the beating and empty heart. With the heart decompressed, the RVOT tract was dissected out and noted to be severely dilated and aneurysmal [**Variation:** The Transventricular patch was noted to be severely calcified]. There was also significant dilation of the right ventricle.

A longitudinal incision was made on the anterior aspect of the main pulmonary artery patch and carried proximally onto the right ventricular outflow tract and distally to the level of the bifurcation. [**Variation:** RVOT was opened transversely at the level of the pulmonary valve annulus]. TEE confirmed no air in the left heart. There were no remnants of native pulmonary valve. The branch pulmonary arteries easily accepted a Hegar dilator several millimeters larger than normal based on body surface area. Given the massive size of the right ventricular outflow tract, a [**BLANK**] mm bioprosthesis/mechanical valve could easily be placed in an orthotopic position. Prior to placing the valve, the size of the right ventricular outflow tract and main pulmonary artery was reduced by excising a portion of the redundant anterior wall [**Variation:** The aneurysmal calcified outflow patch was completely excised]. The posterior aspect of the valve was then secured in place using multiple horizontal mattress pledgeted 2-0 Ticron/Ethibond sutures (multifilament braided suture) which were placed at the level of the annulus and then passed through the sewing ring of the prosthetic valve. Valve was positioned into the annulus and sutures were tied and divided. Anteriorly, non-pledgeted sutures were taken through the valve sewing ring and then brought through the pulmonary artery and tied exterior to the pulmonary artery [**Variation:** Posteriorly the sewing ring of the valve was secured to the muscular right ventricular outflow tract at the level of the pulmonary annulus with running 2-0 polyproplyene. Anteriorly, the sewing ring was incorporated into the closure of the arteriotomy]. The edges of the main pulmonary artery and right ventricular outflow tract were then closed using running 4-0 polyproplyene suture. [**Variation:** A bovine pericardial/CorMatrix/GORE-TEX/Dacron patch was used to augment the MPA/RVOT being sewn in place with running polypropylene suture. Anteriorly, non-pledgeted sutures were taken through the valve sewing ring and then brought through the patch and tied exterior to the neo-pulmonary artery].

The patient was fully rewarmed and weaned from cardiopulmonary bypass without difficulty and with good hemodynamics. Protamine was administered to reverse the heparin and the patient was sequentially decannulated. The suture lines and cannulation sites were inspected and found to be hemostatic. A mediastinal chest tube and right/left pleural drains were placed. The mediastinum was irrigated with copious amounts of warm antibiotic saline irrigation. The sternal edges were re-approximated using stainless steel wires. The soft tissues were closed in multiple layers using running absorbable suture. The skin edges were re-approximated using a running absorbable subcuticular stitch.

The patient tolerated the procedure well. The patient was extubated in the operating room and transported to the Pediatric Cardiac Intensive Care Unit in a satisfactory condition. Sponge, needle and instrument counts were correct.

Cardiopulmonary bypass time was [**BLANK**] minutes.

Dr. [**BLANK**] was present and scrubbed for [**BLANK**] elements of this procedure.

Suggested Readings:

1. Khonsari S, Sintek CF. Cardiac Surgery: Safeguards and Pitfalls in Operative Technique. 4th ed. Philadelphia, PA: Lippincott Williams & Wilkins; 2008, p 276-287.
2. B.E. Kogon, K.A. Rodby, P.M. Kirshbom et al. Adult congenital pulmonary valve replacement: a simple, effective, and reproducible technique, Congenit Heart Dis, 2 (2007), pp. 314–318.

III. Congenital Cardiac Surgery

25. Repair of Truncus Arteriousus (TA)

Joshua L. Hermsen, MD and D. Michael McMullan, MD

Seattle Children's Hospital, Seattle, WA

Essential Operative Steps

1. General endotracheal anesthesia
2. Standard lines and monitors
3. Review of transesophageal echocardiogram (TEE)
4. "Time-out" pre-surgical check
5. Median Sternotomy
6. Thymectomy
7. Harvest pericardium and treat with gluteraldehyde
8. Pericardial well
9. Dissect, control and snare right pulmonary artery between aorta and SVC
10. Dissect truncus/ascending aorta/aortic arch to allow high cannulation
11. Complete circumferential dissection of RPA to hilum
12. Circumferentially dissect LPA to hilum and control with tape
13. Identify coronary origins and coronaries crossing RVOT
14. Systemic Heparinization (3mg/kg)
15. Bicaval - high ascending aortic cannulation
16. Initiate CPB when ACT > 400s
17. Systemic hypothermia (cooling to 32°C).
18. Snare LPA
19. Place antegrade cardioplegia cannula
20. Cross clamp ascending aorta
21. Administer antegrade cardioplegia with topical cooling
22. Consider ostial cardioplegia depending upon truncal valve regurgitation.
23. Administer maintenance cardioplegia per institutional protocol
24. Place vent to capture return to left heart
25. Transect ascending aorta just superior to PA's
26. Excise PA's as a "Carrel patch" using the posterior truncal wall. This is done even for type 1 truncus to aid reconstruction of the aorta
27. Perform right ventriculotomy guided by a right angle clamp passed through the truncal valve and VSD.
28. Patch close the VSD through the ventriculotomy and/or atrium
29. An appropriately sized RV-PA conduit is selected and the distal conduit is anastomosed to the PA confluence
30. Truncal valve repair is performed as needed
31. Truncus (proximal) is anastomosed end-to-end to the ascending aorta (distal)
32. Begin rewarming to 36°C
33. The proximal conduit is anastomosed to the ventricle.
34. De-air and remove aortic cross-clamp. Continue deairing through cardioplegia site

35. Inspect for hemostasis
36. Remove LA vent and ensure LV contracting well
37. Evaluate deairing, ventricular function, VSD closure, conduit/PA flow and truncal valve function with TEE
38. Address residual shunts, anastomotic or valve problems as needed
39. Wean from CPB
40. Assess RV pressures with direct measure by needle.
41. Venous decannulation
42. Modified Ultrafiltration
43. Heparin reversal with protamine
44. Aortic decannulation
45. Place atrial and ventricular epicardial pacing wires
46. Place drains as needed
47. Assure hemostasis
48. Pericardial reconstruction with 0.1 mm goretex membrane **[Optional]**
49. Sternal Closure

Potential Complications and Pitfalls

1. Hemodynamic instability pre-bypass. Due to systemic and coronary hypoperfusion from pulmonary overcirculation and diastolic runoff. Hypoventilation (to increase PVR), vasopressors (to increase BP) and snaring of the RPA (to shunt blood to the systemic circulation) are simple, common methods to address the mismatch between systemic and pulmonary circulations.
2. An absent or hypoplastic thymus likely indicates 22q11 deletion. Resulting hypocalcemia may impair ventricular function, especially post-bypass and in response to blood product transfusions. This finding should be shared with the anesthesia and perfusion providers so they can adjust calcium replacement strategies.
3. Inadequate myocardial protection. Most truncal valves are insufficient to some degree, which may compromise delivery of truncal root antegrade cardioplegia. Manual compression of the ventricle may suffice for mildly insufficient valves. More severely regurgitant valves necessitate handheld ostial cardioplegia to ensure good delivery and avoid ventricular distension.
4. Post-Bypass RV hypertension. RV pressures greater than 75% systemic require treatment. RV outflow obstruction related to reconstruction must be revised to provide unobstructed pulmonary flow. Residual VSD's causing RV hypertension must be closed (the influence of an echocardiographically evident residual defect can be assessed by the Qp:Qs using simultaneous SVC and PA blood samples and Qp:Qs > 1.5 indicates need for closure).
5. Pulmonary hypertension should be treated with inhaled nitric oxide. Elevated PVR not responsive to medical treatment may require fenestration of the VSD patch. RV diastolic dysfunction that increases

III. Congenital Cardiac Surgery

CVP will resolve with time but may require creation of a small ASD to: minimize morbidity associated with early post-operative systemic venous congestion and maintain cardiac output at the expense of mild cyanosis.

Template Dictation

Preoperative Diagnosis: Truncus arteriosus (type 2), DiGeorge Syndrome

Post-operative diagnoses: Same

Procedure(s) Performed: Repair of truncus arteriosus

Attending Surgeon: [BLANK]

Secondary Surgeon: [BLANK]

Assistants: [BLANK]

Anesthesia: [BLANK]

Indication(s) for Procedure: [Age] year old [Weight] neonate with pre-natal diagnosis of truncus arteriosus. The aortic arch is intact and the baby is well saturated with very mild failure symptoms while feeding. Informed consent for neonatal repair was obtained from the parents to limit progression of pulmonary vascular disease and enable long-term survival.

Description of Procedure: A time-out was performed per institutional protocol. General endotracheal anesthesia was induced and appropriate therapeutic and monitoring lines were placed. A transesophageal echocardiographic exam was performed. The chest was prepped and draped in a sterile fashion.

A median sternotomy was performed. There was no thymus gland present. A patch of pericardium was excised and treated with glutaraldehyde. A pericardial well was fashioned.

The right pulmonary artery was circumferentially dissected between the aorta and superior vena cava, encircled with a silicone tape and occlusively snared which increased the systemic blood pressure. Saturations dipped slightly but remained above 90%.

The truncus, ascending aorta and aortic arch were completely mobilized. The pulmonary arteries were mobilized to the hila and the anatomy was consistent with a type II truncus. A silicone tape was placed around the left pulmonary artery. The coronary origins were normal and no major coronary branches crossed the right ventricular outflow tract.

The patient was anticoagulated with 3mg/kg unfractionated heparin and connected to the heart-lung machine with bicaval to distal ascending aortic cannulation. ACT was confirmed to be > 480 s, bypass was initiated with adequate drainage and flows and the tape around the LPA was snared. The patient was cooled to

32°C. A vent was placed through the tip of the right atrial appendage and the cavae were snared. An antegrade cardioplegia needle was placed.

The distal ascending aorta was cross-clamped under low-flow conditions and antegrade cardioplegia delivered with prompt arrest and no appreciable ventricular distension. A small incision was made in the right atrium and the vent redirected through a patent foramen ovale.

The ascending aorta was divided just distal to the origin of the pulmonary arteries. The pulmonary arteries were then separated from the truncus as a single unit with a cuff of truncal/aortic wall.

A right ventriculotomy was made guided by a right angle clamp passed through the truncal valve and ventricular septal defect. Care was taken to not injure any coronary branches. The ventricular edges were slightly undermined. The VSD was closed with a dacron patch sewn with a running 5-0 polypropylene suture.

A 12 mm bovine jugular valved conduit was opened, appropriately rinsed and trimmed. The distal conduit was anastomosed to the pulmonary artery cuff with running 6-0 polypropylene suture. The ascending aorta was anastomosed to the divided truncus with running 6-0 polypropylene suture. Rewarming to 36°C was begun and the proximal conduit was trimmed and anastomosed to the right ventriculotomy with 5-0 polypropylene suture. The vent was removed and replaced via the left atrial appendage. The PFO was not closed. The right atriotomy was closed with double layer running 6-0 polypropylene sutures.

The heart was thoroughly deaired through the cardioplegia needle site and the cross clamp removed under low-flow conditions. Deairing was continued allowing the cardioplegia needle site to bleed into the field. The heart appeared well perfused and sinus rhythm resumed spontaneously within several minutes. TEE confirmed adequate deairing and the needle site snared. Ventricular function was vigorous and the LA vent was removed. Hemostasis appeared adequate at all suture lines. Cardiopulmonary bypass was weaned uneventfully.

Post-bypass TEE revealed normal ventricular function, truncal valve function was unchanged and there was no residual VSD. RV outflow appeared to be unobstructed with low velocity flow in the conduit and PA's. RV pressures were directly measured with a needle and found to be 40% systemic. Venous cannulae were removed and modified ultrafiltration was performed. Protamine sulfate was given and well tolerated. The aortic cannula was removed without incident. Blood and blood products were administered as needed per anesthesia. Hemostasis was achieved throughout the operative field. Atrial and ventricular epicardial pacing wires were placed. A single mediastinal drain was placed. The anterior pericardium was reconstructed with a 0.1 mm goretex membrane [Optional]. Sternal wires were placed to approximate the sternum and the soft tissues were closed in 3 layers with absorbable suture. Dermabond was used to dress the skin and occlusive dressings were placed at tube and wire sites.

III. Congenital Cardiac Surgery

Sponge, needle and instrument counts were correct. The patient was transferred intubated, in expected condition, to the cardiac intensive care unit.

Cardiopulmonary bypass time was **[BLANK]** minutes, with a cross-clamp period of **[BLANK]** minutes.

Dr. **[BLANK]** was present and scrubbed for **[BLANK]** elements of this procedure.

26. Cone Repair for Ebstein Malformation

Sameh M. Said, MD, and Joseph A. Dearani, MD

Mayo Clinic, Rochester, MN

Essential Operative Steps

1. Lines and Monitoring
2. General endotracheal anesthesia
3. Intraoperative transesophageal echocardiogram (TEE)
4. Median sternotomy
5. Open pericardium, pericardial well
6. Systemic heparinization (400 U/Kg)
7. CO_2 in the operative field
8. Arterial cannulation
9. Bicaval venous cannulation with caval snares
10. Aortic root vent/cardioplegia needle
11. Check ACT (>400 sec)
12. Initiate cardiopulmonary bypass
13. Maintain normothermia or mild hypothermia
14. Aortic cross clamp (reduce pump flow rate, apply cross clamp, increase pump flow rate to 2.0-2.5 L/min/m^2); include pulmonary artery in cross clamp
15. Antegrade cold blood cardioplegia induction and every 20 minutes
16. Iced slush saline applied to right ventricle
17. Caval tapes are snared
18. Oblique right atriotomy
19. Closure of patent foramen ovale
20. Assess the tricuspid valve (evaluate each component of the anterior, inferior and septal leaflets) and right ventricle (area of atrialization)
21. Start the surgical delamination process - anterior, inferior (when present) and septal leaflets
22. Augmentation of the shallow anterior leaflet, if needed
23. Delamination (360°) with subsequent rotation of the delaminated anterior leaflet towards the septal leaflet to form the cone
24. Plication of the atrialized portion of the right ventricle
25. Annular plication
26. Inspection of epicardial surface of heart to confirm no coronary artery compromise
27. Anchoring the delaminated leaflets to the true annular level
28. Check valve competence with saline installation
29. Close residual leaflet fenestrations
30. Annuloplasty band from the anteroseptal to the inferoseptal commissure anchored in coronary sinus
31. Release the aortic cross clamp
32. Right reduction atrioplasty

III. Congenital Cardiac Surgery

33. Closure of the right atriotomy
34. De-airing maneuvers
35. Check for hemostasis
36. Placement of epicardial atrial and ventricular pacing wires
37. Chest tube placement
38. Wean from cardiopulmonary bypass
39. Evaluate tricuspid valve with transesophageal echocardiogram
40. Venous decannulation
41. Ensure adequate de-airing of the heart prior to removal of aortic root vent
42. Protamine administration for heparin reversal
43. Aortic decannulation (systolic blood pressure 90 mmHg)
44. Assess hemostasis
45. Sternotomy closure

Potential Complications and Pitfalls

1. Injury to sinoatrial node during SVC cannulation or during placement of the SVC snare
2. Injury of the pulmonary artery during cross clamp application
3. Poor venous drainage (incorrect choice of cannula size, advancing the two-stage cannula too far in so it is obstructing hepatic veins)
4. Buttonhole the right ventricular wall or the tricuspid valve leaflets during the surgical delamination process
5. Injury to the right coronary artery during plication of the atrialized right ventricle or the annulus
6. Injury to the atrioventricular node during reattachment of the septal leaflet of the tricuspid valve
7. Failure to recognize shallow leaflets which require patch augmentation
8. Missed residual fenestrations which contribute to residual valve regurgitation
9. Improper placement of the annuloplasty sutures with risk of injury to the right coronary artery

Template Dictation

Preoperative Diagnosis:

1. Ebstein malformation
2. Severe tricuspid valve regurgitation
3. Patent foramen ovale

Postoperative Diagnosis: Same

Procedure(s) Performed:

1. Complete repair of Ebstein's malformation
2. Suture closure patent foramen ovale
3. Tricuspid valve repair, with placement of flexible annuloplasty ring
4. Plication of atrialized right ventricle

5. Right reduction atrioplasty
6. Establishment of temporary extracorporeal circulation
7. Cardioplegic arrest (blood) 4:1
8. Intraoperative transesophageal echocardiography

Drainage: 2 No. 28 Argyle chest tubes

Attending Surgeon: [BLANK]

Secondary Surgeon: [BLANK]

Assistants: [BLANK]

Anesthesia: [BLANK]

Indication(s) for Procedure: [AGE] year old [GENDER] with [DURATION] history of [COMPLAINT] –e.g. increasingly shortness of breath]. Preoperative transthoracic echocardiography reveals [FINDINGS - e.g. severe tricuspid valve regurgitation in the setting of Ebstein malformation].

Description of the Procedure: After informed consent, patient identification and surgical site confirmation, the patient was brought to the operating room and placed on the operating table in a supine position. Single lumen general endotracheal tube anesthesia was induced and all the necessary monitoring lines were placed. Precardiopulmonary bypass transesophageal echocardiography demonstrated severe tricuspid regurgitation with anatomy consistent with Ebstein's malformation. There was marked displacement of the diminutive septal leaflet. The height of anterior leaflet was [Blank]. There were multiple muscular attachments between the body of the anterior leaflet and the free wall of the right ventricle. There was inferior leaflet that was also displaced apically. The right ventricle was enlarged (Grade xx/6). The patient was prepped and draped in a surgical sterile fashion and a primary median sternotomy was performed. The pericardium was opened in the midline. Heparin was administered. The ascending aorta was cannulated with a 20-French DLP cannula, and the superior and inferior venae cavae were cannulated separately with right-angle venous cannulae. Cardiopulmonary bypass was commenced at 2.4 L/min/m^2 for [Blank] minutes, and the perfusate was maintained at normothermia. An aortic tack vent was placed on aspiration, and a CO2 line was maintained in the operative field. The aorta was cross-clamped and [Blank] cc of cold blood cardioplegia was infused in the aortic root obtaining satisfactory asystolic arrest. Additional cold blood cardioplegia was administered antegrade via the aortic root at 20-minute intervals during the cross-clamp period. Iced slush saline was applied topically to the right ventricle. Caval tapes were snared. An oblique right atriotomy was performed. The patent foramen ovale was closed with a mattress suture of polypropylene backed with felt pledgets. The anterior annulus was suspended at 10 o'clock and 2 o'clock with fine polypropylene sutures. The anterior leaflet was incised above the annulus. A surgical delamination process was performed of muscular and chordal attachments to the anterior leaflet. The inferior leaflet was surgically delaminated. The septal leaflet was surgically delaminated. The inferior leaflet was rotated to meet the proximal edge of the septal leaflet and was approximated in two layers with fine polypropylene suture. The atrialized right ventricle was then plicated in a triangular fashion from apex to base with continuos 4/0 polypropylene suture taking care not to injure or distort the right coronary artery. The tricuspid valve annulus was severely dilated and was plicated in multiple spots around the annulus, avoiding an exaggerated plication in one location, that would potentially distort the right coronary artery. We then reanchored the newly reconstructed septal leaflet to the ventricular septum with continuous polypropylene suture in two layers. This was done to the ventricular side of the conduction tissue. The anterior leaflet was reanchored to the true annulus with two layers of 5-0 polypropylene. The anterior leaflet reattachment to the Cor Matrix membrane was done using continuous 6-0 polypropylene in two layers. Instillation of saline into the right ventricle demonstrated mild residual central regurgitation. Next, a [Blank] mm annuloplasty ring was placed and secured in position with multiple interrupted 4/0 Prolene sutures from the anteroseptal clockwise to the inferoseptal commissure and anchored in the coronary sinus. The cross-clamp was released after [Blank] minutes with suction on the aortic root vent. Normal sinus rhythm resumed. The redundant right atrium was excised and the atriotomy was oversewn in two layers of running polypropylene suture. Air was evacuated through the suture line prior to securing it. Cardiopulmonary bypass was gradually discontinued with satisfactory hemodynamics on low-dose epinephrine and milrinone infusions. Postcardiopulmonary bypass transesophageal echo demonstrated [Blank]. There was no gradient across the tricuspid valve, and the atrial septum was intact. Decannulation was accomplished and surgical sites oversewn with polypropylene suture. Protamine was administered. Hemostasis was achieved, and chest tubes were left in the mediastinum and the right hemithorax. The sternum was closed with interrupted wire in the usual manner and the wound closed in layers with absorbable sutures. The patient was transferred to the Cardiac Surgical Intensive Care Unit in a stable hemodynamic condition.

All the instruments, sponges and needles counts were correct twice at the conclusion of the procedure.

Cardiopulmonary bypass time was [BLANK] minutes, with a cross-clamp period of [BLANK] minutes.

Dr. [BLANK] was present and scrubbed for [BLANK] elements of this procedure.

27. Pediatric Lung Transplantation: Bilateral Sequential Lung Transplantation

Muhammad Aftab, MD, Magdy M. El-Sayed Ahmed[ϵ] MD, Ramanan Umakanthan* MD, Jeffrey S. Heinle*, MD

Baylor College of Medicine/Texas Heart Institute, Houston, TX,

[ϵ]Department of Cardiovascular Surgery, Texas Heart Institute, Houston, TX, USA

*Texas Children's Hospital/Baylor College of Medicine, Houston, TX

Essential Operative Steps

1. Lines and Monitoring.
2. General endotracheal anesthesia.
3. Intra-operative Transesophageal Echocardiogram (TEE)
4. Inspection of donor lungs by the procurement team.
5. Confirm the good quality of donor lungs.
6. Administer induction immunosuppressives and steroids
7. Start the recipient operation.
8. Bilateral transverse (clamshell) thoracosternotomy [**Variation:** Median Sternotomy].
9. Lysis of adhesions.
10. Systemic heparinization (3-4 mg/Kg).
11. Direct aortic cannulation.
12. Dual stage venous cannulation. (unless need to close PFO)
13. Establish Cardiopulmonary bypass (CPB) circuit.
14. Check ACT >450.
15. Initiate Cardiopulmonary bypass.
16. Systemic hypothermia (cooling to 32°C).
17. Vent the main Pulmonary artery (PA).
18. Deflate both lungs, aspirate bronchial secretions.
19. Tobramycin irrigation of airways [**Optional for colonized airways**]
20. Start hilar dissection for recipient pneumonectomy.
21. Control the branch pulmonary arteries with atraumatic snares
22. Dissect pulmonary arteries in the pleural space and ligate distally beyond the first order bifurcation.
23. Transect the pulmonary arteries.
24. Ligate large bronchial collaterals.
25. Divide the pulmonary veins with vascular staples.
26. Aspirate instilled tobramycin irrigation and divide the bronchus.
27. Avoid any bronchial contents spillage in the pleural space.
28. Irrigate the pleural space with copious antibiotic irrigation.
29. Perform contralateral pneumonectomy in a similar fashion.
30. Confirm the donor-recipient ABO compatibility and size matching.
31. Prepare the donor lung.

32. Divide the main PA and transect the branch PA's to the appropriate length. Divide left atrium and prepare the left atrial cuff.
33. Staple and divide the left bronchus and place the right lung in the ice preservative solution.
34. Trim the donor bronchus up to one tracheal ring (within several mm) proximal to the bifurcation.
35. Lung in pleural space and keep cold with iced saline sponges.
36. Perform an end-to-end bronchial anastomosis using running absorbable fine monofilament suture on membranous portion and interrupted on cartilaginous portion.
37. Clamp the base of donor pulmonary veins and the left atrial cuff, excise staple lines and create common orifice.
38. Construct an end-to-end left atrium to recipient pulmonary veins anastomosis using running fine monofilament polypropylene suture.
39. De-air the pulmonary vein by instilling the cold preservative solution into the pulmonary artery.
40. Remove the clamp and snare the pulmonary veins.
41. Create an end to end pulmonary artery anastomosis using running fine monofilament polypropylene suture.
42. Keep the implanted lung cold and reprefuse both lungs at the same time [**Variation:** Re-perfuse the implanted lung. We don't use this technique].
43. Perform contralateral lung implantation in a similar fashion.
44. Start rewarming during the final anastomosis.
45. Remove snares and discontinue the PA vent
46. Aortic root vent to deair
47. Ventilate the donor lungs and perform bronchoscopy to clear the airway.
48. To avoid the reperfusion injury, slowly wean from cardiopulmonary bypass
49. [Note: Also avoid high FiO2, high PEEP and high airway pressures to avoid reperfusion/lung injury].
50. Use Inotropes, vasopressors, prostaglandins infusion and inhaled nitric oxide as needed [**Optional**].
51. Confirm the graft function, check the ABG and wean supplemental oxygen as tolerated.
52. Administer protamine and sequentially decannulate.
53. Ensure excellent hemostasis.
54. Place bilateral anterior and posterior chest tubes.
55. Re-approximate the ribs and sternal edges.
56. Standard wound closure.

Potential Complications and Pitfalls

1. Special attention should be paid to identify and preserve bilateral phrenic and vagal nerves.
2. The hilar dissection is extended into the pericardium by creating a pericardial slit posterior to phrenic nerves and anterior to pulmonary

veins. This exposure necessary in order to secure clamps and snares on the left atrium and pulmonary arteries for creating the anastomosis.
3. Hilar vessels should be dissected to the branch pulmonary arteries into the lung parenchyma and securely ligated beyond the first order bifurcation.
4. Any skeletonization of recipient bronchus by dissecting the area of bronchial bifurcation is avoided. The peri-bronchial fat is preserved to maintain the blood supply of main-stem bronchus for new bronchial anastomosis.
5. Bilateral recipient pneumonectomy should be performed first before starting the donor lung implantation to avoid any spillover of secretions into the implanted lung.
6. Avoid contaminaton of pleural space with bronchial secretions
7. During preparation of donor lung for the anastomosis, a careful attention should be paid to the anastomotic size, identifying and orienting the hilar structures.
8. The appropriate donor to recipient size matching is crucial to early and long term successful outcomes of pediatric lung transplantation. While the oversizing of the donor lung can cause compression atelectasis and pneumonia, under sizing of the donor lung may result in chronic space problems.
9. During the entire process of implantation the lung should be kept cold within the thoracic cavity, wrapped in ice cold saline sponges/laparotomy pads.
10. Both donor bronchi should be cultured, and all the secretions should be aspirated prior to performing the bronchial anastomosis.
11. An end-to-end bronchial anastomosis is performed using running absorbable monofilament PDS (polydioxanone) suture for the membranous portion and interrupted PDS sutures on the anterior cartilaginous portion. (Note: In case of significant size discrepancy, consider telescoping Optional). I will sometimes telescope if there is a significant size discrepancy
12. To create the left atrium to recipient pulmonary veins anastomoses, the pulmonary veins are cut open and intervening tissue between two orifices is incised. Both vascular anastomoses are performed using fine monofilament, non-absorbable sutures.
13. At the completion of suture lines both pulmonary artery and veins should be deaired and forward flushed and/or cold saline should be instilled.
14. Special attention should be paid to presence of any pulmonary artery emboli which should be removed and completely flushed out prior to completing the anastomoses.

Template Dictation

Preoperative Diagnosis:

1. Cystic fibrosis

III. Congenital Cardiac Surgery

2. End-stage lung disease

Postoperative Diagnosis: Same

Procedure(s) Performed:

1. Bilateral sequential lung transplantation with cardiopulmonary bypass support.

Drainage: Bilateral anterior and posterior chest tubes

Attending Surgeon: [BLANK]

Secondary Surgeon: [BLANK]

Procuring Surgeon: [BLANK]

Assistants: [BLANK]

Anesthesia: [BLANK]

Indication(s) for Procedure: This is a [AGE]-year-old Caucasian boy with [DURATION] history of [COMPLAINT – eg cystic fibrosis with progressive and now end-stage lung disease.] He was listed for bilateral lung transplantation. Suitable donor lungs have become available and he is felt to be an acceptable candidate for transplantation at this time.

The donor suffered a head injury following an ATV accident. There is good gas exchange in the donor lungs.

Operative Findings: There were minimal adhesions in the pleural spaces. The donor lungs were hyperexpanded. There was mediastinal lymphadenopathy. The donor lungs were of good quality and good size match. The hilar structures were only slightly larger than the recipient.

There was excellent early graft function, with PaO2 of greater than 200 on an FIO2 of 0.40 Both lungs inflated well and appeared to be a good size match.

Description of the Procedure: After informed consent and patient identification, the patient was brought to the operating room and placed on the operating table in a supine position. After induction of general anesthesia with single lumen endotracheal tube intubation, arterial and central venous monitoring lines were placed. The patient was positioned supine with the arms at the side and the chest and abdomen were prepped and draped. After the donor lungs were visualized and confirmed to be of good quality, we began the recipient operation.

A bilateral transverse thoracosternotomy incision was performed in the 4th intercostals space [**Variation:** 5th Intercostal space], dividing the mammary pedicles bilaterally. The thymus was divided and a pericardial well was created. The ascending aorta was mobilized. The patient was then systemically heparinized and cannulated for the cardiopulmonary bypass using an arterial cannula in the distal ascending aorta and a dual-stage venous cannula inserted through the right atrial appendage. Total cardiopulmonary bypass was established and there was good venous return. The patient was cooled to a nasopharyngeal temperature of 32 degrees centigrade. An active vent was placed in the main pulmonary artery. After instituting bypass both lungs were deflated, the bronchial secretions were aspirated and tobramycin irrigation was instilled into the airways.

Bilateral recipient pneumonectomies were then carried out. The hilar dissections were performed, with care being taken to identify and avoid injuring the phrenic nerves. The right pneumonectomy was performed first. The branch pulmonary arteries were controlled with atraumatic snares. Within the pleural space, the pulmonary arteries were further dissected and ligated distally beyond the first order bifurcation. The pulmonary artery was transected. The pulmonary veins were then divided between vascular staples. The tobramycin irrigation was aspirated and the bronchus divided using electrocautery. Bronchial vessels were controlled with hemoclips. Care was taken to avoid spilling bronchial contents into the pleural space. The lung was removed from the field. Hemostasis was assured in the hilum. The pleural space was irrigated with copious amounts of warm antibiotic saline irrigation. The left pneumonectomy was carried out in a similar fashion. Again, hemostasis was assured, and the pleural space was irrigated with warm antibiotic saline irrigation.

By this point in time, the donor lungs were in the operating suite. ABO compatibility was verified. The donor lungs were brought onto the field and prepared. Atrial cuffs were created. The main pulmonary artery was divided and the branch pulmonary arteries were transected at an appropriate length. The left bronchus was stapled proximally and divided distally. The right lung was placed back in the iced preservative solution. The left donor bronchus was trimmed to one tracheal ring proximal to the bifurcation. The lung was placed in the left pleural space and kept cold with iced saline sponges. An end-to-end bronchial anastomosis was performed using running 4-0 PDS suture for the membranous portion and interrupted 4-0 PDS sutures on the anterior cartilaginous portion. Prior to completing the suture line, a suction catheter was advanced into the left bronchus and placed on low continuous suction. A large vascular clamp was placed across the base of the donor pulmonary veins, the staple lines were excised and the recipient pulmonary veins were opened creating a common orifice. An end-to-end left atrium to recipient pulmonary vein anastomosis was then performed using running 4-0 polypropylene suture. Prior to completing the suture line, cold preservative solution was instilled into the pulmonary artery to de-air the pulmonary veins. The suture line was then completed. An atraumatic snare was passed around the pulmonary veins and the vascular clamp was removed. An end-to-end pulmonary artery anastomosis was then performed using running 5-0 polypropylene suture. The suture line was completed. The lung was packed in ice and attention was then turned to the right side. In a similar fashion, the right lung was implanted. During the final anastomosis, the patient was rewarmed. A bronchoscopy was carried out by the anesthesia team to clear the airway of secretions and confirm patency of the airways. The lungs were then ventilated. After complete rewarming and institution of prostaglandin infusion and inotropic agents, the patient was slowly weaned from cardiopulmonary bypass over approximately 15 minutes to avoid re-perfusion injury [**Variation:** Inhaled nitric oxide was administered]. Both lungs inflated well and appeared to be a good size match. There was excellent early graft function, with PaO2 of greater than 200 on an FIO2 of 0.40 [**Variation:** Initial saturations were in the high 80s to low 90s, but with time, these improved, and prior to leaving the operating room, the PaO2 was greater than 120 mmHg on an FiO2 of 0.50]. Protamine was administered and the patient was sequentially decannulated. Hemostasis was assured. The pleural spaces and mediastinum were irrigated with copious amounts of warm antibiotic saline irrigation. The pericardial edges were loosely reapproximated. Bilateral anterior and posterior chest tubes were placed. The sternal edges were reapproximated using stainless steel wires. The rib edges were reapproximated using interrupted absorbable pericostal sutures. The muscle and soft tissues were closed in multiple layers using running absorbable suture. The skin edges were reapproximated using a running absorbable subcuticular stitch. Sterile dressings were applied.

Cardiopulmonary bypass time was [BLANK] minutes. Donor ischemic time was [BLANK] hours and [BLANK] minutes.

Dr. [BLANK] was present and scrubbed for [BLANK] elements of this procedure.

Suggested Readings:

1. Michler RE, Pediatric Lung Transplantation. In Kapoor AS, Laks H (eds). Atlas of Heart-Lung Transplantation; McGraw-Hill, New York, NY; 1994, p 141-157.
2. Spray TL, Mallory G, Canter CE, et al. Pediatric lung transplantation: indications, techniques and early results. J Thorac Cardiovasc Surg 1994; 107: 990.

28. Pediatric Heart Transplantation

Brody Wehman, MD, MSc and Sunjay Kaushal, MD, PhD

University of Maryland Medical Center, Baltimore, MD

Essential Operative Steps

1. Confirm suitability of donor organ
2. Lines and monitoring
3. General endotracheal anesthesia
4. Intraoperative transesophageal echocardiogram
5. Median sternotomy
6. Open pericardium, create pericardial well
7. Systemic heparinization (400U/kg)
8. Arterial cannulation
9. Bicaval venous cannulation
10. Myocardial protection cannula placement in aortic root
11. Confirm ACT > 400 sec
12. Initiate CPB (goal 2.0-2.5L/min/m2)
13. Moderate hypothermia (28° C)
14. Cross-clamp aorta
15. Recipient cardiectomy
16. Divide SVC
17. Divide IVC
18. Divide great vessels
19. Create left atrial cuff
20. Donor heart brought to the field
21. Inspection for injury
22. Atrial cuff and great vessels appropriately trimmed
23. Left atrial anastomosis
24. IVC anastomosis
25. Aortic anastomosis
26. LV vent placed via left atrial appendage to de-air left heart
27. Aortic cross-clamp removed
28. Pulmonary artery anastomosis
29. SVC anastomosis
30. Rewarm
31. Ensure hemostasis
32. Wean from CPB
33. Venous decannulation
34. Protamine administration
35. Aortic decannulation
36. Placement of atrial and ventricular temporary pacer wires
37. Blake drainage tube placement
38. Sternal closure

III. Congenital Cardiac Surgery

Potential Complications and Pitfalls

1. Cardiac injury during the sternal re-entry can result into massive hemorrhage (if re-do sternotomy).
2. PA should be appropriately trimmed and kinking of PA from excess donor PA
3. SVC stenosis from purse-string of anastomoses
4. Bleeding from posterior anastomoses
5. Injury to SA nodal tissue from excessive manipulation or short donor SVC
6. Inability to wean from CPB (consider ischemia-reperfusion injury, elevated recipient PA pressures, hyperacute rejection/graft failure)

Template Dictation

Preoperative Diagnosis: [INDICATION – e.g. End-stage dilated cardiomyopathy]

Post-operative Diagnosis: Same

Procedure(s) Performed: Bicaval, orthotopic heart transplantation

Attending Surgeon: [BLANK]

Secondary Surgeon: [BLANK]

Procuring Surgeon: [BLANK]

Assistants: [BLANK]

Anesthesia: [BLANK]

Indication(s) for Procedure: The patient is a [AGE] year old [GENDER] with [DURATION] history of [COMPLAINT or DIAGNOSIS e.g. worsening shortness of breath, history of dilated cardiomyopathy]. The patient was initially treated medically yet has developed progressively worse left ventricular dysfunction as evidenced by echocardiogram (ejection fraction 20%) and cardiac magnetic resonance imaging which has been refractory to inotropic therapy. A suitable donor heart is now available for heart transplantation.

Description of Procedure: The patient was taken to the operating room on [DATE]. The patient's identity and planned procedure were verified, and the patient was placed on the operating room table in the supine position. General anesthesia was obtained. Monitoring lines were secured. The patient was prepped and draped in the usual sterile fashion. Median sternotomy was performed and the mediastinum was entered without any complications. Systemic heparin was administered. Cannulation sutures were placed in the distal ascending aorta, the SVC and the IVC. The aortic cannula was then inserted, secured and de-aired. The venous cannulae were then inserted and secured. Cardiopulmonary bypass was then initiated and we cooled the patient to 28° Celsius. An aortic cross-clamp was applied and snares were secured around the SVC and IVC cannulae. The recipient heart was next excised starting with division of the SVC, IVC, left atrium and finally the great vessels.

The donor heart was then brought to the field, inspected and appropriately trimmed. An ice pack was placed around the heart. The left atrial anastomosis was performed with a running #5-0 polypropylene suture. Next, the IVC anastomosis was performed with a running #5-0 polypropylene suture. The aorta was then anastomosed with a running #5-0 polypropylene suture. Once completed, an LV vent was then placed in the left atrial appendage. The left side of the heart was subsequently de-aired and the aortic cross-clamp was removed. The pulmonary artery anastomosis was next performed with a running #5-0 polypropylene suture followed by the SVC anastomosis, which was performed with a #6-0 polypropylene suture.

Upon completion of anastomoses the patient was completely rewarmed. Normal sinus rhythm was regained. Hemostasis was ensured at each anastomosis prior to weaning from cardiopulmonary bypass. We separated from cardiopulmonary bypass with low inotropic support. A test dose of protamine was administered and patient was monitored for adverse reaction before the full protamine dose was resumed. Decannulation was performed and the cannulation sutures tied down. Hemostasis was achieved. Temporary atrial and ventricular wires were placed and tested for appropriate capture. A total of [NUMBER] Blake tubes were placed in the mediastinum and the [LEFT/RIGHT] pleural space. The sternum was re-approximated with a total number of [BLANK] stainless steel sternal wires. The wound was irrigated with Betadine and antibiotic saline solution. The fascia was closed with a running #1 Vicryl suture and the deep dermal layer with a running #2-0 Vicryl suture. The skin and subcuticular layer was closed with a running #3-0 Monocryl. The skin was cleansed with sterile saline and dressed with a Primapore dressing.

All instrument, sponge and needle counts were confirmed to be correct x2 at the end of the operation. The patient was subsequently transferred to the post-operative cardiac surgical intensive care unit in critical condition.

Ischemic donor time was [BLANK] minutes and and cardiopulmonary bypass time was [BLANK] minutes.

Dr. [BLANK] was present and scrubbed for [BLANK] elements of this procedure.

Size considerations: #5-0 polypropylene suture is used for left atrial, IVC and great vessel anastomoses and 6-0 polypropylene is used for the SVC anastomosis in infants and small children. However, the larger children and adolescents generally required #4-0 and #5-0 polypropylene for the above-mentioned anastomoses, respectively.

Made in the USA
Coppell, TX
11 January 2020